Critical Care

Editors

JACQUELINE M. KRUSER
GREGORY A. SCHMIDT

CLINICS IN
CHEST MEDICINE

www.chestmed.theclinics.com

September 2022 • Volume 43 • Number 3

ELSEVIER

1600 John F. Kennedy Boulevard • Suite 1800 • Philadelphia, Pennsylvania, 19103-2899

http://www.theclinics.com

CLINICS IN CHEST MEDICINE Volume 43, Number 3
September 2022 ISSN 0272-5231, ISBN-13: 978-0-323-89682-5

Editor: Joanna Collett
Developmental Editor: Karen Justine Solomon

Clinics in Chest Medicine (ISSN 0272-5231) is published quarterly by Elsevier Inc., 360 Park Avenue South, New York, NY 10010-1710. Months of issue are March, June, September, and December. Periodicals postage paid at New York, NY and additional mailing offices. Subscription prices are $408.00 per year (domestic individuals), $1049.00 per year (domestic institutions), $100.00 per year (domestic students/residents), $436.00 per year (Canadian individuals), $1091.00 per year (Canadian institutions), $499.00 per year (international individuals), $1091.00 per year (international institutions), $100.00 per year (Canadian Students), and $230.00 per year (International Students). International air speed delivery is included in all Clinics subscription prices. All prices are subject to change without notice. **POSTMASTER:** Send address changes to Clinics in Chest Medicine, Elsevier Health Sciences Division, Subscription Customer Service, 3251 Riverport Lane, Maryland Heights, MO 63043. **Customer Service: Telephone: 1-800-654-2452** (U.S. and Canada); **1-314-447-8871** (outside U.S. and Canada). **Fax: 1-314-447-8029. E-mail: journalscustomerservice-usa@elsevier.com (for print support); journalsonlinesupport-usa@elsevier.com (for online support).**

Reprints. For copies of 100 or more of articles in this publication, please contact the Commercial Reprints Department, Elsevier Inc., 360 Park Avenue South, New York, NY 10010-1710. Tel.: 212-633-3874; Fax: 212-633-3820; E-mail: reprints@elsevier.com.

Clinics in Chest Medicine is covered in *MEDLINE/PubMed (Index Medicus), Current Contents/Clinical Medicine, EMBASE/ Excerpta Medica, Science Citation Index,* and *ISI/BIOMED.*

Contributors

EDITORS

JACQUELINE M. KRUSER, MD, MS
Assistant Professor, Division of Allergy,
Pulmonary, and Critical Care Medicine,
Department of Medicine, University of
Wisconsin-Madison School of Medicine and
Public Health, Madison, Wisconsin, USA

GREGORY A. SCHMIDT, MD
Professor, Division of Pulmonary and Critical
Care, Department of Occupational Medicine,
Department of Internal Medicine, Associate
Chief Medical Officer, Critical Care, Director of
Critical Care Programs, University of Iowa
Hospitals & Clinics, University of Iowa Carver
College of Medicine, Iowa City, Iowa, USA

AUTHORS

GHADA BOURJEILY, MD
Professor, Department of Medicine, Divisions
of Pulmonary, Critical Care and Sleep Medicine
and Obstetric Medicine, The Warren Alpert
Medical School of Brown University,
Providence, Rhode Island, USA

KRISTIN M. BURKART, MD, MSc
Professor of Medicine, Division of Pulmonary,
Allergy, and Critical Care Medicine,
Department of Medicine, Columbia University
Vagelos College of Physicians & Surgeons,
New York, New York, USA

LEIGH M. CAGINO, MD, MSc
Division of Pulmonary and Critical Care
Medicine, University of Michigan, Ann Arbor,
Michigan, USA

**ERIC W. CUCCHI, MS, PA-C, CAQ-HM,
DFAAPA**
Digital Medicine Program, Director of eICU
Operations, UMass Memorial Medical Center,
Instructor of Nursing, University of
Massachusetts Medical School, Graduate
School of Nursing, Faculty, University of
Massachusetts, Worcester, Massachusetts,
USA

KEVIN C. DOERSCHUG, MD, MS, FCCP
Clinical Professor of Internal Medicine, Division
of Pulmonary Diseases, Critical Care, and

Occupational Medicine, University of Iowa
Carver College of Medicine, Iowa City, Iowa,
USA

TIMOTHY D. GIRARD, MD, MSCI
Associate Professor, Department of Critical
Care Medicine, The Clinical Research,
Investigation, and Systems Modeling of Acute
Illness (CRISMA) Center, University of
Pittsburgh, Pittsburgh, Pennsylvania, USA

JOHN GRANTON, MD, FRCPC
Professor of Medicine, Faculty of Medicine,
University of Toronto, Consultant, Pulmonary
and Critical Care Medicine, University Health
Network, Toronto, Ontario, Canada

YONATAN Y. GREENSTEIN, MD, FCCP
Associate Professor, Department of Medicine,
Division of Pulmonary and Critical Care
Medicine, Rutgers – New Jersey Medical
School, Newark, New Jersey, USA

KELLY M. GRIFFIN, MD
Assistant Professor, Department of Medicine,
Division of Pulmonary and Critical Care, Weill
Cornell Medical College, New York, New York,
USA

KEITH GUEVARRA, DO, FCCP
Associate Professor, Department of Medicine,
Division of Pulmonary and Critical Care

Medicine, Rutgers – New Jersey Medical School, Newark, New Jersey, USA

MATTHEW K. HENSLEY, MD, MPH
Department of Internal Medicine, Division of Pulmonary and Critical Care, University of Pittsburgh Medical Center, Pittsburgh, Pennsylvania, USA

KAREN E. JACKSON, MD
Assistant Professor of Medicine, Division of Pulmonary, Critical Care and Sleep Medicine, Rush University Medical Center, Chicago, Illinois, USA

SCOTT E. KOPEC, MD
Director, Internal Medicine Residency Program, Associate Professor of Medicine, University of Massachusetts Medical School, Worcester, Massachusetts, USA

JACQUELINE M. KRUSER, MD, MS
Assistant Professor, Division of Allergy, Pulmonary, and Critical Care Medicine, Department of Medicine, University of Wisconsin-Madison School of Medicine and Public Health, Madison, Wisconsin, USA

CRAIG M. LILLY, MD
Professor of Medicine, Surgery and Anesthesia, University of Massachusetts Medical School, Worcester, Massachusetts, USA

JAKOB I. McSPARRON, MD
Division of Pulmonary and Critical Care Medicine, University of Michigan, Ann Arbor, Michigan, USA

LAVEENA MUNSHI, MD, MSc
Interdepartmental Division of Critical Care Medicine, Department of Medicine, Sinai Health System, University of Toronto, Mount Sinai Hospital, Toronto, Ontario, Canada

BOULOS S. NASSAR, MD, MPH, FCCP
Department of Internal Medicine, Division of Pulmonary, Critical Care and Occupational Medicine, University of Iowa Hospital & Clinics, Iowa City, Iowa, USA

ALEXANDER S. NIVEN, MD
Division of Pulmonary and Critical Care Medicine, Associate Professor, Department of Medicine, Mayo Clinic, Rochester, Minnesota, USA

CORRINA OXFORD-HORREY, MD
Assistant Professor of Clinical Obstetrics and Gynecology, Department of Obstetrics and Gynecology, Division of Maternal Fetal Medicine, Weill Cornell Medical College, New York, New York, USA

ALYSSA A. PEREZ, MD, MEd
Division of Pulmonary and Critical Care Medicine, Assistant Professor of Medicine, University of California, San Francisco, San Francisco, California, USA

CHIAGOZIE I. PICKENS, MD
Department of Medicine, Pulmonary and Critical Care Division, Northwestern University Feinberg School of Medicine, Chicago, Illinois, USA

NIALL T. PRENDERGAST, MD
Instructor, Division of Pulmonary, Allergy, and Critical Care Medicine, Department of Medicine, University of Pittsburgh, Pittsburgh, Pennsylvania, USA

HALLIE C. PRESCOTT, MD, MSc
Department of Internal Medicine, University of Michigan, VA Center for Clinical Management Research, HSR&D Center of Innovation, Ann Arbor, Michigan, USA

MATTHEW RISCINTI, MD
Director of Emergency Ultrasound, Emergency Medicine, Denver Health Medical Center, Denver, Colorado, USA, Assistant Professor, Emergency Medicine, University of Colorado School of Medicine, Aurora, Colorado, USA

GREGORY A. SCHMIDT, MD
Professor, Division of Pulmonary and Critical Care, Department of Occupational Medicine, Department of Internal Medicine, Associate Chief Medical Officer, Critical Care, Director of Critical Care Programs, University of Iowa Hospitals & Clinics, University of Iowa Carver College of Medicine, Iowa City, Iowa, USA

KATHARINE S. SEAGLY, PhD
Division of Rehabilitation Psychology and Neuropsychology, Department of Physical Medicine and Rehabilitation, University of Michigan, Ann Arbor, Michigan, USA

KATHARINE E. SECUNDA, MD
Department of Medicine, Division of Pulmonary
and Critical Care, University of Pennsylvania

MATTHEW W. SEMLER, MD, MSc
Assistant Professor of Medicine, Division of
Allergy, Pulmonary and Critical Care Medicine,
Vanderbilt University Medical Center,
Nashville, Tennessee, USA

CURTIS N. SESSLER, MD
Orhan Muren Distinguished Professor of
Medicine, Division of Pulmonary and Critical
Care Medicine, Department of Internal
Medicine, Virginia Commonwealth University,
Richmond, Virginia, USA

RUPAL J. SHAH, MD, MSCE
Division of Pulmonary and Critical Care
Medicine, Associate Professor of Medicine,
University of California, San Francisco, San
Francisco, California, USA

BRIANA SHORT, MD
Assistant Professor of Medicine, Division of
Pulmonary, Allergy, and Critical Care Medicine,
Department of Medicine, Columbia University
Vagelos College of Physicians & Surgeons,
New York, New York, USA

MICHAEL C. SKLAR, MD
Interdepartmental Division of Critical Care
Medicine, Department of Anesthesiology and
Pain Medicine, St. Michael's Hospital, Unity
Health Toronto, Department of Anesthesiology
and Pain Medicine, University of Toronto,
Toronto, Canada

RICARDO TEIJEIRO-PARADIS, MD
Interdepartmental Division of Critical Care,
University of Toronto, University Health
Network, Toronto, Ontario, Canada

MOLLY E.W. THIESSEN, MD, FACEP
Attending Physician, Emergency Medicine,
Denver Health Medical Center, Denver,
Colorado, USA

PERRY J. TIBERIO, MD, PhD
Fellow, Division of Pulmonary, Allergy, and
Critical Care Medicine, Department of
Medicine, University of Pittsburgh, Pittsburgh,
Pennsylvania, USA

RICHARD G. WUNDERINK, MD
Department of Medicine, Pulmonary and
Critical Care Division, Northwestern University
Feinberg School of Medicine, Chicago, Illinois,
USA

Contents

Preface: Evolution in Critical Care Medicine: Technology, Humanity, and a Global Pandemic   xiii

Jacqueline M. Kruser and Gregory A. Schmidt

Point-of-Care Ultrasound in the Intensive Care Unit: Applications, Limitations, and the Evolution of Clinical Practice   373

Yonatan Y. Greenstein and Keith Guevarra

 Video content accompanies this article at http://www.chestmed.theclinics.com.

The use of point-of-care ultrasonography in the intensive care unit has been rapidly advancing over the past 20 years. This review will provide a broad overview of the discipline spanning lung ultrasonography to advanced critical care echocardiography. It will highlight new research that questions the utility of the inferior vena cava for determining volume responsiveness and will introduce the reader to cutting-edge technology including artificial intelligence, which is likely to revolutionize ultrasound teaching and image interpretation, increasing the reach of this modality for the frontline clinician.

Application of Focused Assessment with Sonography for Trauma in the Intensive Care Unit   385

Molly E.W. Thiessen and Matthew Riscinti

 Video content accompanies this article at http://www.chestmed.theclinics.com.

The Extended-Focused Assessment with Sonography for Trauma (E-FAST) allows clinicians to rapidly diagnose traumatic thoracoabdominal injuries at the bedside without ionizing radiation. It has high specificity and is extremely useful as an initial test to rule in dangerous diagnoses such as hemoperitoneum, pericardial effusion, hemothorax, and pneumothorax. Its moderate sensitivity means that it should not be used alone as a tool to rule out dangerous thoracoabdominal injuries. In patients with a concerning mechanism or presentation, additional imaging should be obtained despite a negative FAST examination.

Capnography for Monitoring of the Critically Ill Patient   393

Boulos S. Nassar and Gregory A. Schmidt

Capnography has been widely adopted in multiple clinical areas. The capnogram and end-tidal carbon dioxide offer a wealth of information, in the right clinical setting, and when properly interpreted. In this article, the authors aim to review the most common clinical scenarios during which capnography has been shown to be of benefit. This includes the areas of fluid responsiveness, cardiopulmonary resuscitation, and conscious sedation. They review the published literature, highlighting its pitfalls and identifying its limitations.

Novel and Rapid Diagnostics for Common Infections in the Critically Ill Patient   401

Chiagozie I. Pickens and Richard G. Wunderink

There are several novel platforms that enhance detection of pathogens that cause common infections in the intensive care unit. These platforms have a sample to answer time of a few hours, are often higher yield than culture, and have the potential to improve antibiotic stewardship.

Pharmacologic Management of Delirium in the Intensive Care Unit   411

Perry J. Tiberio, Niall T. Prendergast, and Timothy D. Girard

Delirium, often underdiagnosed in the intensive care unit, is a common complication of critical illness that contributes to significant morbidity and mortality. Clinicians should be aware of common risk factors and triggers and should work to mitigate these as much as possible to reduce the occurrence of delirium. This review first provides an overview of the epidemiology, pathophysiology, evaluation, and consequences of delirium in critically ill patients. Presented next is the current evidence for the pharmacologic management of delirium, focusing on prevention and treatment of delirium in the intensive care unit. It concludes by outlining some emerging treatments of delirium.

Management of the Critically Ill Patient with Pulmonary Arterial Hypertension and Right Heart Failure   425

John Granton and Ricardo Teijeiro-Paradis

Right ventricular (RV) failure is a recognized complication of pulmonary hypertension (PH). Pregnancy and surgery represent unique challenges to the patient with PH and require input from an interprofessional team. Approach to treatment must embrace sound physiologic principles that are based on optimization of RV preload, contractility, and afterload to improve cardiac function and tissue perfusion before the onset of multiorgan dysfunction. Failure of medical therapy needs to be recognized before the onset of irreversible shock. When appropriate, eligible patients should be considered for mechanical circulatory support as a bridge to recovery or transplantation.

Caring for the Critically Ill Patient with COVID-19   441

Matthew K. Hensley and Hallie C. Prescott

The COVID-19 pandemic has resulted in unprecedented numbers of critically ill patients. Critical care providers have been challenged to increase the capacity for critical care, prevent the spread of syndrome coronavirus 2 in hospitals, determine the optimal treatment approaches for patients with critical COVID-19, and to design and implement systems for fair allocation of scarce life-saving resources when capacity is exhausted. The global burden of COVID-19 highlighted disparities, across geographic regions and among minority patient populations. Faced with a novel pathogen, critical care providers grappled with the extent to which conventional supportive critical care practices should be followed versus adapted to treat patients with COVID-19. Fiercely debated practices included the use of awake prone positioning, the timing of intubation, and optimal approach to sedation. Advances in clinical trial design were necessary to rapidly identify appropriate therapeutics for the critically ill patient with COVID-19. In this article, we review the epidemiology, outcomes, and treatments for the critically ill patient with COVID-19.

Critical Care of the Lung Transplant Patient   457

Alyssa A. Perez and Rupal J. Shah

> Lung transplantation is a therapeutic option for end-stage lung disease that improves survival and quality of life. Prelung transplant admission to the intensive care unit (ICU) for bridge to transplant with mechanical ventilation and extracorporeal membrane oxygenation (ECMO) is common. Primary graft dysfunction is an important immediate complication of lung transplantation with short- and long-term morbidity and mortality. Later transplant-related causes of respiratory failure necessitating ICU admission include acute cellular rejection, atypical infections, and chronic lung allograft dysfunction. Lung transplantation for COVID-19-related ARDS is increasingly common.

Obstetric Disorders and Critical Illness   471

Kelly M. Griffin, Corrina Oxford-Horrey, and Ghada Bourjeily

> In this article, we discuss some of the more common obstetric-related conditions that can lead to critical illness and require management in an ICU. These include the hypertensive disorders of pregnancy, postpartum hemorrhage, hemolysis, elevated liver enzymes, and low platelet syndrome, acute fatty liver of pregnancy, amniotic fluid embolism, and peripartum cardiomyopathy. We also discuss pulmonary embolism and Covid-19. Despite not being specific to obstetric patients, pulmonary embolism is a common, life-threatening diagnosis in pregnancy with particular risks and management aspects. Covid-19 does not seem to occur with higher frequency in pregnant women, but it leads to higher rates of ICU admissions and mechanical ventilation in pregnant women than in their nonpregnant peers. Its prevalence during our current global pandemic makes it important to discuss in this article. We provide a basis for critical care physicians to be engaged in informed conversations and management in a multidisciplinary manner with other relevant providers in the care of critically ill pregnant and postpartum women.

Advances in Sepsis Care   489

Karen E. Jackson and Matthew W. Semler

> This review article summarizes current scientific evidence regarding the treatment of sepsis. We highlight recent advances in sepsis management with a focus on antibiotics, fluids, vasopressors, and adjunctive therapies such as corticosteroids and renal replacement therapy.

Advances in Ventilator Management for Patients with Acute Respiratory Distress Syndrome   499

Michael C. Sklar and Laveena Munshi

> The ventilatory care of patients with acute respiratory distress syndrome (ARDS) is evolving as our understanding of physiologic mechanisms of respiratory failure improves. Despite several decades of research, the mortality rate for ARDS remains high. Over the years, we continue to expand strategies to identify and mitigate ventilator-induced lung injury. This now includes a greater understanding of the benefits and harms associated with spontaneous breathing.

Patient-Ventilator Synchrony   511

Kevin C. Doerschug

Patient-ventilator asynchrony develops when the ventilator output does not match the efforts of the patient and contributes to excess work of breathing, lung injury, and mortality. Asynchronies are categorized as trigger (breath initiation), flow (delivery of the breath), and cycle (transition from inspiration to expiration). Clinicians should be skilled at ventilator waveform analysis to detect patient-ventilator asynchronies and make informed ventilator adjustments. Ventilator overdrive suppresses respiratory drive and reduces asynchrony, while other adjustments specific to the asynchrony are also useful.

Extracorporeal Life Support in Respiratory Failure   519

Briana Short and Kristin M. Burkart

Extracorporeal life support (ECLS) has a role in different types of respiratory failure including acute respiratory distress syndrome (ARDS), decompensated pulmonary hypertension, bridge to lung transplantation, and primary graft dysfunction after lung transplantation. ECLS in ARDS allows for lung-protective ventilation with the goal to reduce the risk of ventilator-induced lung injury. ECLS use in severe ARDS should be considered when conventional management strategies are not sufficient to safely support gas exchange. More research is needed to identify optimal mechanical ventilation during ECLS, weaning ECLS support, strategies for mobilization, sedation and anticoagulation, and long-term outcomes post-ECLS.

COVID-19 and the Transformation of Intensive Care Unit Telemedicine   529

Eric W. Cucchi, Scott E. Kopec, and Craig M. Lilly

The concept of telecritical care has evolved over several decades. ICU Telemedicine providers using both the hub-and-spoke ICU telemedicine center and consultative service delivery models offered their services during the COVID-19 pandemic. Telemedicine center responses were more efficient, timely, and widely used than those of the consultative model. Bedside nurses, physicians, nurse practitioners, physician assistants, and respiratory therapists incorporated the use of ICU telemedicine tools into their practices and more frequently requested critical care specialist telemedicine support.

Patient-Centered and Family-Centered Care in the Intensive Care Unit   539

Katharine E. Secunda and Jacqueline M. Kruser

Patient-centered and family-centered care (PFCC) is widely recognized as integral to high-quality health-care delivery. The highly technical nature of critical care puts patients and families at risk of dehumanization and renders the delivery of PFCC in the intensive care unit (ICU) challenging. In this article, we discuss the history and terminology of PFCC, describe interventions to promote PFCC, highlight limitations to the current model, and offer future directions to optimize PFCC in the ICU.

Survivorship After Critical Illness and Post-Intensive Care Syndrome   551

Leigh M. Cagino, Katharine S. Seagly, and Jakob I. McSparron

> Improvements in critical care medicine have led to a marked increase in survivors of the intensive care unit (ICU). These survivors encounter many difficulties following ICU discharge. The term post -intensive care syndrome (PICS) provides a framework for identifying the most common symptoms which fall into three domains: cognitive, physical, and mental health. There are numerous risk factors for the development of PICS including premorbid conditions and specific elements of ICU hospitalizations. Management is complex and should take an individualized approach with interdisciplinary care. Future research should focus on prevention, identification, and treatment of this unique population.

Supporting Professionals in Critical Care Medicine: Burnout, Resiliency, and System-Level Change   563

Alexander S. Niven and Curtis N. Sessler

> Burnout is occurring in epidemic proportions among intensive care unit physicians and other health-care professionals—accelerated by pandemic-driven stress. The impact of burnout is far-reaching, threatening the health of individual workers, the safety and quality of care our patients receive, and eroding the infrastructure of health care in general. Drivers of burnout include excessive quantity of work (nights, weekends, and acuity surges); excessive menial tasks; incivility, poor communication, and challenges to team success; and frequent moral distress and end-of-life issues. This article provides system-based practice and individual strategies to address these drivers and improve the well-being of our team and our patients.

CLINICS IN CHEST MEDICINE

FORTHCOMING ISSUES

December 2022
Cystic Fibrosis in the Era of Highly Effective CFTR Modulator Therapy
Clemente J Britto and Jennifer L. Taylor-Cousar, *Editors*

March 2023
Lung Transplantation
Luis Angel and Stephanie M. Levine, *Editors*

June 2023
COVID-19 lung disease: Lessons Learned
Charles Dela Cruz and Guang-Shing Cheng, *Editors*

RECENT ISSUES

June 2022
Sleep Deficiency and Health
Melissa P Knauert, *Editor*

March 2022
Bronchiectasis
James D. Chalmers, *Editor*

December 2021
Pleural Disease
David Feller-Kopman and Fabien Maldonado, *Editors*

SERIES OF RELATED INTEREST

Cardiology Clinics
Available at: https://www.cardiology.theclinics.com/
Sleep Medicine Clinics
Available at: https://www.sleep.theclinics.com/

THE CLINICS ARE AVAILABLE ONLINE!
Access your subscription at:
www.theclinics.com

Preface
Evolution in Critical Care Medicine: Technology, Humanity, and a Global Pandemic

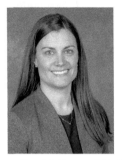
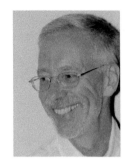

Jacqueline M. Kruser, MD, MS   Gregory A. Schmidt, MD
Editors

The evolution of critical care medicine is often marked and even led by technological advances in the diagnosis, monitoring, and treatment of life-threatening illness. This special issue of *Clinics in Chest Medicine* highlights major and recent technological advances in critical care—from bedside evaluation with ultrasound and capnography to novel diagnostic technology for common infections in the intensive care unit (ICU) to extracorporeal life support. Technological advances have changed not only bedside care but also the organization of critical care delivery—highlighted in a provocative account of the importance of ICU telemedicine in the pandemic era.

This issue also includes comprehensive reviews that evaluate recent evidence and provide practical guidance in managing hallmark critical care syndromes, including sepsis, acute respiratory distress syndrome, and right heart failure. In addition to a focus on these common syndromes, this special issue addresses the unique (and sometimes not so unique) features of critical care management in less common populations, such as lung transplant recipients and pregnant patients.

Despite (or perhaps because of) the focus on technological advancement, this issue of *Clinics*

in Chest Medicine simultaneously highlights how the evolution of critical care has impacted the human experiences of those within its reach—including patients with life-threatening illness, their families, and ICU clinicians. Given the growing potential of critical care technology to extend and save lives, articles in this issue convey an urgent need to focus on patient survivorship, the support of patients and families throughout the increasingly prolonged periods of critical illness, and the well-being of our ICU clinicians and interprofessional team members.

The broad and human impact of critical illness is only underscored by our shared experiences during the ongoing pandemic caused by severe acute respiratory syndrome coronavirus 2 (SARS-CoV-2). The influence of and leading-edge knowledge about COVID-19 is documented and evaluated across most of the articles contained in this special issue of *Clinics in Chest Medicine*, including a dedicated review on critical care of the patient with COVID-19. Our hope is that by the next special issue of *Clinics in Chest Medicine* focused on the critical care, the pressing issues raised by these contributing authors and by this global pandemic will be considered in hindsight, from

Clin Chest Med 43 (2022) xiii–xiv
https://doi.org/10.1016/j.ccm.2022.06.001
0272-5231/22/© 2022 Published by Elsevier Inc.

yet another horizon of advancement in the technology and humanity of critical care medicine.

Jacqueline M. Kruser, MD, MS
Division of Allergy, Pulmonary
and Critical Care Medicine
Department of Medicine
University of Wisconsin School of Medicine
and Public Health
H4/612 Clinical Science Center
600 Highland Avenue
Madison, WI 53792-0001, USA

Gregory A. Schmidt, MD
Division of Pulmonary and Critical Care
Department of Internal Medicine
Department of Occupational Medicine
Critical Care
University of Iowa Hospitals and Clinics
University of Iowa Carver College of Medicine
C33-K General Hospital
Iowa City, IA 52242, USA

E-mail addresses:
jkruser@wisc.edu (J.M. Kruser)
gregory-a-schmidt@uiowa.edu (G.A. Schmidt)

Point-of-Care Ultrasound in the Intensive Care Unit
Applications, Limitations, and the Evolution of Clinical Practice

Yonatan Y. Greenstein, MD, FCCP[a],*, Keith Guevarra, DO, FCCP[a]

KEYWORDS

• Ultrasonography • Echocardiography • Point-of-care ultrasonography • POCUS • Intensivist

KEY POINTS

• POCUS has application for diagnostic, management, and procedural guidance purposes in the intensive care unit. Its use has increased dramatically over the past 20 years.
• Artificial intelligence is a promising technology that will likely increase the diagnostic yield of POCUS. Deep learning has recently been applied to lung ultrasonography.
• Successful POCUS programs generate formal reports of performed studies with clinically relevant conclusions and store these reports and images in the electronic health record.

 Video content accompanies this article at http://www.chestmed.theclinics.com.

INTRODUCTION

Point-of-care ultrasonography (POCUS) is widely used by frontline clinicians taking care of critically ill patients. The intensivist images the heart, lungs, abdomen, kidneys, and vascular system, enabling the clinician to guide the management of patients, quickly identify life-threatening entities, and enhance procedure success and safety. This review highlights the uses of POCUS and focuses on innovations in this field.

TRAINING

Most stakeholders agree that POCUS is a basic competency for intensivists.[1,2] Despite this, many fellowship programs do not offer robust training and thus many graduating fellows do not possess competence in POCUS. Recent studies of academic critical care training programs show a discrepancy between the recognition of the importance of POCUS and the allotment of resources and faculty time to its implementation.[3–5]

Universal use of POCUS requires effective training programs. For intensivists or trainees who do not have expertise in POCUS, national and regional courses can provide training. Studies show that these courses are effective with the main disadvantages being the cost to operate them and travel expenses for the participants and faculty.[6]

Travel and gathering restrictions during the COVID-19 pandemic disrupted traditional teaching avenues and opened opportunity for innovation because of new demand for distanced learning.

Some national courses adjusted their formats to fit a hybrid approach, by converting live didactics to prerecorded lectures to maximize

The authors have nothing to disclose.
[a] Department of Medicine, Division of Pulmonary and Critical Care Medicine, Rutgers – New Jersey Medical School, University Hospital Building, Room I-354, 150 Bergen Street, Newark, NJ 07103, USA
* Corresponding author.
E-mail address: yonatan@njms.rutgers.edu

Clin Chest Med 43 (2022) 373–384
https://doi.org/10.1016/j.ccm.2022.04.001
0272-5231/22/© 2022 Elsevier Inc. All rights reserved.

hands-on scanning and mentored image interpretation time. Companies like SonoSim offer remote hands-on ultrasound training, didactic instruction, and assessment from the comfort of a laptop computer and a plug and play ultrasound probe with an accelerometer that detects probe manipulation. Robust studies testing this remote simulator device do not exist, but small studies suggest utility in its use as an adjunct to traditional ultrasound learning paradigms.[7,8] Ultrasound manikin simulators have been in use for many years. We previously published the usefulness of using these simulators to assess competency in high-risk, low-frequency scenarios.[9] Multiple studies have demonstrated the role of simulation training for intensivist-performed transesophageal echocardiography (TEE).[10,11] Some companies are touting the integration of augmented reality to simulators to create a more immersive experience for the scanner and the group of learners training with an instructor. The inclusion of augmented reality in ultrasound training has yet to be reported.

BASIC CRITICAL CARE ECHOCARDIOGRAPHY

Basic critical care echocardiography (CCE) aims to answer limited questions, focused on target-oriented, qualitative assessments that help guide management.[1] The views included in a basic CCE examination are shown in **Table 1** and Video 1. Scanning can be repeated to assess the effects of therapeutic interventions. Cognitive skills required for basic CCE include the visual assessment of global left ventricular (LV) size and function, identification of segmental versus global wall motion abnormalities, right ventricular (RV) size and function, and identification of severe valvular dysfunction using color Doppler.

Basic CCE can narrow the differential diagnosis and may help identify reversible life-threatening causes of shock.[12] Hypovolemic shock may be deduced by visualizing end-systolic effacement of the LV cavity and a small, fully collapsible inferior vena cava (IVC) in a hypotensive patient (Video 2). When clinical evidence of tamponade exists, the presence of a pericardial effusion with right atrial or RV collapse clinches the diagnosis. Acute cor pulmonale causing obstructive shock manifests as RV dilation with septal flattening (Video 3). We previously reported on a patient admitted with septic shock presumed from a urinary tract infection, on a continuous norepinephrine infusion, in whom POCUS revealed severe RV dilatation and a common femoral vein (CFV) deep vein thrombosis (DVT). The POCUS examination rapidly changed the diagnosis, and management immediately shifted to the administration of thrombolytics for massive pulmonary embolism (PE).[13] The intensivist performing basic CCE uses this modality on critically ill, hemodynamically unstable patients, as some of the findings may not represent actionable pathology in an otherwise stable patient. For example, severe LV systolic dysfunction or RV dilatation may be chronic and may not be the primary etiology of the patient's clinical presentation. The intensivist with basic CCE capability must fully understand the shortcomings of the assumptions made when performing basic CCE.

ADVANCED CRITICAL CARE ECHOCARDIOGRAPHY

Advanced CCE distinguishes itself from a consultative echocardiogram by focusing on emergent findings and the hemodynamic assessment rather than findings that contribute to the long-term management of the patient. Advanced CCE allows the intensivist to assess shock and contributing cardiac pathologies and guide therapy in a more comprehensive way compared with basic CCE. **Table 2** lists the common views and

Table 1
The basic critical care echocardiogram

View	Main Utility
Parasternal long axis	General assessment; identification of valvular dysfunction with color Doppler
Parasternal short axis (papillary muscle level)	Overall LV systolic function; segmental wall motion analysis; septal motion
Apical 4-chamber	RV:LV ratio; identification of valvular dysfunction with color Doppler
Subcostal long axis	Overall assessment; identification of valvular dysfunction with color Doppler
Inferior vena cava long axis	Assessment of volume status

Abbreviations: LV, left ventricle; RV, right ventricle.

Table 2
The advanced critical care echocardiogram

View	Points of Assessment
Parasternal long axis	Overall assessment; color Doppler MV, AV; EPSS; LVOT diameter
RV inflow	Color Doppler TV; PASP estimation
Parasternal short axis (all levels)	Wall motion analysis; color Doppler, CW, PW of valves; septal motion analysis; PA acceleration time
Apical 4-chamber	RV:LV ratio; assessment of MR and TR; PASP estimation; TAPSE; S' velocity; wall motion; pulmonary venous flow analysis
Apical 5-chamber	LVOT$_{VTI}$
Apical 3-chamber	LVOT$_{VTI}$; assessment of MR; wall motion
Apical 2-chamber	Assessment of MR; wall motion
Subcostal long axis	Overall assessment; RV:LV ratio; color Doppler MV, TV
Subcostal short axis (all levels)	Wall motion analysis; color Doppler, CW, PW of valves; septal motion analysis; PA acceleration time
IVC longitudinal	Assessment of volume status; hepatic venous flow analysis

Abbreviations: AV, aortic valve; CW, continuous wave; EPSS, end-point septal separation; IVC, inferior vena cava; LV, left ventricle; LVOT, left ventricular outflow tract; LVOT$_{VTI}$, left ventricular outflow tract velocity time integral; MR, mitral regurgitation; MV, mitral valve; PA, pulmonary artery; PASP, pulmonary artery systolic pressure; PW, pulsed wave; RV, right ventricle; TAPSE, tricuspid annular plane systolic excursion; TR, tricuspid regurgitation; TV, tricuspid valve.

measurements that are obtained with advanced CCE. Several assessments are highlighted:

Assessment of Right Ventricular Function and Pulmonary Hypertension

RV dysfunction is common in the intensive care unit (ICU).[14] Fluid loading can have deleterious effects on patients with compromised RV function making identification of at-risk patients crucial. Useful measurements include tricuspid annular plane systolic excursion (TAPSE) with a normal value $\geq$ 16 mm (**Fig. 1**) and tissue Doppler S-wave velocity with a normal value $\geq$ 10 cm/s (**Fig. 2**).[15]

Measurement of the pulmonary artery acceleration time (AT) (**Fig. 3**) allows the intensivist to detect pulmonary hypertension. Vieillard-Baron and colleagues found the AT in patients with acute cor pulmonale from acute respiratory distress syndrome (ARDS) and from massive PE to be 76 ms $\pm$ 27 ms and 68 ms $\pm$ 36 ms, respectively.

A biphasic pulmonary artery velocity envelope is also consistent with acute cor pulmonale.[16] Coupling of these findings with the clinical scenario helps the intensivist make important, management-changing decisions.

Assessment of Cardiac Tamponade

Cardiac tamponade is a challenging diagnosis to make with echocardiography. Intensivists with advanced CCE expertise incorporate spectral Doppler to assess for significant tricuspid and mitral inflow variation, which supports the diagnosis. Ultrasound-assisted pericardiocentesis via an apical or subxiphoid approach can be performed by the intensivist.

Assessment of Cardiac Output

The intensivist needs to judge cardiac output to categorize the type of shock state and guide

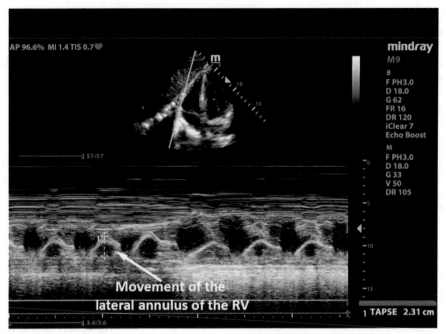

Fig. 1. TAPSE. M-mode analysis of the lateral annulus of the tricuspid valve. Pictured here is a value of 23 mm which is normal.

therapy. The left ventricular outflow tract (LVOT) diameter is measured via a parasternal long axis view (**Fig. 4**). The LVOT velocity time integral (VTI) is measured via the apical 5-chamber or 3-chamber views (**Fig. 5**).

Using the following formula, cardiac output is estimated:

Cardiac Output = $(\pi \ (Diameter_{LVOT}/2)^2 \times VTI_{LVOT}) \times$ heart rate.

When cardiogenic shock is identified, inotropes are titrated to the VTI_{LVOT} in addition to clinical

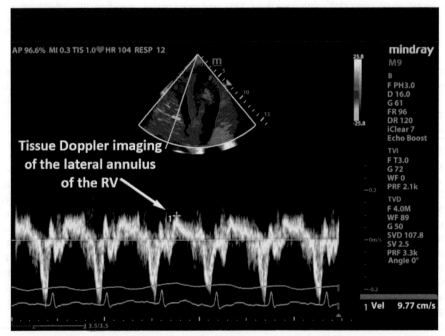

Fig. 2. S velocity. Tissue Doppler analysis of velocity of the lateral annulus of the tricuspid valve. The value of 9.77 cm/s is slightly less than the normal velocity of 10 cm/s.

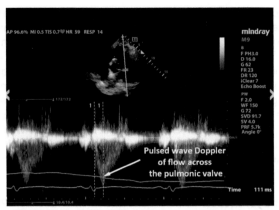

Fig. 3. Pulmonary artery AT. Pulsed wave Doppler analysis of blood flow across the pulmonic valve. The AT denotes the amount of time it takes for ejection to reach maximal velocity. The value of 111 ms depicted here is normal and is not consistent with pulmonary hypertension.

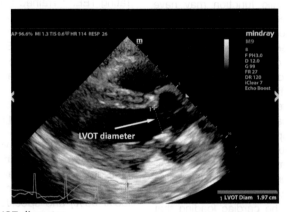

Fig. 4. Measurement of LVOT diameter.

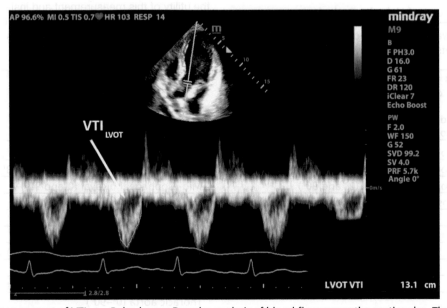

Fig. 5. Measurement of VTI_{LVOT}. Pulsed wave Doppler analysis of blood flow across the aortic valve. The depicted value of 13.1 cm is reduced.

parameters. Accurate Doppler angle is essential to reduce error. Whereas these measures are not always feasible in critically ill patients, the existing literature supports their use.[17,18] The intensivist may forgo formal calculation and instead make decisions based on the VTI_{LVOT} alone, understanding that 18 to 22 cm is normal. An average of two to three cardiac cycles should be used for patients with normal cardiac rhythms. When an irregular rhythm exists, such as in atrial fibrillation, a single VTI_{LVOT} may not accurately reflect the stroke volume and the clinician should average additional cardiac cycles.

Assessment of Diastolic Dysfunction

Diastolic dysfunction occurs in 20% to 57% of patients with sepsis and is associated with increased mortality.[19–22] Patients with bilateral pulmonary infiltrates and normal systolic function may have cardiogenic pulmonary edema from LV diastolic dysfunction. The advanced CCE-capable intensivist is familiar with the American Society of Echocardiography guidelines on diastolic dysfunction but also considers the utility of simplifying the assessment with a reliance on the E/e' ratio.[23,24] A new elevation of left atrial pressure during a spontaneous breathing trial indicates a load-related failure of the trial and may prompt the intensivist to focus on rate control and reducing preload and afterload.[25–27] The intensivist may opt to extubate a patient with diastolic dysfunction and elevated left atrial pressure to noninvasive positive pressure ventilation to ameliorate the cardiac loading that occurs immediately after extubation.[28]

Assessment of Valvular Pathology

Pulsed wave and continuous wave Doppler measurements are used to assess valvular stenosis and regurgitation. Pulmonary artery systolic pressure and aortic valve area are often estimated in critically ill patients. The degree of regurgitation can be assessed by jet area or the vena contracta width; however, other quantitative methods using spectral Doppler inform the final quantification.[29] Since many patients have preexisting pulmonary hypertension or aortic stenosis, these findings must be integrated with the history, prior echocardiographic results, and other clinical information to judge their contribution to the acute episode of critical illness.

Transesophageal Echocardiography

When transthoracic echocardiography is not feasible, the American College of Cardiology and the American Heart Association support incorporating TEE.[30] Trained intensivists and emergency physicians can safely and accurately perform critical care TEE.[31–35] Some critical care physicians perform a focused TEE with four views, while others perform a more comprehensive examination, dependent on the stability of the patient (**Table 3**).

ASSESSMENT OF VOLUME STATUS

Assessing a patient's volume status and determining the expected hemodynamic response after infusion of intravascular volume are challenging. Recent studies demonstrate poor sensitivity (38%–55%) and specificity (61%–70%) with IVC size and respiratory variation to guide fluid resuscitation.[36–38] As a result, we have de-emphasized the utility of this measurement and instead assess for extremes. If the IVC is < 1 cm and there is no evidence of pulmonary edema, there is increased probability that the patient will be fluid

Table 3
Critical care transesophageal echocardiography

Focused Examination Views (Rotation in Degrees)	Standard Examination Views (Rotation in Degrees)
Mid-esophageal 4-chamber (0°)	Mid-esophageal AV short-axis (30°–45°)
Mid-esophageal AV long-axis (120°–135°)	Mid-esophageal AV long-axis (120°–135°)
Mid-esophageal bicaval (0° and 90°)	Mid-esophageal bicaval (0° and 90°)
Transgastric midpapillary short-axis (0°)	SVC M mode (90°)
	Mid-esophageal 4-chamber (0°)
	Mid-esophageal long-axis (90°–120°)
	Transgastric mid-papillary short-axis (0°)
	Transgastric long-axis (120°)
	Mid-esophageal ascending aorta short-axis (0°)
	Thoracic aorta (0°–90°)

Abbreviations: AV, aortic valve; SVC, superior vena cava.

responsive.[12] Measurement of the respiratory variation of the superior vena cava via TEE is validated. Using a cutoff of 21%, this measure has a sensitivity of 63% and a specificity of 81% for predicting fluid responsiveness.[37]

Assessing the stroke volume or cardiac output via Doppler before and after a passive leg raise maneuver has a sensitivity of 63%–77% and a specificity of 89%–100% for predicting volume responsiveness.[39,40]

In the 1950s, Guyton recognized the importance of venous return to cardiovascular physiology. Despite this, the venous system—which contains approximately 70% of total blood volume—is often ignored by intensivists. Studies demonstrate that venous overdistension is harmful to patients and researchers have proposed incorporating venous return concepts in the management of critically ill patients.[41] Beaubien-Souligny and colleagues[42] described a constellation of extracardiac ultrasonography findings associated with fluid overload. Subsequently, they developed the Venous Excess Ultrasound (VExUS) Grading System.[43] This paradigm incorporates 2D imaging of the IVC and pulsed wave Doppler imaging of the hepatic, portal, and intrarenal veins. The system was derived via a post-hoc analysis of a data set of noncritically ill patients before and after the cardiac surgery. Exclusion criteria included critical illness, acute kidney injury (AKI), severe chronic kidney disease, and cirrhosis. The authors found that the VExUS grade 3, severe congestion, was associated with the increased risk of developing AKI (aHR 2.82, CI 1.21–6.55, $P = .02$). We look forward to reviewing prospective studies using VExUS to guide clinical care in a generalizable population and applaud the authors on this innovative concept.

PROCEDURAL GUIDANCE

The intensivist uses ultrasonography for procedural guidance, generally relying on a high-resolution linear transducer. Routine use of this modality has elucidated areas for improvement, and the technology is rapidly advancing.

Being aware of the exact position of the needle tip compared with the shaft of the needle is challenging, especially during procedures where the needle insertion is out-of-plane to the ultrasound beam. The experienced clinician moves the probe and needle in harmony, maintaining visualization of the needle tip (Video 4). Preliminary research suggests that electronic needle tip tracking integrated into the insertion needle and interfaced with the ultrasound device may improve procedural outcomes by reducing procedure time, the number of hand movements, and the length of

the needle path.[44–46] Many US devices have modes designed to enhance needle visualization while performing in-plane procedures.

The Butterfly IQ + offers a Biplane Imaging mode, which allows for the simultaneous display of the transverse and longitudinal axis. This allows the clinician to simultaneously see the in-plane and out-of-plane view. Further research is needed to determine whether this results in meaningful improvements to the procedure.

LUNG ULTRASONOGRAPHY

Lung ultrasonography is used for diagnosing and managing acute respiratory failure.[47,48] It can identify interstitial syndrome, consolidations, pleural effusions, and pneumothoraces.[49] It has preferable diagnostic accuracy compared with auscultation and chest radiography and is superior in the evaluation of the dyspneic patient.[50,51] Given the ability to easily repeat a scan to monitor the disease process and observe effects of treatment, ultrasound has clear benefits over ionizing radiation. The COVID-19 pandemic further solidified the importance of lung ultrasonography as the portability and repeatability was of paramount importance in the adverse and constantly changing conditions faced throughout the world.[52]

The ultrasonographic findings of the normal lung include the presence of A-lines and lung sliding (Video 5). A-lines are reverberation artifacts of the pleura that appear as regularly-spaced, horizontal lines separated by the same distance as that of the skin and the pleural line distance. Lung sliding is the dynamic movement of the visceral and parietal pleura sliding opposite each other with respiration.[53]

Pneumothorax

Lung ultrasonography can rapidly assess for pneumothoraces which are frequently on the differential diagnosis in patients who develop acute hypoxemia or hemodynamic collapse. As the COVID-19 pandemic swept across the world, many intensivists saw an increase in pneumothoraces secondary to the high prevalence of associated fibrotic lung disease. Lung sliding rules out the presence of pneumothorax in the scanned area with a 100% negative predictive value (Video 5).[53,54] Lung pulse is seen in a lung with limited respiratory excursion such as the left lung after right mainstem bronchus intubation or in endobronchial obstruction from a large mucus plug resulting in complete atelectasis.[55] Although lung sliding has a high negative predictive value for pneumothorax, its absence is not specific for pneumothorax. Bullous emphysema, pleural adhesions, consolidation, or prior pleurodesis can obliterate lung sliding. Video 6 shows the absence of lung sliding due to a pneumothorax. The "lung point" is the fleeting appearance of lung sliding (or B-lines) that replaces an area of absent lung sliding during inspiration. This finding has 100% specificity and 66% sensitivity for pneumothorax (Video 7).[56]

Interstitial Syndrome

Lung ultrasonography's utility for evaluating interstitial syndrome is well-established.[57] In contrast to the normal aeration pattern comprised of A-lines with lung sliding, interstitial syndrome is represented by reverberation artifacts called B-lines (Video 8). B-lines have five characteristics: (1) vertical in orientation, (2) originate from the pleural line, (3) extend to the bottom of the image, (4) hyperechoic, and (5) move with respiration. Three or more B-lines at an interspace are consistent with interstitial syndrome at that location. The etiology of B-lines must be determined by the clinician based on the clinical picture, the location and distribution of the B-lines, and the pleural morphology.

Diffuse B-lines with systolic or diastolic dysfunction are typical of cardiogenic pulmonary edema. Studies show that the number of B-lines and the wet-to-dry ratio are strongly correlated; additionally, the number of B-lines is reduced after fluid removal from hemodialysis.[58,59]

B-lines may be caused by cardiogenic pulmonary edema, inflammation, infection, or fibrosis. Lung ultrasonography gained widespread attention during the COVID-19 pandemic as there was significant interest in using it to diagnose pulmonary involvement and for prognostication. In a study by Arntfield and colleagues, deep learning technology involving a convolutional neural network was used to identify subvisible ultrasound features. The model significantly outperformed ultrasound-trained clinicians in distinguishing COVID, non-COVID, and hydrostatic pulmonary edema as the cause of B-lines (overall area under the curve (AUC) 0.789 for humans vs 0.978 for the model) and the ability to distinguish between COVID-19 ARDS and non-COVID-19 ARDS ($P < .01$).[60]

Pleural Effusion

A simple pleural effusion appears as an anechoic pocket of fluid (Video 9). Ultrasonography can also detect cellular material or septations in the pleural space (Videos 10 and 11). The sonographic appearance of pleural fluid can help the clinician determine its etiology. Echogenic material or septations within the pleural fluid typically signal

exudative cause, while anechoic effusions may be transudative or exudative.[61–63] Ultrasonography should be used to identify a safe path for thoracentesis. In our institution, we use linear transducers with color Doppler to identify aberrant blood vessels along the needle path before the procedure to avoid inadvertent puncture or laceration (Video 12).[64]

Consolidation

Consolidated lung is easily seen as it is airless and both transmits and reflects ultrasound (Video 13). Lung consolidation is seen in pneumonia, atelectasis, tumor, or pulmonary infarct. The clinician must combine the clinical context with the imaging findings to deduce the etiology of the consolidation.

LOWER EXTREMITY DEEP VEIN THROMBOSIS STUDIES

DVTs occur in approximately 12% of ICU patients despite thromboprophylaxis.[65,66] Acute PE is often part of the differential diagnosis for patients with acute hemodynamic instability and the presence of a DVT with echocardiographic evidence of acute cor pulmonale makes the diagnosis of PE likely. During the COVID-19 pandemic, a high incidence of DVT was found despite pharmacologic thromboprophylaxis (7%–13.6%).[67,68] Intensivist-performed compression ultrasonography studies have a diagnostic accuracy of 95% compared with radiology-performed duplex ultrasonography studies.[69] The addition of color Doppler has not been shown to increase sensitivity.[70] A normal vein is easily compressible (Video 14). A DVT is confirmed when a thrombus is seen within a vein (Video 15) or the vein is not fully compressible (Video 16). A five-point compression study of each leg at the following locations is adequate: (1) CFV at the common femoral artery, (2) CFV at the greater saphenous intake, (3) CFV at the bifurcation of the common femoral artery to the superficial and deep femoral artery, (4) bifurcation of the CFV into the superficial and deep femoral vein, and (5) popliteal vein.

ABDOMINAL AND RETROPERITONEAL ULTRASONOGRAPHY

Abdominal and retroperitoneal ultrasonography is performed for multiple indications.

Aortic Dissection

Intensivists do not perform screening abdominal aortic aneurysm examinations; when the clinical presentation dictates, thoracic and abdominal aortic aneurysms and dissections may be identified with ultrasonography. Identification of an aortic aneurysm or dissection should be further evaluated by computed tomography (CT) imaging if the patient is stable enough for the study.

Hypotension

In trauma patients or patients who recently underwent an abdominal procedure, free fluid in the abdomen may represent hemoperitoneum. Intensivists apply the focused assessment with sonography for trauma examination when searching for free fluid in the abdomen.[71] Video 17 demonstrates hemorrhagic ascites after an abdominal paracentesis called a "hematocrit sign."[72] The layering echogenicity suggests the accumulation of cellular material such as blood or pus. If the clinician strongly suspects abdominal pathology, even a normal abdominal ultrasound does not have sufficient sensitivity, so that CT or angiography should be pursued.

Acute Kidney Injury

AKI occurs in up to 38% of critically ill patients, and a rapid assessment assists in its management.[73] Video 18 demonstrates the sonographic appearance of a normal kidney. Unilateral hydronephrosis generally requires CT imaging to further elucidate the etiology, although sonographers may identify an obstructing ureteral stone prompting urgent removal.[74] Patients with obstructive uropathy may have bilateral hydronephrosis, which is easily identified with POCUS. This finding mandates assessment of the bladder for distension. When the two are both present, bladder outlet obstruction is the leading diagnosis. Videos 19 and 20 demonstrate hydronephrosis and a markedly distended bladder, respectively.

The use of bladder ultrasonography to assess urine volume qualitatively or quantitatively can help clinicians avoid the placement of indwelling foley catheters and thus reduce catheter associated urinary tract infections.[75]

COMPETENCE AND CREDENTIALING

There is no national-level board certification for POCUS. Fellowship-trained intensivists typically have their competence documented by the Program Director. Many non-fellowship trained clinicians have opted to pursue certificate programs. The most robust program to our knowledge is the certificate of completion program offered by CHEST. This longitudinal program includes didactic, hands-on ultrasound scanning sessions with human models, an image portfolio, and a summative written and hands-on examination. Several assessment tools

have been developed and validated and should be considered for use.[76,77]

Credentialing is done at the local hospital level. Intensivists have had success with local credentialing based on letters from fellowship Program Directors or completion of training courses and certificate of completion programs. Creating national standards that individual institutions could use for this process is a worthwhile endeavor.

The National Board of Echocardiography has offered the ability to be board certified in advanced CCE since 2019 via the Examination of Special Competence in Critical Care Ultrasonography. This board examination is one component toward a pathway to becoming board certified in Advanced CCE. In addition to passing this examination, the applicant must complete 150 full critical care echocardiograms that are reviewed by a qualified physician. We expect that most academic medical centers will have at least one intensivist with this board certification in the coming years.

QUALITY ASSURANCE, QUALITY IMPROVEMENT, AND BILLING

Successful POCUS programs share similar traits. They have multiple ultrasound machines available for clinical use, generate formal reports of performed studies with clinically relevant conclusions, store the reports and images in the electronic health record, and perform routine quality assurance of the captured images and interpretations.

Physicians with appropriate training can bill for and be reimbursed for ultrasound studies.[78] Billing is a meaningful way to justify the cost of new machines, probes, image management software, and the maintenance of equipment. Koenig and colleagues[79] have published a thorough review of this topic.

CLINICS CARE POINTS

- Point-of-care ultrasonography (POCUS) has application for diagnostic, management and procedural guidance purposes in the intensive care unit.
- Artificial intelligence is a promising technology that will likely increase the diagnostic yield of POCUS.
- Successful POCUS programs generate formal reports of performed studies with clinically relevant conclusions and store these reports and images in the electronic health record.

SUPPLEMENTARY DATA

Supplementary data related to this article can be found online at https://doi.org/10.1016/j.ccm.2022.04.001.

REFERENCES

1. Mayo PH, Beaulieu Y, Doelken P, et al. American college of chest physicians/La Societe de Reanimation de Langue Francaise statement on competence in critical care ultrasonography. Chest 2009;135:1050–60.
2. Expert Round Table on Ultrasound in ICU. International expert statement on training standards for critical care ultrasonography. Intensive Care Med 2011;37:1077–83.
3. Chulani S, Greenstein Y, Patrawalla A, et al. Critical care ultrasonography use at academic training programs: a survey of critical care program directors. Chest 2019;156(4):A916.
4. Chulani S, Greenstein Y, Patrawalla A, et al. Critical care ultrasonography use at academic training programs: a survey of critical care fellows. Chest 2019;156(4):A846.
5. Brady AK, Spitzer CR, Kelm D, et al. Pulmonary critical care fellows' use of and self-reported barriers to learning bedside ultrasound during training. Results of a national survey. Chest 2021;160(1):231–7.
6. Greenstein YY, Littauer R, Narasimhan M, et al. Effectiveness of a critical care ultrasonography course. Chest 2017;151(1):34–40.
7. Silva JP, Plescia T, Molina N, et al. Randomized study of effectiveness of computerized ultrasound simulators for an introductory course for residents in Brazil. J Educ Eval Health Prof 2016;13:16.
8. Frere A, Samba E, Lejus-Bourdeau C. SonoSim ultrasound simulator training for novice residents. A randomised study [letter]. Eur J Anaesthesiol 2021;38:785–97.
9. Greenstein YY, Martin TJ, Rolnitzky L. Goal-directed transthoracic echocardiography during advanced cardiac life support. A pilot study using simulation to assess ability. Simul Healthc 2015;10(4):193–201.
10. Garcia YA, Quintero L, Singh K, et al. Feasibility, safety, and utility of advanced critical care transesophageal echocardiography performed by pulmonary/critical care fellows in a medical ICU. Chest 2017;152(4):736–41.
11. Jujo S, Nakahira A, Kataoka Y, et al. Transesophageal echocardiography simulator training. A systematic review and meta-analysis of randomized controlled trials. Simul Healthc 2021;16(5):341–52 [ahead of print].
12. Schmidt GA, Koenig S, Mayo PH. Shock. Ultrasound to guide diagnosis and therapy. Chest 2012;142(4):1042–8.
13. Abbasi M, Greenstein YY, Mayo PH. Point-of-care ultrasonography for the evaluation of life-threatening hypotension. Ann Am Thorac Soc 2016;13(12):2272–4.
14. Krishnan S, Schmidt GA. Acute right ventricular dysfunction. Real-time management with echocardiography. Chest 2015;147(3):835–46.
15. Rudski LG, Lai WW, Afilalo J, et al. Guidelines for the echocardiographic assessment of the right heart in adults: a report from the American society of echocardiography. Endorsed by the European association of echocardiography, a registered branch of the European society of cardiology, and the Canadian society of echocardiography. J Am Soc Echocardiogr 2010;23:685–713.
16. Vieillard-Baron A, Prin S, Chergui K, et al. Echo-Doppler demonstration of acute cor pulmonale at the bedside in the medical intensive care unit. Am J Respir Crit Care Med 2002;166:1310–9.
17. Porter TR, Shillcutt SK, Adams MS, et al. Guidelines for the use of echocardiography as a monitor for therapeutic intervention in adults: a report from the American Society of Echocardiography. J Am Soc Echocardiogr 2015;28:40–56.
18. Vignon P, Begot E, Mari A, et al. Hemodynamic assessment of patients with septic shock using transpulmonary thermodilution and critical care echocardiography. A comparative study. Chest 2018;153(1):55–64.
19. Etchecopar-Chevreuil C, Francois B, Clavel M, et al. Cardiac morphological and functional changes during early septic shock: a transesophageal echocardiographic study. Intensive Care Med 2008;34:250–6.
20. Sturgess DJ, Marwick TH, Joyce C, et al. Prediction of hospital outcome in septic shock: a prospective comparison of tissue Doppler and cardiac biomarkers. Crit Care 2010;14:R44.
21. Landesberg G, Gilon D, Meroz Y, et al. Diastolic dysfunction and mortality in severe sepsis and septic shock. Eur Heart J 2020;33:895–903.
22. Brown SM, Pittman JE, Hirshberg EL, et al. Diastolic dysfunction and mortality in early severe sepsis and septic shock: a prospective observational echocardiography study. Crit Ultrasound J 2012;4:8.
23. Nagueh SF, Smiseth OA, Appleton CP, et al. Recommendations for the evaluation of left ventricular diastolic function by echocardiography: an update from the American Society of Echocardiography and the European Association of Cardiovascular Imaging. J Am Soc Echocardiogr 2016;29:277–314.
24. Greenstein YY, Mayo PH. Evaluation of left ventricular diastolic function by the intensivist. Chest 2018;153(3):723–32.
25. Lamia B, Maizel J, Ochagavia A, et al. Echocardiographic diagnosis of pulmonary artery occlusion pressure elevation during weaning from mechanical ventilation. Crit Care Med 2009;37:1696–701.

26. Moschietto S, Doyen D, Grech L, et al. Transthoracic echocardiography with Doppler tissue imaging predicts weaning failure from mechanical ventilation: evolution of the left ventricle relaxation rate during a sponteaneous breathing trial is the key factor in weaning outcome. Crit Care 2012;16:R81.

27. Sanfilippo F, Di Falco D, Noto A, et al. Association of weaning failure from mechanical ventilation with transthoracic echocardiography parameters: a systematic review and meta-analysis. Br J Anaesth 2021;126(1):319–30.

28. Michard F, Teboul JL. Using heart-lung interactions to assess fluid responsiveness during mechanical ventilation. Crit Care 2000;4:282–9.

29. Zoghbi W, Adams D, Bonow R, et al. Recommendations for noninvasive evaluation of native valvular regurgitation. A report from the American Society of Echocardiography developed in collaboration with the Society for Cardiovascular Magnetic Resonance. J Am Soc Echocardiogr 2017;30:303–71.

30. Quinones MA, Douglas PS, Foster E, et al. American College of Cardiology/American Heart Association clinical competence statement on echocardiography. Circulation 2003;107:1068–89.

31. Benjamin E, Griffin K, Leibowitz AB, et al. Goal-directed transesophageal echocardiography performed by intensivists to assess left ventricular function: comparison with pulmonary artery catheterization. J Cardiothorac Vasc Anesth 1998;12(1):10–5.

32. Huttemann E. Transoesophageal echocardiography in critical care. Minerva Anestesiol 2006;72: 891–913.

33. Arntfield R, Pace J, Hewak M, et al. Focused transesophageal echocardiography by emergency physicians is feasible and clinically influential: observational results from a novel ultrasound program. J Emerg Med 2016;50(2):286–94.

34. Lau V, Priestap F, Landry Y, et al. Diagnostic accuracy of critical care transesophageal echocardiography vs cardiology-led echocardiography in ICU patients. Chest 2019;155(3):491–501.

35. Ramalingam G, Choi SW, Agarwal S, et al. Complications related to peri-operative transesophageal echocardiography – a one-year prospective national audit by the Association of Cardiothoracic Anaesthesia and Critical Care. Anaesthesia 2020; 75:21–6.

36. Charbonneau H, Riu B, Faron M, et al. Predicting preload responsiveness using simultaneous recordings of inferior and superior vena cavae diameters. Crit Care 2014;18:473.

37. Vignon P, Repesse X, Begot E, et al. Comparison of echocardiographic indices used to predict fluid responsiveness in ventilated patients. Am J Respir Crit Care Med 2017;195(8):1022–32.

38. Kory P. Counterpoint: should acute fluid resuscitation be guided primarily by inferior vena cava ultrasound for patients in shock? No. Chest 2017; 151(3):533–6.

39. Lamia B, Ochagavia A, Monnet X, et al. Echocardiographic prediction of volume responsiveness in critically ill patients with spontaneously breathing activity. Intensive Care Med 2007;33:1125–32.

40. Maizel J, Airapetian N, Lorne E, et al. Diagnosis of central hypovolemia by using passive leg raising. Intensive Care Med 2007;33:1133–8.

41. Funk DJ, Jacobsohn E, Kumar A. The role of venous return in critical illness and shock – Part 1: Physiology. Crit Care Med 2013;41:255–62.

42. Beaubien-Souligny W, Bouchard J, Desjardins G, et al. Extracardiac signs of fluid overload in the critically ill cardiac patient: a focused evaluation using bedside ultrasound. Can J Cardiol 2017;33:88–100.

43. Beaubien-Souligny W, Rola P, Haycock K, et al. Quantifying systemic congestion with point-of-care ultrasound: development of the venous excess ultrasound grading system. Ultrasound J 2020;12:16.

44. Xia W, West SJ, Finlay MC, et al. Looking beyond the imaging plane: 3D needle tracking with a linear array ultrasound probe. Sci Rep 2017;7:3674.

45. Kasine T, Romundstad L, Rosseland LA, et al. Needle tip tracking for ultrasound-guided peripheral nerve block procedures – an observer blinded, randomised, controlled, crossover study on a phantom model. Acta Anaesthesiol Scand 2019;63:1055–62.

46. Kasine T, Romundstad L, Rosseland LA, et al. The effect of needle tip tracking on procedural time of ultrasound-guided lumbar plexus block: a randomised controlled trial. Anaesthesia 2020;75:72–9.

47. Lichtenstein D. Lung ultrasound in the critically ill. J Med Ultrasound 2009;17(3):125–42.

48. Lichtenstein D, Meziere G, Biderman P, et al. The comet-tail artifact. An ultrasound sign of alveolar-interstitial syndrome. Am J Respir Crit Care Med 1997;156:1640–6.

49. Koenig SJ, Narasimhan M, Mayo PH. Thoracic ultrasonography for the pulmonary specialist. Chest 2011;140:1332–41.

50. Zanobetti M, Poggioni C, Pini R. Can chest ultrasonography replace standard chest radiography for evaluation of acute dyspnea in the ED? Chest 2011;139(5):1140–7.

51. Maw AM, Hassanin A, Ho PM, et al. Diagnostic accuracy of point-of-care lung ultrasonography and chest radiography in adults with symptoms suggestive of acute decompensated heart failure. A systematic review and meta-analysis. JAMA Netw Open 2019;2(3):e190703.

52. Buonsens D, Pata D, Chiaretti A. COVID-19 outbreak: less stethoscope, more ultrasound. Lancet Respir Med 2020;8(5):E27.

53. Lichtenstein DA, Menu Y. A bedside ultrasound sign ruling out pneumothorax in the critically ill. Lung sliding. Chest 1995;108:1345–8.

54. Sartori S, Tombesi P, Trevisani L, et al. Accuracy of transthoracic sonography in detection of pneumothorax after sonographically guided lung biopsy: prospective comparison with chest radiography. AJR Am J Roentgenol 2007;188:37–41.

55. Lichtenstein DA, Lascols N, Prin S, et al. The "lung pulse": an early ultrasound sign of complete atelectasis. Intensive Care Med 2003;29:2187–92.

56. Lichtenstein D, Meziere G, Biderman P, et al. The "lung point": an ultrasound sign specific to pneumothorax. Intensive Care Med 2000;26:1434–40.

57. Volpicelli G, Elbarbary M, Blaivas M, et al. International evidence-based recommendations for point-of-care lung ultrasound. Intensive Care Med 2012; 38(4):577–91.

58. Jambrik Z, Gargani L, Adamicza A, et al. B-lines quantify the lung water content: a lung ultrasound versus lung gravimetry study in acute lung injury. Ultrasound Med Biol 2010;36(12):2004–10.

59. Trezzi M, Torzillo D, Ceriani E, et al. Lung ultrasonography for the assessment of rapid extravascular water variation: evidence from hemodialysis patients. Intern Emerg Med 2013;8;409–15.

60. Arntfield R, VanBerlo B, Alaifan T, et al. Development of a convulational neural network to differentiate among the etiology of similar appearing pathological B lines on lung ultrasound: a deep learning study. BMJ Open 2021;11:e045120.

61. Yang PC, Luh KT, Chang DB, et al. Value of sonography in determining the nature of pleural effusion: analysis of 320 cases. AJR 1992;159:29–33.

62. Sajadieh H, Afzali F, Sajadieh V, et al. Ultrasound as an alternative to aspiration for determining the nature of pleural effusion, especially in older people. Ann N Y Acad Sci 2014;1019:585–92.

63. Shkolnik B, Judson MA, Austin A, et al. Diagnostic accuracy of thoracic ultrasonography to differentiate transudative from exudative pleural effusion. Chest 2020;158(2):692–7.

64. Sekiguchi H, Suzuki J, Daniels CE. Making paracentesis safer. A proposal for the use of bedside abdominal and vascular ultrasonography to prevent a fatal complication. Chest 2013;143(4):1136–9.

65. Marik PE, Andrews L, Maini B. The incidence of deep venous thrombosis in ICU patients. Chest 1997;111:661–4.

66. Malato A, Dentali F, Siragusa S, et al. The impact of deep vein thrombosis in critically ill patients: a meta-analysis of major clinical outcomes. Blood Transfus 2015;13:559–68.

67. Hill JB, Garcia D, Crowther, et al. Frequency of venous thromboembolism in 6513 patients with COVID-10: a retrospective study. Blood Adv 2020; 4(21):5373–7.

68. Bilaloglu S, Aphinyanaphongs Y, Jones S, et al. Thrombosis in hospitalized patients with COVID-19 in a New York city health system [letter]. JAMA 2020;324(8):799–801.

69. Kory PD, Pellecchia CM, Shiloh AL, et al. Accuracy of ultrasonography performed by critical care physicians for the diagnosis of DVT. Chest 2011;139(3): 538–42.

70. Lensing AW, Doris I, McGrath FP, et al. A comparison of compression ultrasound with color Doppler ultrasound for the diagnosis of symptomless postoperative deep vein thrombosis. Arch Intern Med 1997;157:765–8.

71. Patel NY, Riherd JM. Focused assessment with sonography for trauma: methods, accuracy, and indications. Surg Clin North Am 2011;91:195–207.

72. Subbaiah TC, Greenstein Y. A 75-year old woman with cirrhosis and shock. Chest 2019;155(4):e87–9.

73. Koeze J, Dieperink W, van der Horst IC, et al. Incidence, timing and outcome of AKI in critically ill patients varies with the definition used and the addition of urine output criteria. BMC Nephrol 2017;18:70.

74. Greenstein YY, Koenig SJ. A woman in her 60s with septic shock, abdominal pain, and a positive urinalysis. Chest 2014;145(3):e7–9.

75. Lee YY, Tsay WL, Lou MF, et al. The effectiveness of implementing a bladder ultrasound programme in neurosurgical units. J Adv Nurs 2006;57(2): 192–200.

76. Patrawalla P, Eisen LA, Shiloh A, et al. Development and validation of an assessment tool for competency in critical care ultrasound. J Grad Med Educ 2015; 7(4):567–73.

77. Millington SJ, Arntfield RT, Guo RJ, et al. The assessment of competency in thoracic sonography (ACTS) scale: validation of a tool for point-of-care ultrasound. Crit Ultrasound J 2017;9:25.

78. American medical association res. H-230.960. Privileging for ultrasound imaging. 2010. Available at: https://policysearch.ama-assn.org/policyfinder/detail/Ultrasound%20imaging?uri=%2FAMADoc%2FHOD.xml-0-1591.xml. Accessed July 28, 2021.

79. Koenig SJ, Lou BX, Moskowitz Y, et al. Ultrasound billing for intensivists. Chest 2019;156(4):792–801.

Application of Focused Assessment with Sonography for Trauma in the Intensive Care Unit

Molly E.W. Thiessen, MD[a,b,1,*], Matthew Riscinti, MD[a,b,1]

KEYWORDS

- FAST • E-FAST • Focused abdominal sonography for trauma • Point-of-care ultrasound
- Critical care • Trauma • Emergency medicine • Ultrasound

KEY POINTS

- The Focused Assessment with Sonography for Trauma (FAST) and Extended-FAST (E-FAST) examinations allow clinicians to rapidly diagnose hemoperitoneum, pericardial effusion, hemothorax, and pneumothorax at the bedside.
- The traditional FAST examination is highly specific and has an excellent ability to quickly diagnose life-threatening injuries and prompt immediate action.
- It is moderately sensitive and should not be used alone to rule out dangerous thoracoabdominal trauma in patients with a significant mechanism or presentation.
- The E-FAST includes evaluation for hemothorax and pneumothorax. Lung ultrasound has been found to have better diagnostic accuracy than supine chest radiograph for pneumothorax.

Video content accompanies this article at http://www.chestmed.theclinics.com.

INTRODUCTION
History of the Focused Assessment with Sonography for Trauma

The Focused Assessment with Sonography for Trauma (FAST) examination has evolved from one of the first point-of-care ultrasound modalities to a key component of the Advanced Trauma Life Support primary survey. The FAST examination emerged in the literature in the 1990s to provide a rapid, noninvasive method of evaluating blunt abdominal trauma for free intraperitoneal fluid in unstable trauma patients at the bedside. This utility allowed it to replace the more invasive diagnostic peritoneal lavage (DPL).[1,2] Initial studies by Tso and Rozycki described its use and accuracy in diagnosing hemoperitoneum and hemopericardium.[3,4]

Rozycki and *colleagues* recommended that it is the initial diagnostic modality for patients in the setting of trauma and the patients with hemopericardium or hemoperitoneum and hypotension should receive immediate surgical intervention.[4] In the setting of penetrating cardiac injury, it was found to decrease the time to diagnosis and improve survival and quality of life in survivors.[5] Numerous studies followed, and in 1999, an international consensus conference coined the term "Focused Assessment with Sonography for Trauma" and described the clinical integration for

The author has nothing to disclose.
[a] Department of Emergency Medicine, Denver Health Medical Center, Denver, CO, USA; [b] Department of Emergency Medicine, University of Colorado School of Medicine, Aurora, CO, USA
[1] Denver Health Medical Center, MC 0108, 777 Bannock Street, Denver, CO 80204, USA
* Corresponding author.
E-mail address: Molly.Thiessen@dhha.org
Twitter: @ermama1979 (M.E.W.T.); @thepocusatlas (M.R.)

Clin Chest Med 43 (2022) 385–392
https://doi.org/10.1016/j.ccm.2022.05.004
0272-5231/22/© 2022 Elsevier Inc. All rights reserved.

the FAST examination: hemodynamically unstable patients with free intra-abdominal fluid should go for immediate laparotomy; hemodynamically unstable patients without demonstrable free fluid should have an alternative etiology of shock pursued; and hemodynamically stable patients who have free fluid should be evaluated with computed tomography (CT).[6] The FAST examination has evolved to include imaging of the thorax in what is known as the "Extended-FAST" (E-FAST).

DISCUSSION

Literature Support for Focused Assessment with Sonography for Trauma/Extended-Focused Assessment with Sonography for Trauma

Since the FAST emerged as an imaging modality for the evaluation of trauma patients, it has been rigorously studied. Netheron and colleagues performed a systematic review and meta-analysis that included 75 studies and 24,350 patients spanning 28 years. The pooled sensitivities and specificities were 74% and 98% for intraperitoneal free fluid, 91% and 94% for pericardial effusion, and 69% and 99% for pneumothorax.[7] The E-FAST has been shown to change management in a significant number of trauma patients, reducing the use of CT and DPL.[8,9] A positive FAST examination has been shown to be highly associated with a need for laparotomy, even in normotensive patients.[10] A recent large Cochrane review found the pooled sensitivity of 74% and specificity of 96%, which is consistent with multiple previous studies. The authors concluded that the E-FAST is helpful for guiding treatment in patients who have experienced trauma.[11]

The supportive evidence tends to be even stronger for the thoracic applications of the E-FAST examination. POCUS is more accurate than a supine chest radiograph for the diagnosis of pneumothorax.[12–15] In a recent Cochrane review, Chan and *colleagues* found the pooled sensitivity and specificity of ultrasound for pneumothorax to be 91% and 99%, respectively. The superiority of ultrasound over chest radiograph was persistent regardless of the type of trauma, the experience of the sonographer, or the type of transducer.[16] In addition, ultrasound has been found to have good accuracy in detecting hemothorax.[17–19]

More recently, its predictive value in the setting of traumatic cardiac arrest has been evaluated. Multiple studies indicate that if a patient presents in cardiac arrest has no cardiac activity on ultrasound and no pericardial effusion or tamponade, the likelihood of survival to hospital discharge is so low that further resuscitative efforts are not warranted.[20–23] Israr and colleagues demonstrated that cardiac activity on ultrasound is associated with survival to hospital admission, but subsequent survival to hospital discharge is not likely. Because of the possibility of survival through organ donation, some investigators recommend continuing resuscitative efforts in the patients with organized cardiac activity.[23,24]

The E-FAST carries a long-term clinical experience as well as an extensive literature base to support its use. The American College of Surgeons lists it in the "Best Practice in Imaging Guidelines," and the American College of Emergency Physicians lists it as a "core" ultrasound skill for emergency physicians. Its use is described in numerous critical care publications.[1,25–27] Although its traditional application is the evaluation of patients with trauma for immediately intervenable injuries, its ability to rapidly identify intraperitoneal fluid, hemothorax, pneumothorax, and pericardial effusion can provide the intensivist with invaluable information to guide patient management.

Indications

Indications for the E-FAST examination are traditionally abdominal or thoracic trauma. This allows for an assessment of free intraperitoneal fluid, pericardial effusion, pneumothorax, and hemothorax in the setting of blunt or penetrating trauma, with a goal of identifying immediately intervenable causes of shock. Traditionally, patients who are hypotensive and have free intraperitoneal fluid should have immediate surgical intervention. Pericardial effusion can be treated with thoracotomy when indicated, and tube thoracostomy can be performed to relieve pneumothorax or hemothorax. Patients with a positive E-FAST examination, normal vital signs, and no indication for immediate intervention should undergo definitive imaging with CT to further delineate the nature of their injuries. Given the known sensitivities and limitations of the E-FAST, it is essential that clinicians do not use the E-FAST alone to rule out injuries in the patients whereby the mechanism or presentation is concerning for significant thoracoabdominal trauma. In these patients, a negative E-FAST should be followed by definitive imaging. In the general intensive care unit (ICU) setting, these modalities can be used to evaluate for other sources of free intraperitoneal fluid (ie, ascites), pleural effusion, pericardial effusion, and so forth.

Imaging Technique

Probe selection

The E-FAST examination can use the full complement of ultrasound probes. The curvilinear probe has appropriate depth for visualization of deep abdominal structures. The phased array probe trades off resolution for a smaller footprint that allows easier access to the subxiphoid cardiac view and visualization between ribs in the upper quadrant views. Both of these probes can be used for the thoracic portion of the E-FAST, or the operator can switch to the high-frequency linear probe to specifically assess for pneumothorax.

Views and Scanning Technique

Traditionally, the first view obtained in an E-FAST examination is the right upper quadrant (RUQ) view, as it is known to be the most sensitive in detecting free intraperitoneal fluid.[28] The examination then proceeds to the evaluation of the left upper quadrant (LUQ), the pelvis, the heart, and finally the lungs. This is by convention, and the examination can be carried out in any order, depending on the clinical situation. In cases of penetrating thoracic trauma, the operator may wish to obtain the cardiac and lung views initially, as pericardial tamponade and pneumothorax may be more immediately life-threatening and require immediate intervention.

To obtain the RUQ view, the probe is placed in the coronal plane in the mid-axillary line (**Fig. 1**). In this view, the liver, kidney, and Morrison's pouch are easily visualized (Video 1). In this position, sliding towards the head a few inches will allow visualization of the right hemithorax over the diaphragm. Free intraperitoneal fluid seems as an anechoic stripe in any of these areas (Video 2). Free fluid may accumulate in Morison's pouch, but once this view is obtained, the operator should fan the probe anteriorly and posteriorly to evaluate the entire area, making special note of any fluid under the diaphragm or at the inferior tip of the liver, keeping in mind that the most sensitive location is at the inferior tip of the liver[28] (Video 3).

The LUQ view is obtained by placing the probe in the coronal plane in the mid-posterior axillary line in the LUQ. As opposed to the RUQ view, this view is more easily obtained by aiming the probe from posterior to anterior, as the spleen is a retroperitoneal organ (**Fig. 2**). This orientation will also mitigate gas in the stomach and splenic flexure of the colon obstructing the view. In this view, the spleen, kidney, and diaphragm are visualized (Video 4). Sliding towards the head will again allow for visualization of the left hemithorax over the diaphragm. Of note, because of the attachment of the phrenicocolic ligament, fluid in the LUQ may accumulate more readily under the diaphragm or at the inferior tip of the spleen (**Fig. 3**), and special attention must be paid to these areas. Although the RUQ is the most sensitive view, a significant number of patients may have fluid accumulation in the LUQ as well.[29]

The pelvic view is obtained by placing the probe just above the pubic symphysis in the transverse orientation, with the indicator to the patient's right (**Fig. 4**). The probe then fans through the entire bladder, which will appear as a round, anechoic structure (Video 5). Following this view, the probe should be rotated to the sagittal plane, and the bladder should be visualized while fanning left to right, looking again for the presence of free fluid. Free fluid will appear as an anechoic stripe deep to the bladder in anatomic males or in the pouch of Douglas in anatomic females (Video 6).

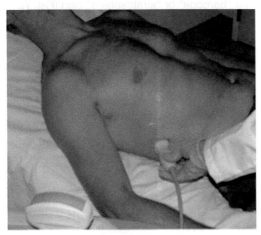

Fig. 1. Right upper quadrant probe placement. (*From* Williams, Sarah, et al. "The FAST and E-FAST in 2013: Trauma Ultrasonography," Crit Care Clin 30 (2014): 119-150.)

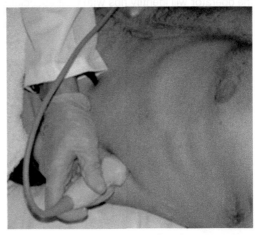

Fig. 2. Left upper quadrant probe placement. (*From* Williams, Sarah, et al. "The FAST and E-FAST in 2013: Trauma Ultrasonography," Crit Care Clin 30 (2014): 119-150.)

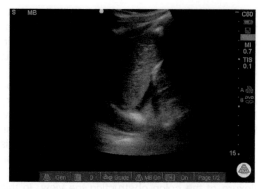

Fig. 3. Free fluid in the left upper quadrant. (*Courtesy of* M Macias, MD, La Jolla, California.)

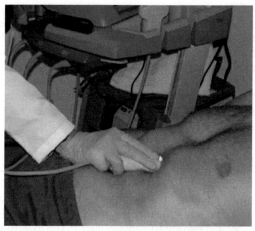

Fig. 5. Subxiphoid cardiac probe placement. (*From* Williams, Sarah, et al. "The FAST and E-FAST in 2013: Trauma Ultrasonography," Crit Care Clin 30 (2014): 119-150.)

The cardiac view can be obtained with any of the traditional echocardiography views, subxiphoid, parasternal long axis, or apical. Many operators find the subxiphoid view the most efficient while providing excellent information. In the subxiphoid view, the probe is placed in the transverse plane in the subxiphoid region, and the heart is scanned deep to the sternum (**Fig. 5**). The normal anatomic structures are visualized (Video 7), and the operator should make a note of overall cardiacactivity and evaluate for the presence of pericardial effusion that seems as an anechoic stripe between the liver and right atria and right ventricle (Video 8).

To complete the E-FAST, the lungs are visualized for pneumothorax. This is best obtained with the patient supine, and the probe should be placed in the sagittal plane in the mid-clavicular line (**Fig. 6**) or in the least-dependent area in a patient who is not supine. This is to ensure the probe is placed on the area of the patient's chest where the air is most likely to be present. In this view, the operator will identify ribs with their associated shadows and look for lung sliding on the pleural line at the base of the ribs (Video 9). Lung sliding appears as a scintillating appearance or "ants on a log" appearance of movement along the pleural line, indicating that the visceral and parietal pleura are sliding against each other. Alternatively, lungs motion can be visualized using the M-Mode functionality of the ultrasound. The M-Mode cursor is placed over the pleural line, and in a normal lung, a "seashore sign" appears, in which there is a sharp demarcation at the level of the pleural line and the lines going across the screen change from smooth to grainy. When a pneumothorax is present and there is air under the probe, lung sliding will not be present, and the M-Mode view will lose the sharp demarcation seen and appear as a "barcode" or "stratosphere" sign (**Fig. 7**).

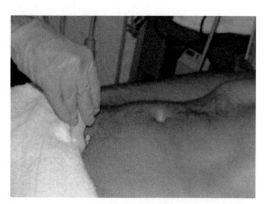

Fig. 4. Transverse pelvic view probe placement. (*From* Williams, Sarah, et al. "The FAST and E-FAST in 2013: Trauma Ultrasonography," Crit Care Clin 30 (2014): 119-150.)

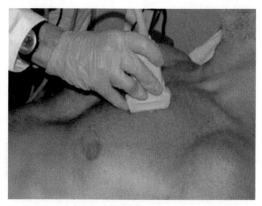

Fig. 6. Probe placement for lung ultrasound for pneumothorax. (*From* Williams, Sarah, et al. "The FAST and E-FAST in 2013: Trauma Ultrasonography," Crit Care Clin 30 (2014): 119-150.)

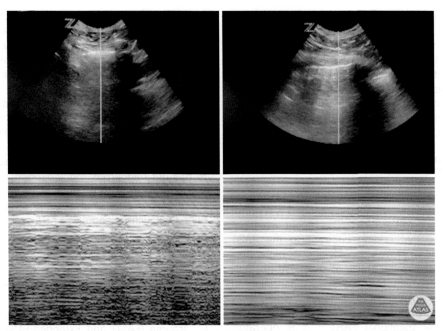

Fig. 7. Seashore sign (left) versus the barcode sign (right). (*Courtesy of* E Roseman, MD, Brooklyn, New York.)

Pitfalls

Although the literature base for the E-FAST is robust, there are pitfalls and limitations that clinicians should be aware of to use the test appropriately. Most importantly, the E-FAST is traditionally a highly specific and moderately sensitive test. It is best used to rule in a diagnosis in question, and a single negative E-FAST should not be used to rule out significant injury. Depending on the rate of hemorrhage and the timing of presentation, patients will have variable amounts of free intraperitoneal fluid. A study performed by Branney and colleagues found that sensitivity increased as the volume of fluid increased. In their study, the smallest amount of fluid detected was 225 mL, but fewer than 10% of sonographers were able to detect volumes of less than 400 mL. That number increased to 85% when 850 mL of fluid was present.[30] As such, clinicians must not assume that a negative FAST conclusively rules out hemoperitoneum and pursue further workup. In addition, when a patient who has experienced trauma becomes hypotensive, a repeat FAST examination may reveal free intraperitoneal fluid that was not visualized previously. An evaluation of false-negative FAST examinations showed that head injuries were highly associated with false-negative FASTs (odds ratio [OR] 4.9; 95% confidence interval [CI] 1.5–15.7), whereas severe intra-abdominal injury was negatively associated (OR 0.3; 95% CI 0.1–0.5). False-negative FASTs were not associated with increased mortality, prolonged ICU stay or overall length of stay.[31]

The FAST was traditionally designed to detect free intraperitoneal fluid. As such, it has limited application with respect to the diagnosis of solid organ injury, hollow viscus injury with minimal or no hemoperitoneum, diaphragmatic injury, retroperitoneal hemorrhage, and pelvic fractures.[2,32] Although the sensitivity improves with the grade of solid organ injury, and it is highly specific for solid organ injury, additional imaging with CT is recommended to further evaluate for this when the FAST is negative, and there is a clinical suspicion of significant abdominal trauma.[1,33] Retroperitoneal hemorrhage is difficult to evaluate with FAST, given the nature of the examination. Pelvic fractures may result in significant hypotension without detection of free fluid on the FAST, and pelvic radiographs are still indicated in patients with trauma at risk for these injuries.[1]

False-positive E-FAST examinations also occur. Classic pitfalls are misidentifying fluid in the abdomen as intraperitoneal when it is actually contained within the bowel, the bladder, the gallbladder, or renal cysts. The fluid that is appropriately contained within another structure will have a round and regular appearance, the walls surrounding the fluid will be concave, and in the case of the bowel, it may exhibit peristalsis. The fluid that is not contained will have irregular borders that are convex to the fluid (Video 10).

Perinephric fat and epicardial fat can also be misinterpreted as clotted blood, which takes on a more echogenic or gray-to-white appearance. Some patients will have intraperitoneal free fluid that is not blood, such as ascites or urine, in the case of bladder rupture. In these instances, a diagnostic peritoneal aspirate may help in the rapid evaluation of the nature of the fluid within the abdomen.[1]

Future/Emerging Applications

As the E-FAST has evolved, there have been emerging additional applications to improve on its use. Contrast-enhanced ultrasound is a promising addition to the FAST. The recent investigations show that adding contrast to the FAST examination improves sensitivities to more than 90%.[34–36] It has the ability to diagnose not only active hemorrhage but also solid organ injury of the liver, spleen, and kidneys, significantly improving on the known limitations in the sensitivity of the traditional FAST.[37] It is operator-dependent and requires specialized equipment to perform, in addition to the actual contrast media. However, it shows promise, especially as a method to follow injuries initially diagnosed on a computed tomography (CT) scan while avoiding additional ionizing radiation.[34]

There is a rapidly growing literature base describing the utility of E-FAST in the prehospital setting.[38–40] This has been studied in the hands of physicians and other prehospital providers[39] and has the potential to guide the prehospital care of injured patients.

The addition of the resuscitative endovascular balloon occlusion of the aorta (REBOA) device has added an additional tool to treat shock in the setting of trauma. In a recent study, Christian and *colleagues* found that the FAST performed overall well (96% sensitive and specific) in patients with pelvic fractures and hemorrhagic shock who required pelvic packing. The authors suggest that in this select group of patients, the FAST examination can help guide management. For patients who are hemodynamically unstable in the setting of pelvic fractures, a positive FAST should prompt laparotomy, whereas a negative FAST should prompt the consideration of the placement of a REBOA device.[41]

SUMMARY

The E-FAST is a minimally invasive tool that allows clinicians to rapidly diagnose significant trauma at the bedside without ionizing radiation. It has high specificity and is extremely useful as an initial test to rule in dangerous diagnoses, such as hemoperitoneum, pericardial effusion, hemothorax, and pneumothorax. Patients with significant trauma who are hypotensive and have a positive FAST examination should be taken for immediate laparotomy. Pericardial effusion, pneumothorax, and hemothorax should be treated as the patient's condition indicates. Patients who have a positive FAST and are stable should undergo definitive imaging to further delineate the nature of their injuries. Its moderate sensitivity means that it should not be used alone as a tool to rule out dangerous thoracoabdominal injuries, and in patients with a concerning mechanism or presentation, additional imaging should be obtained following a negative FAST examination.

CLINICS CARE POINTS

- The Focused Assessment with Sonography for Trauma (FAST) and Extended-FAST (E-FAST) examinations allow clinicians to rapidly diagnose hemoperitoneum, pericardial effusion, hemothorax, and pneumothorax at the bedside.

- The traditional FAST examination is highly specific and has an excellent ability to quickly diagnose life-threatening injuries and prompt immediate treatment.

- It is moderately sensitive and should not be used alone to rule out dangerous thoracoabdominal trauma in patients with a concerning mechanism or presentation.

- The E-FAST adds the evaluation of the thorax for hemothorax and pneumothorax. Lung ultrasound has been found to have better diagnostic accuracy than supine chest radiograph for pneumothorax.

SUPPLEMENTARY DATA

Supplementary data related to this article can be found online at https://doi.org/10.1016/j.ccm.2022.05.004.

REFERENCES

1. Williams SR, Perera P, Gharahbaghian L. The FAST and E-FAST in 2013: trauma ultrasonography. CritCareClin 2014;30(1):119–50.
2. Montoya J, Stawicki SP, Evans DC, et al. From FAST to E-FAST: an overview of the evolution of ultrasound-based traumatic injury assessment. Eur J TraumaEmerg Surg 2016;42(2):119–26.

3. Tso P, Rodriguez A, Cooper C, et al. Sonography in blunt abdominal trauma: a preliminary progress report. J Trauma Inj Infect CritCare 1992;33(1):39–44.
4. Rozycki GS, Ballard RB, Feliciano DV, et al. Surgeon-performed ultrasound for the assessment of truncal injuries: lessons learned from 1540 patients. Ann Surg 1998;228(4):557–67.
5. Plummer D, Brunette D, Asinger R, et al. Emergency department echocardiography improves outcome in penetrating cardiac injury. Ann Emerg Med 1992;21(6):709–12.
6. Scalea TM, Rodriguez A, Chiu WC, et al. Focused assessment with sonography for trauma (FAST): results from an international consensus conference. J Trauma Inj Infect CritCare 1999;46(3):466–72.
7. Netherton S, Milenkovic V, Taylor M, et al. Diagnostic accuracy of eFAST in the trauma patient: a systematic review and meta-analysis. CJEM 2019;21(6):727–38.
8. Ollerton JE, Sugrue M, Balogh Z, et al. Prospective study to evaluate the influence of FAST on trauma patient management. J Trauma Inj Infect CritCare 2006;60(4):785–91.
9. Branney SW, Moore EE, Cantrill SV, et al. Ultrasound based key clinical pathway reduces the use of hospital resources for the evaluation of blunt abdominal trauma. J Trauma Inj Infect CritCare 1997;42(6):1086–90.
10. Moylan M, Newgard CD, Ma OJ, et al. Association between a positive ED FAST Examination and therapeutic laparotomy in normotensive blunt trauma patients. J Emerg Med 2007;33(3):265–71.
11. Stengel D, Leisterer J, Ferrada P, et al. Point-of-care ultrasonography for diagnosing thoracoabdominal injuries in patients with blunt trauma. Cochrane Injuries Group. In: Stengel D, editor. Cochrane database of systematic reviews12. John Wiley & Sons, Ltd; 2018:CD012669.
12. Alrajab S, Youssef AM, Akkus NI, et al. Pleural ultrasonography versus chest radiography for the diagnosis of pneumothorax: review of the literature and meta-analysis. CritCare 2013;17(5):R208.
13. Alrajhi K, Woo MY, Vaillancourt C. Test characteristics of ultrasonography for the detection of pneumothorax. Chest 2012;141(3):703–8.
14. Blaivas M. A prospective comparison of supine chest radiography and bedside ultrasound for the diagnosis of traumatic pneumothorax. AcadEmerg Med 2005;12(9):844–9.
15. Soldati G, Testa A, Sher S, et al. Occult traumatic pneumothorax. Chest 2008;133(1):204–11.
16. Chan KK, Joo DA, McRae AD, et al. Chest ultrasonography versus supine chest radiography for diagnosis of pneumothorax in trauma patients in the emergency department. Cochrane Emergency and Critical Care Group. In: Chan KK, editor. Cochrane database of systematic reviews7. John Wiley & Sons, Ltd; 2020:CD013031.
17. Brooks A. Emergency ultrasound in the acute assessment of haemothorax. Emerg Med J 2004;21(1):44–6.
18. Ma OJ, Mateer JR. Trauma ultrasound examination versus chest radiography in the detection of hemothorax. Ann Emerg Med 1997;29(3):312–6.
19. Staub LJ, Biscaro RRM, Kaszubowski E, et al. Chest ultrasonography for the emergency diagnosis of traumatic pneumothorax and haemothorax: a systematic review and meta-analysis. Injury 2018;49(3):457–66.
20. Cureton EL, Yeung LY, Kwan RO, et al. The heart of the matter: utility of ultrasound of cardiac activity during traumatic arrest. J Trauma Acute Care Surg 2012;73(1):102–10.
21. Inaba K, Chouliaras K, Zakaluzny S, et al. FAST ultrasound examination as a predictor of outcomes after resuscitative thoracotomy: a prospective evaluation. Ann Surg 2015;262(3):512–8.
22. Moore EE, Knudson MM, Burlew CC, et al. Defining the limits of resuscitative emergency department thoracotomy: a contemporary western trauma association perspective. J Trauma Inj Infect CritCare 2011;70(2):334–9.
23. Schuster KM, Lofthouse R, Moore C, et al. Pulseless electrical activity, focused abdominal sonography for trauma, and cardiac contractile activity as predictors of survival after trauma. J Trauma Inj Infect CritCare 2009;67(6):1154–7.
24. Israr S, Cook A, Chapple K, et al. Pulseless electrical activity following traumatic cardiac arrest: sign of life or death? Injury 2019;50(9):1507–10.
25. Balmert N, Espinosa J, Arafeh M-O, et al. Integration of bedside ultrasound into the ICU—a review of indications, techniques and interventions. J EmergCritCare Med 2018;2:17.
26. Beaulieu Y, Marik PE. Bedside ultrasonography in the ICU. Chest 2005;128(3):1766–81.
27. Cardenas-Garcia J, Mayo PH. Bedside ultrasonography for the intensivist. CritCareClin 2015;31(1):43–66.
28. Lobo V, Hunter-Behrend M, Cullnan E, et al. Caudal edge of the liver in the right upper quadrant (RUQ) view is the most sensitive area for free fluid on the FAST exam. WestJEM 2017;18(2):270–80.
29. O'Brien KM, Stolz LA, Amini R, et al. Focused assessment with sonography for trauma examination: reexamining the importance of the left upper quadrant view. J Ultrasound Med 2015;34(8):1429–34.
30. Branney SW, Wolfe RE, Moore EE, et al. Quantitative sensitivity of ultrasound in detecting free intraperitoneal fluid. J Trauma Inj Infect CritCare 1995;39(2):375–80.
31. Laselle BT, Byyny RL, Haukoos JS, et al. False-negative FAST examination: associations with injury

characteristics and patient outcomes. Ann Emerg Med 2012;60(3):326–34.e3.

32. Miller MT, Pasquale MD, Bromberg WJ, et al. Not so fast. J Trauma Inj Infect CritCare 2003;54(1):52–60.

33. Schnüriger B, Kilz J, Inderbitzin D, et al. The accuracy of FAST in relation to grade of solid organ injuries: a retrospective analysis of 226 trauma patients with liver or splenic lesion. BMC Med Imaging 2009;9(1):3.

34. Miele V, Piccolo CL, Galluzzo M, et al. Contrast-enhanced ultrasound (CEUS) in blunt abdominal trauma. BJR 2016;89(1061):20150823.

35. Sessa B, Trinci M, Ianniello S, et al. Blunt abdominal trauma: role of contrast-enhanced ultrasound (CEUS) in the detection and staging of abdominal traumatic lesions compared to US and CE-MDCT. Radiol Med 2015;120(2):180–9.

36. Zhang Z, Hong Y, Liu N, et al. Diagnostic accuracy of contrast enhanced ultrasound in patients with blunt abdominal trauma presenting to the emergency department: a systematic review and meta-analysis. Sci Rep 2017;7(1):4446.

37. Cagini L, Gravante S, Malaspina CM, et al. Contrast enhanced ultrasound (CEUS) in blunt abdominal trauma. CritUltrasound J 2013;5(S1):S9.

38. El Zahran T, El Sayed M. Prehospital ultrasound in trauma: a review of current and potential future clinical applications. J EmergTraumaShock 2018; 11(1):4.

39. Mercer CB, Ball M, Cash RE, et al. Ultrasound use in the prehospital setting for trauma: a systematic review. PrehospEmergCare 2021;25(4):566–82.

40. van der Weide L, Popal Z, Terra M, et al. Prehospital ultrasound in the management of trauma patients: systematic review of the literature. Injury 2019; 50(12):2167–75.

41. Christian NT, Burlew CC, Moore EE, et al. The focused abdominal sonography for trauma examination can reliably identify patients with significant intra-abdominal hemorrhage in life-threatening pelvic fractures. J TraumaAcuteCare Surg 2018;84(6): 924–8.

Capnography for Monitoring of the Critically Ill Patient

Boulos S. Nassar, MD, MPH, FCCP[a],*, Gregory A. Schmidt, MD, FCCP[b]

KEYWORDS

- Capnography • Shock • Cardiac arrest • Cardiopulmonary resuscitation • Fluid responsiveness
- Conscious sedation

KEY POINTS

- Capnography and the value of end-tidal carbon dioxide (ETco_2) depend on cardiac output, alveolar ventilation, and co_2 production.
- Changes in ETco_2 can be used to predict fluid responsiveness.
- Capnography plays a significant role during cardiac arrest by reflecting the adequacy of chest compressions and signaling return of spontaneous circulation.
- Capnography can be used to monitor high-risk patients receiving procedural sedation.
- ETco_2 is not a reliable indicator of partial pressure of co_2 in mechanically ventilated patients.

Capnography has become ubiquitous in critical care, presenting new opportunities and challenges in interpretation.[1] Carbon dioxide (co_2) measurement uses infrared spectroscopy, relying on the unique property of co_2 to absorb infrared radiation at a specific wavelength. The amount of infrared light absorbed correlates with co_2 concentration, plotted as the partial pressure of co_2 (Paco_2).

Capnometry refers to the measurement and numerical display of the co_2 value. Capnography refers to the measurement and graphical display of co_2 concentration throughout the breath. Plotting expired co_2 versus time yields a time capnogram; versus volume (using a pneumotachograph to measure flow), a volume-capnogram. A time capnogram plot is made up of 4 phases, as illustrated in **Fig. 1**. Phase I is flat with a zero value, as it reflects inspiration of fresh gas and early exhaled gas from the anatomic dead space. Phase II refers to the transition from anatomic dead space to alveolar gas, hence represented by a sharply rising value. Phase III, or the alveolar plateau, occurs when the exhaled breath is solely from alveoli. It

typically has a small upwards slope, which is due largely to (1) physiologic degree of VQ mismatch, as alveoli with low VQ (and higher alveolar co_2) empty later in the breath, (2) co_2 being presented to the lungs throughout expiration. The end-tidal carbon dioxide (ETco_2) refers to the maximum value at the end of phase III. Phase IV consists of a rapid decrease in Pco_2 as freshly inspired gas is drawn across the sensor.[2]

Volume capnography allows measurement of dead space and total exhaled co_2, but is much less widely used in clinical medicine. Time capnography is the focus of this review as the authors address 5 important questions.

WHAT IS THE RELATIONSHIP BETWEEN END-TIDAL CARBON DIOXIDE AND CARDIAC OUTPUT?

In a steady hemodynamic state, cardiac output has no impact on the Paco_2, which depends solely on co_2 production and elimination. Thus, during

[a] Department of Internal Medicine, Division of Pulmonary, Critical Care and Occupational Medicine, University of Iowa Hospital & Clinics, 200 Hawkins Drive, Iowa City, IA 52242, USA; [b] Pulmonary Diseases, Critical Care, and Occupational Medicine, University of Iowa, Iowa City, IA, USA
* Corresponding author.
E-mail address: Boulos-nassar@uiowa.edu

Clin Chest Med 43 (2022) 393–400
https://doi.org/10.1016/j.ccm.2022.04.002
0272-5231/22/© 2022 Elsevier Inc. All rights reserved.

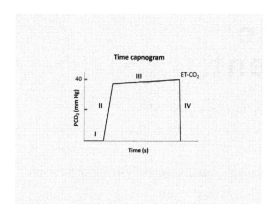

Fig. 1. Plot of time capnogram, showing all 4 phases.

stable conditions, $Paco_2$ can be summarized by the following:

$$P_A CO_2 \propto \dot{V}CO_2/\dot{V}_A$$

where $\dot{V}CO_2$ is co_2 production, and $\dot{V}_A$ is the alveolar ventilation.

It is only during non-steady-state conditions, when there are acute circulatory perturbations and changes in pulmonary perfusion, that the $Paco_2$ value (and, consequently, $ETco_2$) depends on cardiac output.

Early animal studies altered cardiac output and venous return through various techniques, such as ventricular assist devices, inferior vena cava balloon occlusion, or controlled hemorrhage. These experimental studies showed that when shock was induced, the $ETco_2$ correlated closely with cardiac output.[3–6] This relationship was applicable in various types of shock: hemorrhagic, cardiogenic, or vasodilatory. The physiologic explanation for this observation was twofold: (1) When shock occurs, venous return and pulmonary blood flow are reduced. This decreases co_2 delivery to the lungs; (2) The reduction in pulmonary perfusion creates areas with high VQ mismatch or alveolar dead space, which also contributes to a decrease in $ETco_2$.[4,7,8] The clinical application of this relationship has been limited to circumstances whereby the astute clinician can use capnography to recognize hemodynamic changes; one example is using capnography to reflect restoration of native cardiac function as patients are being weaned off pump during cardiac bypass surgery.[8–10]

HOW CAN CAPNOGRAPHY BE USED TO PREDICT FLUID RESPONSIVENESS?

By definition, a fluid responsive (FR) patient will have a $\geq 10\%$ to 15% increase in cardiac output

following an intravenous fluid challenge.[11] In other words, fluids are capable of perturbing the circulation from its steady state, a shift that should be reflected by an increase in $ETco_2$.

Multiple studies of mechanically ventilated patients in shock confirm this hypothesis. FR patients had a significant increase in $ETco_2$ of $\geq 5\%$, or ≥ 2 mm Hg following passive leg raising (PLR) or a fluid challenge,[12–17] a threshold with a sensitivity of 71% to 76% and a specificity of 93% to 100%.[12,18] Despite the low absolute increase of 2 mm Hg, it is higher than the least significant change, validating its role. To confidently detect these small increases, the baseline capnograph must be completely stable, generally requiring controlled mechanical ventilation. The increase in $ETco_2$ in FR patients is explained largely by a transient increase in venous return and co_2 delivery to the lungs, a fact confirmed using volume-capnography to measure total exhaled co_2 in 1 minute.[14] In fact, this measurement correlates even better with FR than the simple $ETco_2$ value. A second contributor to the rising $ETco_2$ in FR patients is recruitment of pulmonary capillaries, lowering the amount of physiologic dead space (co_2 production is assumed stable for the short duration of PLR or fluid bolus).

The physiologic impact of raising positive end-expiratory pressure (PEEP) could be used similarly: PEEP should transiently impede venous return, lowering $ETco_2$. Using volume capnography, Tusman and colleagues[19] found that an 11% decrease in Vco_2 following a PEEP increase from 5 to 10 mm Hg predicted fluid responsiveness with 90% sensitivity and 95% specificity.

PLR-induced changes in $ETco_2$ offer the advantage of being a simple, noninvasive, and repeatable test to predict fluid responsiveness. Unlike pulse pressure variation, capnography is valid in the presence of arrhythmias and does not require raising tidal volume to 8 to 12 mL/kg. Some investigators found $ETco_2$ to remain reliable in the presence of chronic obstructive pulmonary disease,[15] although others have excluded patients with acute lung diseases. The broader application of $ETco_2$ for predicting FR and reliability in those with lung disease requires further study.

WHAT IS THE ROLE OF CAPNOGRAPHY IN MANAGING PATIENTS IN CARDIAC ARREST?

The central role of capnography during cardiopulmonary resuscitation (CPR) stems from its ability to objectively reflect and monitor changes in the circulation.[20–22] **Box 1** summarizes the following discussion.

Box 1
Applications of capnography during cardiac arrest

- Waveform capnography confirms proper endotracheal tube placement
- Capnography guides ventilation rates and volumes (while avoiding hyperventilation)
- Capnography reflects the effectiveness of CPR
- A sustained spike in $ETco_2$ is the first signal of ROSC, reducing unnecessary interruptions
- A precipitous drop in $ETco_2$ could be the first signal of loss of pulse
- Capnography should be included when deciding to terminate resuscitation

End-Tidal Carbon Dioxide Reflects the Adequacy of Cardiopulmonary Resuscitation

As chest compression rate and depth are adjusted to appropriate levels, improving the generated blood flow, $ETco_2$ increases.[23,24] The American Heart Association recommends using capnography as a physiologic parameter, targeting an $ETco_2$ of at least 10 mm Hg.[25] A decreasing $ETco_2$ could signal rescuer fatigue and encourage switching team members.

Capnography Can Be Used to Optimize the Odds of Successful Defibrillation

Prompt defibrillation is the crucial step for shockable rhythms. If the onset of arrhythmia is protracted or unknown, a brief period of chest compression and myocardial perfusion before defibrillation could improve the chances for successful cardioversion.[26] A starving myocardium is unlikely to be converted to sinus rhythm without some degree of reperfusion. Chicote and colleagues[27] found that preshock $ETco_2$ less than 11 mm Hg always led to unsuccessful defibrillation, but $ETco_2$ greater than 40 ensured that 60% of cardioversions was achieved. $ETco_2$ could guide the clinician to delay defibrillation until coronary perfusion has improved.[28]

Capnography Signals Return of Spontaneous Circulation

Chest compressions only generate a fraction of the native cardiac output, but when return of spontaneous circulation (ROSC) is achieved and innate perfusion is restored, $ETco_2$ significantly increases.[24,29] This has important clinical implications: capnography is a much more dependable method to identify ROSC than checking for a pulse. $ETco_2$ is also the first clinical indicator that ROSC is achieved, compared with palpating a pulse, measuring blood pressure, or perceiving patient response.[30] By recognizing that a spike in $ETco_2$ signals ROSC, capnography will also reduce the number of unnecessary interruptions in chest compressions[23] (**Fig 2**A). When ROSC is restored, $ETco_2$ tends to overshoot its prearrest levels, as the lungs are presented with a high CO_2-content venous blood. As a new steady state is reached, $ETco_2$ decreases.[21–23,29–33]

Capnography Can Be Used to Prognosticate

By virtue of reflecting generated blood flow, $ETco_2$ can be used to predict outcomes from resuscitation. A low $ETco_2$ after prolonged resuscitation predicts death. A high $ETco_2$ reflects adequate CPR and greater odds of achieving ROSC.[20] For out of hospital cardiac arrest (OHCA), capnography can help distinguish irreversible cardiac arrest from survival to hospital admission. Using $ETco_2$ less than 10 mm Hg at 20 minutes predicted prehospital death with a sensitivity and specificity approaching 100%.[30,34,35] In the largest prospective study of OHCA, Kolar and colleagues[36] found in 737 patients that $ETco_2$ greater than 14.3 mm Hg predicted ROSC with close to 100% negative predictive value and positive predictive value. Similar observations were made from IHCA studies.[37] It is important to emphasize that patients differ between these studies, and this could impact the absolute value of $ETco_2$. The type of cardiac arrest (cardiac vs asphyxial), the initial rhythm, and the prompt initiation of bystander CPR and ventilation practices all play a role.[38] When including a low $ETco_2$ in terminating resuscitation, the rescuer should be aware of technical failures, such as occluded endotracheal tube or dislodged endotracheal tube, which could falsely reduce $ETco_2$. Although it seems unequivocal that patients who will go on to achieve ROSC will have high $ETco_2$, the cutoff is incompletely defined. Because of these confounders, some have argued to use capnography in conjunction with other factors when deciding to terminate resuscitation.[39,40]

Most published data, including guidelines from the American Heart Association, advocate that the inability to reach 10 mm Hg after 20 minutes of CPR denotes futility, although recognizing that a higher target is more likely to be associated with greater chances for ROSC.[41,42]

CAN CAPNOGRAPHY MAKE CONSCIOUS SEDATION SAFER?

Conscious sedation is used during various procedures to reduce pain, anxiety, and agitation.

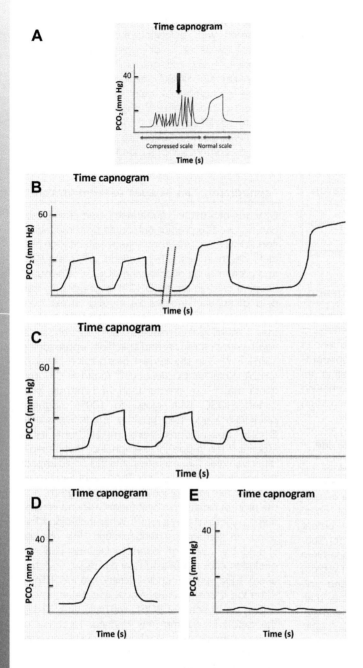

Fig. 2. (*A*) Plot of time capnogram, during CPR using a compressed time scale. Arrow signals ROSC. (*B*) Plot of time capnogram, illustrating bradypneic hypoventilation (owing to a reduction in respiratory rate). The parallel dotted lines represent a time gap. Often seen with opioids, this is associated with a rising $ETco_2$. (*C*) Plot of time capnogram, illustrating hypopneic hypoventilation. Often seen with sedatives (including propofol), the ineffective ventilation leads to a decrease in $ETco_2$ over time. (*D*) Plot of time capnogram, illustrating a steep increase in phase III with a shark fin appearance from bronchospasm, typical of airflow obstruction. (*E*) Plot of time capnogram, illustrating an esophageal intubation.

Conscious sedation relies on a fine balance between achieving patient comfort, without leading to deeper levels of sedation or cardiopulmonary collapse. The various sedatives and anxiolytics used could relax the upper airway muscles, diminish the cough reflex, and restrict the patency of the airway. This can lead to upper airway obstruction or exacerbate obstructive sleep apnea. These drugs can also reduce respiratory drive, causing bradypneic hypoventilation (**Fig. 2**B) or provoking central apneas. They can reduce the tidal volume and lead to ineffective ventilation, precipitating hypopneic hypoventilation (**Fig. 2**C).

Standard monitoring when conscious sedation is used includes pulse oximetry, blood pressure measurement, and electrocardiographic monitoring. Despite o_2 saturation being used to reflect the respiratory function, it is only a late indicator of hypoventilation or an obstructed airway. When these occur, alveolar co_2 increases ($Paco_2$) first, which reduces alveolar and arterial o_2 tension. It is only when Pao_2 drops below a critical level that o_2 desaturation occurs.

Capnography has been touted as an additional tool to detect these events earlier, perhaps leading to timely intervention and reducing the occurrence of respiratory failure. Multiple studies confirmed that pulse oximetry misses 38% to 50% of apneas, hypoventilation, and upper airway obstruction events, when compared with capnography.[43–46] This result is not surprising, but the main clinical question is whether capnography can function as an early warning system, predicting the development of hypoxemia, leading to early interventions and making conscious sedation safer.

A large number of studies demonstrated that the addition of capnography reduced hypoxemia (defined as O_2 saturation <90%) by 13.3% to 23% and severe hypoxemia (defined as O_2 saturation <85%) by 4.1% to 16%.[46–52] This was attributed to various early interventions, which included physical or verbal stimulation, adjusting sedatives, chin lift or jaw thrust maneuvers, or supplementing O_2.[46,48] Capnographic changes were detected 32 to 180 seconds before O_2 desaturation, giving the bedside provider time to intervene.[43,44,47,53,54]

A few studies contradicted these results and revealed that capnography did not reduce hypoxemia in their patient population. The difference in the ability of capnography to influence outcomes could be attributed to a few key differences. Negative studies recruited healthy patients (American Society of Anesthesiologists [ASA] group I–II), occurred in the outpatient setting, included simple procedures of short duration (routine esophagogastroduodenoscopy and colonoscopy), and avoided using propofol.[54–56] Positive studies enrolled sicker patients (ASA group I–IV), monitored more complex procedures (endoscopic ultrasound, endoscopic retrograde cholangiopancreatography, bronchoscopy), and frequently used propofol. Similar to standard short-acting benzodiazepines and narcotics used, propofol is an attractive agent because of its short onset of action and brief duration of action; however, it has a narrow therapeutic range and can precipitate respiratory failure.

These data suggest that capnography might not be warranted for routine outpatient procedures involving healthy patients, and it only incurs additional cost without improving safety.[56] However, most societal guidelines do strongly recommend adding capnography as a monitoring tool during conscious sedation.[57] This is a prudent step, as out-of-the-operating-room procedures have increased, and nonanesthesiologists are often providing conscious sedation. It is imperative that hospitals institute training and educational programs when introducing capnography. This includes recognizing certain waveform abnormalities (such as bronchospasm; **Fig. 2**D) and knowing the limitations of this technology. False positive findings are common, ranging between 17.8% and 27% and attributed to cannula dislocation or tube malfunction and obstruction with secretions.[47,48] False negatives are also common, reported to be around 35% in some studies, and owing to coughing or aspiration during the procedure.[49]

CAN END-TIDAL CARBON DIOXIDE BE USED AS A SURROGATE OF PARTIAL PRESSURE OF CARBON DIOXIDE?

Obtaining an arterial blood gas level requires an arterial puncture and is labor intensive. Capnography is noninvasive and continuous, making it a potentially attractive substitute. In healthy patients, $Paco_2$ is slightly higher than $ETco_2$ by ∼ 4 to 5 mm Hg.[58] This expected gradient is physiologic and attributed to a small amount of dead space.

What is true in health does not apply to mechanically ventilated patients, whereby $Paco_2$ is needed the most. Although the gradient remains within normal limits in healthy patients without significant cardiopulmonary diseases,[59–61] there are high rates of false negatives and positives that make its regular use for patients treacherous.[62] Multiple studies in various clinical settings found $ETco_2$ to not accurately reflect $Paco_2$, whether it is patients with airflow obstruction, acute respiratory failure, trauma, postoperative patients, critically ill patients, or those in the emergency department.[61–67] This normally occurring gap of roughly 5 mm Hg increases to as high as 14 mm Hg in patients with various pulmonary diseases[62,66,68] and is attributed to the development of alveolar dead space. Critically ill patients often have other comorbidities that can also influence $ETco_2$, including hypovolemia, pulmonary embolism, or lung overdistention, all of which increase the fraction of alveolar dead space.[69]

$ETco_2$ also depends on ventilator settings; reducing the rate, especially in patients with airflow obstruction, can increase $ETco_2$ as a reflection of the rising nature of phase III. The $ETco_2$ might actually surpass the $Paco_2$, and the gradient becomes negative.

One might argue that if $ETco_2$ cannot be used to accurately estimate $Paco_2$ in mechanically ventilated patients, would the trends in $ETco_2$ or $Paco_2$ track each other? Here again, multiple studies show the changes went in opposite directions in 18.4% to 32% of cases.[62,67]

SUMMARY

Capnography offers a wealth of information, reflecting the state of the circulation, airway patency, and ventilation. It is available in intensive care units, recovery rooms, and procedural suites. Despite the wide adoption of this technology, it remains critical for hospitals to institute training programs to educate various providers how to fully appreciate the capnographic waveforms and properly interpret ET_{CO_2}.

CLINICS CARE POINTS

- Time capnography is essential during CPR to detect ROSC.
- Time capnography, when appropriately used, can detect fluid responsiveness.
- Time capnography enhances the safety of procedural sedation.
- Capnography should not be routinely used to reflect the partial pressure of CO_2.

DISCLOSURE

The authors have no commercial or financial conflicts of interest, or funding, related to this article.

REFERENCES

1. Kodali BS. Capnography outside the operating rooms. Anesthesiology 2013;118:192–201.
2. Nassar BS, Schmidt GA. Capnography during critical illness. Chest 2016;149(2):576–85.
3. Ornato JP, Garnett AR, Glauser FL, et al. Relationship between cardiac output and the end-tidal carbon dioxide tension. Ann Emerg Med 1990;19:1104–6.
4. Isserles SA, Breen PH. Can changes in end-tidal PCO2 measure changes in cardiac out-put? Anesth Analg 1991;73:808–14.
5. Idris AH, Staples ED, O'Brien DJ, et al. Effect of ventilation on acid-base balance and oxygenation in low blood-flow states. Crit Care Med 1994;22:1827–34.
6. Jin X, Weil MH, Tang W, et al. End-tidal carbon dioxide as a noninvasive indicator of cardiac index during circulatory shock. Crit Care Med 2000;28:2415–9.
7. Dubin A, Murias G, Estenssoro E, et al. End-tidal CO2 pressure determinants during hemorrhagic shock. Intensive Care Med 2000;26(11):1619–23.
8. Shibutani K, Muraoka M, Shirasaki S, et al. Do changes in end-tidal PCO2 quantitatively reflect changes in cardiac output? Anesth Analg 1994;79:829–33.
9. Maslow A, Stearns G, Bert A, et al. Monitoring end-tidal carbon dioxide during weaning from cardiopulmonary bypass in patients without significant lung disease. Anesth Analg 2001;92:306–13.
10. Wahba RW, Tessler MJ, Béïque F, et al. Changes in PCO2 with acute changes in cardiac index. Can J Anaesth 1996;43(3):243–5.
11. Guerin L, Monnet X, Teboul JL. Monitoring volume and fluid responsiveness: from static to dynamic indicators. BestPractResClinAnaesthesiol 2013;27:177–85.
12. Monnet X, Bataille A, Magalhaes E, et al. End-tidal carbon dioxide is better than arterial pressure for predicting volume responsiveness by the passive leg raising test. Intensive Care Med 2013;39:93–100.
13. Monge García MI, Gil Cano A, Gracia Romero M, et al. Non-invasive assessment of fluid responsiveness by changes in partial end-tidal CO2 pressure during a passive leg-raising maneuver. Ann Intensive Care 2012;2:9.
14. Young A, Marik PE, Sibole S, et al. Changes in end-tidal carbon dioxide and volumetric carbon dioxide as predictors of volume responsiveness in hemodynamically unstable patients. J Cardiothorac Vasc Anesth 2013;27:681–4.
15. Toupin F, Clairoux A, Deschamps A, et al. Assessment of fluid responsiveness with end-tidal carbon dioxide using a simplified passive leg raising maneuver: a prospective observational study. Can J Anaesth 2016;63:1033–41.
16. Jacquet-Lagreze M, Baudin F, David JS, et al. End-tidal carbon dioxide variation after a 100- and a 500-ml fluid challenge to assess fluid responsiveness. Ann Intensive Care 2016;6:37.
17. Lakhal K, Nay MA, Kamel T, et al. Change in end-tidal carbon dioxide outperforms other surrogates for change in cardiac output during fluid challenge. Br J Anaesth 2017;118:355–62.
18. Xiao-ting W, Hua Z, Da-wei L, et al. Changes in end-tidal CO2 could predict fluid responsiveness in the passive leg raising test but not in the mini-fluid challenge test: a prospective and observational study. J Crit Care 2015;30:1061–6.
19. Tusman G, Groisman I, Maidana GA, et al. The sensitivity and specificity of pulmonary carbon dioxide elimination for noninvasive assessment of fluid responsiveness. Anesth Analg 2016;122:1404–11.
20. Sanders AB, Ogle M, Ewy GA. Coronary perfusion pressure during cardiopulmonary resuscitation. Am J Emerg Med 1985;3(1):11–4.
21. Weil MH, Bisera J, Trevino RP, et al. Cardiac output and end-tidal carbon dioxide. Crit Care Med 1985;13(11):907–9.

22. Gudipati CV, Weil MH, Bisera J, et al. Expired carbon dioxide: a noninvasive monitor of cardiopulmonary resuscitation. Circulation 1988;77(1):234–9.

23. Falk JL, Rackow EC, Weil MH. End-tidal carbon dioxide concentration during cardiopulmonary resuscitation. N Engl J Med 1988;318(10):607–11.

24. Kalenda Z. The capnogram as a guide to the efficacy of cardiac massage. Resuscitation 1978;6: 259–63.

25. Link MS, Berkow LC, Kudenchuk PJ, et al. Part 7: adult advanced cardiovascular life support: 2015 American Heart Association guidelines update for cardiopulmonary resuscitation and emergency cardiovascular care. Circulation 2015;132:S444–64.

26. Berg KM, Soar J, Andersen LW, et al. Adult advanced life support Collaborators . Adult advanced life support: 2020 International Consensus on cardiopulmonary resuscitation and emergency cardiovascular care Science with Treatment Recommendations. Circulation 2020;142(16):S92–139.

27. Chicote B, Aramendi E, Irusta U, et al. Value of capnography to predict defibrillation success in out-of-hospital cardiac arrest. Resuscitation 2019;138:74–81.

28. Savastano S, Baldi E, Raimondi M, et al. End-tidal carbon dioxide and defibrillation success in out-of-hospital cardiac arrest. Resuscitation 2017;121:71–5.

29. Garnett AR, Ornato JP, Gonzalez ER, et al. End-tidal carbon dioxide monitoring during cardiopulmonary resuscitation. JAMA 1987;257:512–5.

30. Wayne MA, Levine RL, Miller CC. Use of end-tidal carbon dioxide to predict outcome in prehospital cardiac arrest. Ann Emerg Med 1995;25(6):762-767.

31. Pokorná M, Necas E, Kratochví IJ, et al. A sudden increase in partial pressure end-tidal carbon dioxide (PETCO2) at the moment of return of spontaneous circulation. J Emerg Med 2010;38(5):614–21.

32. Steedman DJ, Robertson CE. Measurement of end-tidal carbon dioxide concentration during cardiopulmonary resuscitation. Arch Emerg Med 1990;7: 129–34.

33. Sehra R, Underwood K, Checchia P. End tidal CO2 is a quantitative measure of cardiac arrest. Pacing Clin Electrophysiol 2003;26(1p2):515–7.

34. Levine RL, Wayne MA, Miller CC. End-tidal carbon dioxide and outcome of out-of-hospital cardiac arrest. N Engl J Med 1997;337(5):301–6.

35. Grmec S, Klemen P. Does the end-tidal carbon dioxide (EtCO2) concentration have prognostic value during out-of-hospital cardiac arrest? Eur J Emerg Med 2001;8:263–9.

36. Kolar M, Krizmaric M, Klemen P, et al. Partial pressure of end-tidal carbon dioxide successful predicts cardiopulmonary resuscitation in the field: a prospective observational study. Crit Care 2008;12(5): R115.

37. Ahrens T, Schallom L, Bettorf K, et al. End-tidal carbon dioxide measurements as a prognostic indicator of outcome in cardiac arrest. Am J Crit Care 2001;10:391–8.

38. Heradstveit BE, Sunde K, Sunde GA, et al. Factors complicating interpretation of capnography during advanced life support in cardiac arrest—a clinical retrospective study in 575 patients. Resuscitation 2012;83(7):813–8.

39. Brinkrolf P, Borowski M, Metelmann C, et al. Predicting ROSC in out-of-hospital cardiac arrest using expiratory carbon dioxide concentration: is trend-detection instead of absolute threshold values the key? Resuscitation 2018;122:19–24.

40. T ouma O, Davies M. The prognostic value of end tidal carbon dioxide during cardiac arrest: a systematic review. Resuscitation 2013;84:1470–9.

41. Hartmann SM, Farris RW, Di Gennaro JL, et al. Systematic review and meta-analysis of end-tidal carbon dioxide values associated with return of spontaneous circulation during cardiopulmonary resuscitation. J Intensive Care Med 2015;30:426–35.

42. Paiva EF, Paxton JH, O'Neil BJ. The use of end-tidal carbon dioxide (ETCO2) measurement to guide management of cardiac arrest: a systematic review. Resuscitation 2018;123:1–7.

43. Vargo JJ, Zuccaro G Jr, Dumot JA, et al. Automated graphic assessment of respiratory activity is superior to pulse oximetry and visual assessment for the detection of early respiratory depression during therapeutic upper endoscopy. Gastrointest Endosc 2002;55(7):826–31.

44. Cacho G, Pérez-Calle JL, Barbado A, et al. Capnography is superior to pulse oximetry for the detection of respiratory depression during colonoscopy. Rev Esp Enferm Dig 2010;102(2):86–9.

45. Waugh JB, Epps C, Khodneva Y. Capnography enhances surveillance of respiratory events during procedural sedation: a meta-analysis. J Clin Anesth 2011;23(3):189–96.

46. Friedrich-Rust M, Welte M, Welte C, et al. Capnographic monitoring of propofol-based sedation during colonoscopy. Endoscopy 2014;46:236–44.

47. Deitch K, Miner J, Chudnofsky CR, et al. Does end tidal CO2 monitoring during emergency department procedural sedation and analgesia with propofol decrease the incidence of hypoxic events? A randomized, controlled trial. Ann Emerg Med 2010;55:258–64.

48. Beitz A, Riphaus A, Meining A, et al. Capnographic monitoring reduces the incidence of arterial oxygen desaturation and hypoxemia during propofol sedation for colonoscopy: a randomized, controlled study (ColoCap Study). Am J Gastroenterol 2012;107: 1205–12.

49. Qadeer MA, Vargo JJ, Dumot JA, et al. Capnographic monitoring of respiratory activity improves safety of sedation for endoscopic cholangiopancreatography and ultrasonography. Gastroenterology 2009;136: 1568–76.

50. Schlag C, Wörner A, Wagenpfeil S, et al. Capnography improves detection of apnea during procedural sedation for percutaneous transhepatic cholangiodrainage. Can J Gastroenterol 2013;27:582–6.

51. Klare P, Reiter J, Meining A, et al. Capnographic monitoring of midazolam and propofol sedation during ERCP: a randomized controlled study (EndoBreath Study). Endoscopy 2016;48:42–50.

52. Conway A, Douglas C, Sutherland JR. A systematic review of capnography for sedation. Anaesthesia 2016;71:450–4.

53. Ishiwata T, Tsushima K, Terada J, et al. Efficacy of end-tidal capnography monitoring during flexible bronchoscopy in nonintubated patients under sedation: a randomized controlled study. Respiration 2018;96(4):355–62.

54. Van Loon K, van Rheineck Leyssius AT, van Zaane B, et al. Capnography during deep sedation with propofol by nonanesthesiologists: a randomized controlled trial. Anesth Analg 2014;119(1): 49–55.

55. Mehta PP, Kochhar G, Albeldawi M, et al. Capnographic monitoring in routine EGD and colonoscopy with moderate sedation: a prospective, randomized, Controlled Trial. Am J Gastroenterol 2016;111(3): 395–404.

56. Barnett S, Hung A, Tsao R, et al. Capnographic monitoring of moderate sedation during low-risk screening colonoscopy does not improve safety or patient satisfaction: a prospective cohort study. Am J Gastroenterol 2016;111:388–94.

57. Apfelbaum J, Gross J, Connis R, et al. Practice guidelines for moderate procedural sedation and analgesia 2018: a report by the American Society of Anesthesiologists Task Force on moderate procedural sedation and analgesia, the American Association of Oral and Maxillofacial Surgeons, American College of Radiology, American Dental Association, American society of Dentist Anesthesiologists, and Society of Interventional Radiology. Anesthesiology 2018;128:437–79.

58. Nunn JF, Hill DW. Respiratory dead space and arterial to end- tidal CO, tension difference in anesthetized man. J Appl Phys lol 1960;15:383–9.

59. Sharma SK, McGuire GP, Cruise CJE. Stability of the arterial to end-tidal carbon dioxide difference during anaesthesia for prolonged neurosurgical procedures. Can J Anaesth 1995;42(6):498–503.

60. Lee S-W, Hong Y-S, Han C, et al. Concordance of end-tidal carbon dioxide and arterial carbon dioxide in severe traumatic brain injury. J Trauma 2009; 67(3):526–30.

61. Whitesell R, Asiddao C, Gollman D, et al. Relationship between arterial and peak expired carbon dioxide pressure during anesthesia and factors influencing the difference. Anesth Analg 1981;60: 508–12.

62. Russell GB, Graybeal JM. Reliability of the arterial to end-tidal carbon dioxide gradient in mechanically ventilated patients with multisystem trauma. J Trauma 1994;36:317–22.

63. Heines SJH, Strauch U, Roekaerts PMHJ, et al. Accuracy of end-tidal CO2 capnometers in postcardiac surgery patients during controlled mechanical ventilation. J Emerg Med 2013;45:130–5.

64. Prause G, Hetz H, Lauda P, et al. A comparison of the end-tidal-CO2 documented by capnometry and the arterial pCO2 in emergency patients. Resuscitation Ireland 1997;35:145–8.

65. Warner KJ, Cuschieri J, Garland B, et al. The utility of early end-tidal capnography in monitoring ventilation status after severe injury. J Trauma Inj Infect Crit Care 2009;66(1):26–31.

66. Morley TF, Giaimo J, Maroszan E, et al. Use of capnography for assessment of the adequacy of alveolar ventilation during weaning from mechanical ventilation. Am Rev Respir Dis 1993;148(2):339–44.

67. Russell GB, Graybeal JM. The arterial to end-tidal carbon dioxide difference in neurosurgical patients during craniotomy. Anesth Analg 1995;81:806–10.

68. Jabre P, Jacob L, Auger H, et al. Capnography monitoring in nonintubated patients with respiratory distress. Am J Emerg Med 2009;27:1056–9.

69. Nassar BS, Schmidt GA. Estimating arterial partial pressure of carbon dioxide in ventilated patients: how valid are surrogate measures? Ann Am Thorac Soc 2017;14(6):1005–14.

Novel and Rapid Diagnostics for Common Infections in the Critically Ill Patient

Chiagozie I. Pickens, MD[a],*, Richard G. Wunderink, MD[a]

KEYWORDS

- Rapid diagnostic • Molecular • Antibiotic stewardship • Infection • Critical care

KEY POINTS

- Diagnosing infection in critically ill patients is complex and can be limited by the long turnaround time and poor sensitivity of standard culture.
- Some advantages of rapid diagnostic tests include semiautomated protocols, short turnaround times, and high sensitivity and specificity.
- There are multiple single-target and multiplex culture-independent assays to rapidly detect organisms from respiratory samples.
- Some novel diagnostics for bloodstream infection can be direct from whole blood, bypassing the need for a positive culture.
- Rapid diagnostics for intraabdominal, genitourinary, and neurologic infection exist; however, the impact on clinically important outcomes is unclear.

INTRODUCTION

Infection associated with sepsis is the most common immediate cause of death in the intensive care unit (ICU).[1,2] The ICU mortality rate of critically ill patients with infection ranges from 25% to 60%, more than twice the mortality rate of noninfected critically ill patients.[3,4] Infection in critically ill patients is also an independent risk factor for delirium, acute renal failure, and increased hospital length of stay.[5] The economic burden of hospital-acquired infections in the United States is estimated to be $9.8 billion dollars yearly with infections common in the critically ill, such as ventilator-associated pneumonia (VAP), making up a significant proportion of the cost.[6] For these reasons, a comprehensive understanding of diagnostic tools for common infections in ICU patients is important for clinicians.

Detection of infection in critically ill patients is complex. First, a history localizing infectious symptoms is often difficult to obtain because patients are unable to communicate due to pain, agitation, encephalopathy, and/or intubation. Second, typical signs of infection such as tachypnea, leukocytosis, or tachycardia may not be present in critically ill patients with sepsis.[7] Conversely, these signs may be present in noninfected critically ill patients, often leading to excessive antibiotic use in this population.[8] Third, infection is a continuous threat to a critically ill patient and thus a negative diagnostic workup is only valid for a limited amount of time. The risk of infection increases as ICU length of stay increases, particularly for infection with drug-resistant organisms.[3] This increase creates the challenge of deciding when to repeat an infectious workup and when to initiate or deescalate antibiotic therapy. Fourth, critically ill patients are subject to atypical and opportunistic pathogens that are often difficult to detect with standard diagnostic tests. And lastly,

[a] Department of Medicine, Pulmonary and Critical Care Division, Northwestern University Feinberg School of Medicine, 303 E. Superior Street Simpson Querrey 5th Floor, Suite 5-406, Chicago, IL 60611-2909, USA
* Corresponding author.
E-mail address: chiagozie-ononye@northwestern.edu

Clin Chest Med 43 (2022) 401–410
https://doi.org/10.1016/j.ccm.2022.04.003

chestmed.theclinics.com

the tenuous status of many critically ill patients due to the underlying disease that caused ICU admission often creates a sense of urgency regarding "missing" an infection, leading to greater reliance on empirical antibiotic use. These factors contribute to the challenge of identifying infection in the ICU. Unfortunately, the complexity of detecting infection in critically ill patients is further heightened by the limitations of current diagnostic tools. This review discusses the advantages and disadvantages of current diagnostics tools and describe some of the available novel rapid diagnostic tests (RDT) for evaluating infection in an ICU population.

Traditional Diagnostic Techniques

In the clinical setting, semiquantitative culture is perhaps the test most commonly used to diagnose infection. Culture is prepared by using aseptic technique to inoculate growth media with a tissue or body fluid sample. The sample is then incubated at a specific temperature for 24 to 48 hours. If growth is present, traditionally Gram stain is performed for morphology, and subcultures may be prepared to maintain bacterial growth. Identification of bacteria occurs using a combination of stains, motility testing, rapid biochemical tests, and commercial identification assays. Only after sufficient growth to allow subculturing is antibiotic susceptibility testing performed. The process to culture other pathogens, including viruses, fungi, and *Mycobacterium*, is different.

Quantitative culture remains the gold standard for detecting infection and has several strengths as a diagnostic tool. The unsupervised approach of the test allows many organisms to be identified without the requirement for the clinician to indicate a pathogen of interest *a priori*. Culture is versatile; pertinent pathogens can be cultured from almost any tissue of body fluid specimen as long as the clinical team is able to obtain a sample. Importantly, culture is low cost relative to other diagnostic tests, allowing its use in almost any clinical setting.

However, several limitations of culture exist. The prolonged turnaround time is a significant disadvantage in the ICU setting where delay in appropriate antibiotic therapy directly translates to increases in mortality.[9] The median turnaround time from initial culture preparation to bacterial identification and antibiotic sensitivities ranges from 48 to 72 hours.[10] Any error or delay in the multiple steps from sample collection to final report may prolong the turnaround time.[11–13] The insensitivity of culture is also an important weakness. A culture may be negative for multiple reasons: delay in transport to the microbiology laboratory, errors in preparation, receipt of antibiotics before the sample being cultured, suboptimal growth media, and metabolic impairment of growth of certain bacteria in polymicrobial infections. For fastidious or uncommon organisms, additional subcultures and/or molecular studies for identification may be required.[14] These disadvantages highlight the need for more rapid and sensitive diagnostic tests for common infections in the ICU.

Novel Diagnostics for Pulmonary Infections

Pulmonary infections are the most common infection in the ICU.[15] In a point prevalence study of more than 13,000 ICU patients, the lung was the source of infection 64% of the time.[3] In patients who are admitted to the ICU, the incidence rate of nosocomial pneumonia is 6% to 27%.[16] The mortality associated with pneumonia requiring ICU admission ranges from 15% to 50%.[17] Empirical treatment choices are determined by multiple factors including whether the patient meets criteria for community-acquired pneumonia (CAP), hospital-acquired pneumonia (HAP), or VAP.[18,19] Definitive treatment is determined by the cause of the infection.

Multiplex nucleic amplification tests (NAAT) are an example of a novel, RDT uniquely positioned to improve the diagnosis and management of pneumonia in the ICU. These tests address many of the shortcomings of culture with their rapid turnaround time and excellent sensitivity for the detection of certain pathogens. The operating characteristics of both multiplex and single-target polymerase chain reaction (PCR) assays vary based on the platform but generally have a sensitivity and specificity greater than 90%.[20] However, no test is completely accurate, and the performance characteristics of both single-target and multiplex platforms should be interpreted in the context of disease prevalence; for example, a positive test for influenza is more likely to be a false positive during periods of low influenza infection frequency compared with seasons of high disease prevalence.

Rapid diagnostic tests for viral respiratory infection

Multiplex NAATs for detection of respiratory viruses gained widespread acceptance over the past decade and have largely replaced viral culture. More than 15 NAATs are dedicated to the detection of individual respiratory viruses. The comprehensive list can be found on the Food and Drug Administration (FDA) Web site (https://www.fda.gov/medical-devices/in-vitro-diagnostics/nucleic-acid-based-tests). These tests are semiautomated and can be run on samples obtained by minimally invasive methods, such as nasopharyngeal swab, with a turnaround time less than 2 hours.

Viral pneumonia requiring ICU admission has a mortality rate comparable to severe bacterial pneumonia. Yet no prospective studies report superior clinical outcomes from either earlier or more specific detection of viruses in the lower respiratory tract (LRT) of patients with severe pneumonia. The major limitation is the small armamentarium of antivirals. However, avoidance of empirical antibiotic therapy is also an important therapeutic result. Thus, the decision to test lower respiratory tract (LRT) samples for viruses remains controversial. Multiple studies demonstrate discordance between viral test results from nasopharyngeal swabs and LRT samples.[21–23] Studies also indicate that patients with respiratory failure from nonviral causes may still test positive for a virus.[24,25] Importantly, upper respiratory tract testing is not sufficient to diagnose LRT viral infection in critically ill patients. However, except for the FilmArray Respiratory Panel, most multiplex NAATs for viruses are not FDA approved for use on BAL fluid. Conversely, bacterial superinfection is a major concern for severe viral pneumonia, and distinguishing between the primary viral pneumonia and bacterial superinfection is difficult. The ATS Consensus Statement recommends nucleic-acid-based testing for patients with severe CAP and/or immunocompromised status.[26,27] This recommendation is based on low-quality evidence that suggests a positive NAAT result may reduce antibiotic duration.[28,29]

Rapid diagnostic tests for bacterial pneumonia

The clinical utility of multiplex molecular diagnostic assays for the detection of a bacterial pneumonia is evolving. The BioFire FilmArray Pneumonia Panel and the Unyvero LRT are 2 FDA-approved molecular diagnostic platforms for detection of multiple bacterial pathogens from respiratory samples. **Table 1** compares the 2 platforms.[30,31] The Unyvero LRT panel includes *Pneumocystis jirovecii* and *Stenotrophomonas maltophilia*, which are not present on the FilmArray. Operating characteristics of these tests should be interpreted with the understanding that culture was used as the gold standard. Thus, a high positive predictive value could indicate that the test is generating false-positive results or that the test is accurately detecting a pathogen that did not grow on culture. Independent validation suggests that most discrepant results are false-negative cultures, rather than false-positive NAATs. However, prospective, randomized trials are needed to determine the impact of multiplex bacterial NAATs on

antibiotic management, especially the safety of test-based antibiotic deescalation/discontinuation. Current studies suggest significant opportunities for antibiotic deescalation using NAATs on LRT specimens.[32,33]

The ability of an NAAT to specifically exclude methicillin-resistant *Staphylococcus aureus* (MRSA) pneumonia has unique implications for antibiotic stewardship. Empirical antibiotic regimens for CAP with risk factors or HAP/VAP include anti-MRSA antibiotics because of the increased mortality associated with this infection. The prolonged turnaround time of culture leads to critically ill patients often being exposed to several days of empirical anti-MRSA therapy while awaiting culture results. Use of multiplex or single-target PCR assays for detection of the *mecA* gene, which confers methicillin resistance, can effectively rule out the presence of MRSA pneumonia. Nasal swabs that screen for MRSA colonization have been studied as tools to rule out MRSA pneumonia. The negative predictive value of an MRSA nasal swab for the detection of culture-proven MRSA pneumonia is as high as 99.2%.[34] This excellent negative predictive value suggests that nasal swabs can be used to rule out MRSA pneumonia. Note that the studies investigating MRSA nasal swabs as tools to detect MRSA pneumonia are retrospective. However, the assay used for detecting MRSA from nasopharyngeal samples has been prospectively validated for use on bronchoalveolar lavage samples. In a randomized controlled trial of antibiotic deescalation based on the results of MRSA PCR tests on BAL samples compared with usual care, MRSA PCR tests run on BAL samples had a sensitivity of 95.7%, specificity of 98.2%, and negative predictive value of 99.6% for the detection of culture-positive MRSA pneumonia. In this trial there was a trend toward decreased mortality in patients randomized to antibiotic deescalation based on PCR. Thus, if MRSA is not detected in a respiratory sample, and no suspicion for extrapulmonary MRSA infection exists, clinicians can safely discontinue anti-MRSA antibiotics in critically ill patients without risk of adverse outcomes.[35,36] It is important for clinicians to know that nasopharyngeal colonization with MRSA is a risk factor for MRSA pneumonia, but the positive predictive value of an MRSA nasal swab is still is low, ranging from 17% to 35%. Therefore, a positive test cannot be use to rule-in MRSA pneumonia.[37]

In addition to methicillin resistance, the 2 major multiplex NAATs for bacterial pneumonia also include carbapenem resistance genes. Because many mechanisms of carbapenem resistance

Table 1
Comparison of Two Multiplex PCR Panels for Pneumonia

	BioFire FilmArray Pneumonia Panel	Unyvero Lower Respiratory Tract Panel
Specimen	Bronchoalveolar lavage Sputum Endotracheal aspirate	Bronchoalveolar lavage Sputum Endotracheal aspirate
Bacterial Targets	18	20 (includes *Pneumocystis jirovecii* and *Stenotrophomonas maltophilia*)
Viral Targets	8	0
Resistance Markers	7	10
Quantitation	Semiquantitative	No quantitation
Overall Weighted Sensitivity	96.2% (96.3% for sputum)	94.7%
Specificity	98.3% (97.2% for sputum)	98.4%
Turnaround Time	1.5 h	4.5 h
Technology	Multiplex PCR	Multiplex PCR followed by probe array
Clinical Application	Could allow for antibiotic deescalation in hospitalized patients, could save 6.2 antibiotic days per patient[32]	Could allow for antibiotic deescalation in hospitalized patients[33]

other than resistance genes occur, including efflux pumps, enzymatic deactivation (acquired carbapenemases), and target site mutations,[38] multiplex NAATs cannot reliably exclude carbapenem resistance. However, detection of these carbapenem resistance genes is highly predictive of phenotypic carbapenem resistance. The same is true of detection of the *ctx*M mutation, leading to extended spectrum beta-lactamase resistance in Enterobacterales.

Rapid Diagnosis of Bloodstream Infection

Bloodstream infections (BSI) are common in the ICU. Risk factors for BSI include disruption of anatomic barriers, presence of central venous catheters, immunosuppression, dialysis, and parenteral nutrition.[39] Development of BSI is associated with longer hospital stays, increased in-hospital mortality, and increased hospital expenditures.[40–42] Blood culture is the standard diagnostic tool for the identification of BSI; however, the yield of blood cultures is notoriously low. Two blood cultures can typically detect 80% of BSIs but sensitivity may be lower if antibiotics are administered before collection.[43] Over that past decade multiple RDTs have been developed to improve detection of BSI. Because critically ill patients have multiple risk factors for BSI, these novel diagnostic tools may be particularly useful in the ICU.

Mechanisms by which the novel diagnostics tests detect BSI vary. The first mechanism is matrix-assisted laser desorption ionization–time-of-flight mass spectrometry (MALDI-TOF). With MALDI-TOF, a sample is placed into a mass spectrometer and then ionized to become electrically charged. The charged molecule is accelerated through a tube and lands on a detector. The time taken for the molecule to accelerate, known as "time of flight," is recorded by the detector and compared with a calibrated standard of peptide mass fingerprints to provide identification of the bacteria.[44] Two commercial kits use MALDI-TOF technology for detection of BSI—Vitek MS and Sepsityper. MALDI-TOF has been reported to decrease time to organism identification by 1.5 days and decrease time to appropriate antibiotic therapy.[45] This technology has the advantage of identifying known and unknown organisms, unlike PCR where primers are required to identify an organism. However, MALDI-TOF is only clinically applicable for positive culture samples. Thus, MALDI-TOF is useful for organism identification but not for baseline detection of infection. MALDI-TOF is also unable to reliably differentiate bacteria in a polymicrobial infection because of overlap in spectra.[46–49]

Another technique used by newer diagnostic tools for BSI is gel electrofiltration and fluorescent in-situ hybridization. The Accelerate Pheno system is a fully automated assay that uses this technique to identify bacteria within 2 hours and antimicrobial susceptibility within 7 hours.[50] Accelerate has a reported overall sensitivity and specificity of 95.6% and 99.5%, respectively.[50] When combined with an antibiotic stewardship program, the Accelerate PhenoTest was shown to lead to earlier deescalation of unnecessary antibiotics in greater than 50% of patients.[51] As MALDI-TOF, the major limitation of the Accelerate PhenoTest is current availability only for positive blood cultures.

Several novel diagnostic tools for BSI use standard nucleic acid amplification to detect infection. These assays are either fully automated or semiautomated, have a turnaround time less than 3 hours, and can detect multiple pathogens. Commercially available NAATs for BSI from positive blood cultures include the BioFire FilmArray BCID, Unyvero System, and Verigene BC-GN. Similar to NAATs for LRT infection, randomized controlled trials of NAATs for BSI are lacking in an ICU population. Available data for the BioFire FilmArray BCID demonstrated a decrease in duration of piperacillin-tazobactam therapy when hospitalized patients with BSI were randomized to use of the FilmArray BCID plus an antimicrobial stewardship intervention versus usual care.[52]

Unlike the aforementioned tests for BSI, the T2 Biosystems NAATs can diagnose infection direct from blood and do not require a positive blood culture. The T2 Biosystems platform is also unique in that it uses T2-magnetic resonance biosensing capabilities to detect cellular and nucleic acid targets in whole blood. The instrument concentrates the microbial cells and cellular debris, amplifies DNA using target-specific primers, and detects amplified product by amplicon-induced aggregation of magnetic particles with a turnaround time of 3 to 5 hours. The T2Bacteria Panel is FDA approved for the detection of *Pseudomonas aeruginosa, Escherichia coli, Klebsiella pneumoniae, S aureus*, and *Enterococcus faecium*. The T2Candida Panel NAAT detects 5 *Candida* species with an overall sensitivity of 91% and specificity of 94%.

Next-generation sequencing (NGS) takes an unbiased approach to sequencing DNA or RNA present in a given sample. The Karius test is a commercially available NGS platform approved for use on whole blood samples. The assay is capable of detecting more than 1000 bacteria, viruses, and fungi by sequencing of cell-free DNA, with results potentially available within 24 hours. Clinically, the Karius test has a reported agreement of 100% when the identified organism is compared with conventional diagnostic methods. In addition, Karius testing has been applied to diagnostically challenging scenarios such as febrile neutropenia and culture-negative endocarditis. Clinical trials on the effect of Karius testing on clinical outcomes in critically ill patients are ongoing.

Rapid Diagnosis of Intraabdominal Infections

Intraabdominal infections are the third most common cause of sepsis in the ICU.[53] Many intraabdominal infections can be the primary reason for ICU admission, but other infections such as peritonitis, acalculous cholecystitis, and *Clostridioides* (formerly *Clostridium*) *difficile* infection (CDI) are often acquired during hospitalization. Radiographic imaging and culture of a fluid sample from the site of infection with or without blood culture is the current standard for diagnosis of cholecystitis, cholangitis, intraabdominal fluid collections, and/or peritonitis, with the limitations of culture discussed earlier. No commercially available multiplex molecular diagnostic assays are designed specifically for intraabdominal fluid collections. However, several small studies report use of 16s rRNA sequencing and/or metagenomic shotgun sequencing on intraabdominal fluid samples to detect infection.

Commercially available multiplex NAATs for intraabdominal infection are only applicable to acute diarrheal syndromes. These multiplex gastrointestinal NAATs contrast to the current method of diagnosis, which includes fecal culture, ova and parasite stains, and single-target PCRs. Bacteria on the panels include enteric pathogens such as *E coli, Salmonella*, and *Campylobacter* with a turnaround time of 2 to 5 hours depending on the platform. Some platforms also test for parasites and/or viruses, whereas others do not. The comprehensive list of pathogens can be found on the FDA Web site. In the clinical setting, the Bio-Fire FilmArray Gastrointestinal panel detected pathogens in 54% of cases compared with an 18% detection rate with conventional culture. Importantly, the CDC has emphasized that multiplex NAAT for enteric pathogens may negatively affect public health foodborne disease surveillance. This concern was raised because, once *C difficile* has been excluded, diagnosing the exact cause of acute diarrheal illness may have little impact on clinical course (many acute illnesses self-resolve) and the cost of multiplex NAATs can be substantial.

Although multiplex PCR testing for diarrheal pathogens is controversial, specific testing for *C difficile* is widely accepted as important for critically ill patients. CDI is the most common infectious cause of diarrhea in the ICU.[54] About 20% of patients with symptomatic CDI will develop

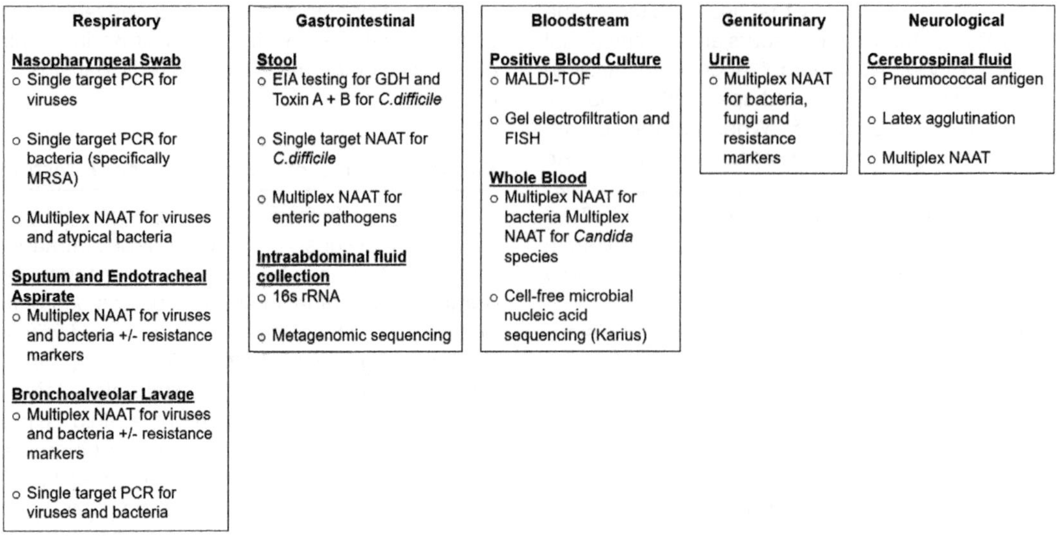

Respiratory	Gastrointestinal	Bloodstream	Genitourinary	Neurological
Nasopharyngeal Swab o Single target PCR for viruses o Single target PCR for bacteria (specifically MRSA) o Multiplex NAAT for viruses and atypical bacteria **Sputum and Endotracheal Aspirate** o Multiplex NAAT for viruses and bacteria +/- resistance markers **Bronchoalveolar Lavage** o Multiplex NAAT for viruses and bacteria +/- resistance markers o Single target PCR for viruses and bacteria	**Stool** o EIA testing for GDH and Toxin A + B for *C.difficile* o Single target NAAT for *C.difficile* o Multiplex NAAT for enteric pathogens **Intraabdominal fluid collection** o 16s rRNA o Metagenomic sequencing	**Positive Blood Culture** o MALDI-TOF o Gel electrofiltration and FISH **Whole Blood** o Multiplex NAAT for bacteria Multiplex NAAT for *Candida* species o Cell-free microbial nucleic acid sequencing (Karius)	**Urine** o Multiplex NAAT for bacteria, fungi and resistance markers	**Cerebrospinal fluid** o Pneumococcal antigen o Latex agglutination o Multiplex NAAT

Fig. 1. Tools for diagnosis of common infections in the ICU.

fulminant infection, which is associated with a mortality of greater than 50%.[55] The diagnosis of *C difficile* can be particularly challenging in the ICU setting. Severe CDI may not present with a classic diarrheal illness but with signs and symptoms of shock indistinguishable from other causes of shock. A variety of diagnostic tools are currently available to detect CDI. Importantly, these tests must be sent in the appropriate clinical setting, as they do not differentiate between asymptomatic colonization and true infection. The gold standard for *C difficile* diagnosis is a culture that first detects growth of *C difficile*, followed by testing to detect toxin production. A second test also considered to be the gold standard is a cell cytotoxicity test to detect toxin A or B. Although both gold-standard tests have excellent sensitivity, they are no longer used in clinical laboratories due to long turnaround time and have been replaced by novel RDTs.

NAATs for *C difficile* may be single-target or part of a multiplex enteropathogen panel with a sensitivity ranging from 87% to 95% and a specificity up to 98% based on multiple systematic analyses.[56] Enzyme immunoassay (EIA) is another RDT currently used by many clinical laboratories. EIA can detect the presence of toxin A or B or the presence of glutamate dehydrogenase (GDH). Note that GDH is an enzyme produced by both toxigenic and nontoxigenic strains of *C difficile*, and thus, GDH testing should be paired with testing for toxins. Many society guidelines recommend a combination of EIA and PCR testing to confirm *C difficile* diagnosis in symptomatic patients. RDTs for *C difficile* in hospitalized patients can significantly decrease empirical antibiotic therapy and decrease duration of isolation.[57,58]

Rapid Detection of Meningitis

Although an uncommon infection, meningitis affects a disproportionate number of ICU admissions. The potential spectrum is very broad, and empirical therapy is usually a complex regimen of multiple antibiotics, antivirals, and occasionally antifungals. Delays in treatment are associated with adverse neurologic outcomes, so empirical therapy is commonly given even before a diagnostic lumbar puncture, markedly compromising the yield of bacterial cultures. This infection is therefore a prime candidate for use of RDTs.

The BinaxNOW test is an immunochromatographic test for rapid detection of the *S pneumoniae* antigen in cerebrospinal fluid (CSF). The sensitivity of the test ranges from 85% to 95% with a specificity of 95% to 100%.[59,60] Clinically, this test has demonstrated enhanced detection of pneumococcal meningitis in culture-negative cases.[60] Latex agglutination (LA) is another rapid test commonly used in bacterial meningitis.[61] This test uses latex beads coated with antibodies to bacterial antigens, and if the antigen is present the beads will agglutinate. Results of the test are typically available in less than 30 minutes. The commercially available LA assays detect *S pneumoniae*, *Haemophilus influenzae*, and *Neisseria meningitidis* with a sensitivity greater than 90%. There are also multiplex NAATs to diagnose meningitis.[62,63] The FilmArray Meningitis/Encephalitis Panel is an example of a multiplex PCR for CSF.

PROCESS TO IMPLEMENT A NOVEL DIAGNOSTIC TEST IN THE ICU   *EXAMPLE*

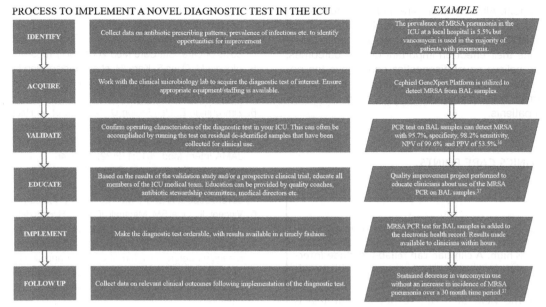

Fig. 2. Novel diagnostics review.

The 14 targets included in this panel cover the spectrum of major viral, bacterial, and fungal pathogens. Clinical application of this test has shown enhanced detection of a pathogen compared with standard diagnostic tools.[61,64] The impact on antibiotic stewardship is unknown.

Rapid Diagnosis of Urinary Tract Infections

Genitourinary tract infection (UTI) is among the most common causes of sepsis and septic shock in critically ill patients. The incidence of nosocomial UTI increases with hospital length of stay, and patients with ICU-acquired UTI have increased mortality. The gold standard for diagnosis of UTI is urine quantitative culture with an organism growing at least 10^5 CFU from a clean catch specimen or 10^3 from a catheterized specimen. Urine cultures have the same limitations as cultures from other fluids, especially inability to distinguish between true infection and colonization or contamination.[65,66] Some single-center studies report multiplex PCR-enhanced detection of polymicrobial infection in symptomatic patients with UTI. 16s rRNA sequencing has also been used as a method of identifying the cause of culture-negative UTIs.[66,67]

DISCUSSION

Fig. 1 lists some commercially available tools for diagnosis of common infections in the ICU. Although there are clear advantages of RDTs in critically ill patients, areas of uncertainty are also present. A positive result from an NAAT may not translate into true infection, given the high sensitivity of many tests. Furthermore, interpretation of a persistently positive test when a patient is clinically improving is unclear. Many NAATs have a limited panel of pathogens they detect, and thus a negative test does not completely exclude infection. These tests should be used in conjunction with culture, not as a replacement for culture. In addition, many NAATs provide limited or no information on resistance patterns, making it difficult to definitively deescalate antibiotics. Finally, the cost-benefit of RDTs in critically ill patients is unclear.

SUMMARY

Our approach to incorporating RDTs into clinical practice is as follows (**Fig. 2**). The platform of choice should be locally validated before implementing the test into routine clinical care. Education on test result interpretation and antibiotic stewardship should be provided to critical care physicians and staff to maximize the potential benefit of the test. We encourage the use of tests that have an excellent negative predictive value and can safely lead to antimicrobial deescalation. Examples of this would be using an RDT to rule out influenza and discontinue empirical oseltamivir or using a rapid test to rule out MRSA pneumonia to avoid or discontinue empirical vancomycin. As with any diagnostic test, the results of rapid diagnostic platforms must be interpreted in the clinical context. Although there are no large, multicenter, prospective, randomized controlled trials on use of RDTs compared with standard of care to determine their effect on important clinical outcomes, we believe novel diagnostics could have the potential to be a powerful adjunct to culture and improve the management of infection in critically ill patients.

CLINICS CARE POINTS

- The negative predictive value of many RDTs, particularly nucleic acid amplification tests, is high. A clinician can reliably exclude infection by a pathogen on panel if the test is negative.
- The yield of a culture-independent test is generally higher than standard culture. Thus, molecular testing should be considered in culture-negative cases.
- Studies demonstrate RDTs may improve antibiotic stewardship but the impact on other clinically important outcomes remains unclear.

FUNDING

This work is supported by the National Institute of Health Institutional Training grant (3T32HL76139–13S2) and by NIH/NIAID grant U19AI135964.

DISCLOSURE

R.G. Wunderink is a consultant for bioMerieux and Accelerate Diagnostics. His institution has received research grants from bioMérieux and Curetis. All other authors declare no conflict of interest.

REFERENCES

1. Rhee C, Jones TM, Hamad Y, et al. Prevalence, underlying causes, and preventability of sepsis-associated mortality in US acute care hospitals. JAMA Netw Open 2019;2(2):e187571.
2. Perner A, Gordon AC, De Backer D, et al. Sepsis: frontiers in diagnosis, resuscitation and antibiotic therapy. Intensive Care Med 2016;42(12):1958–69.
3. Vincent J-L, Rello J, Marshall J, et al. International study of the prevalence and outcomes of infection in intensive care units. JAMA 2009;302(21):2323–9.
4. Angus DC, Linde-Zwirble WT, Lidicker J, et al. Epidemiology of severe sepsis in the United States: analysis of incidence, outcome, and associated costs of care. Crit Care Med 2001;29(7):1303–10.
5. Aldemir M, Özen S, Kara IH, et al. Predisposing factors for delirium in the surgical intensive care unit. Crit Care 2001;5(5):265.
6. Zimlichman E, Henderson D, Tamir O, et al. Health care–associated infections: a meta-analysis of costs and financial impact on the US health care system. JAMA Intern Med 2013;173(22):2039–46.
7. Kaukonen KM, Bailey M, Pilcher D, et al. Systemic inflammatory response syndrome criteria in defining severe sepsis. N Engl J Med 2015;372(17):1629–38.
8. Vincent JL, Opal SM, Marshall JC, et al. Sepsis definitions: time for change. Lancet 2013;381(9868):774–5.
9. Kumar A, Roberts D, Wood KE, et al. Duration of hypotension before initiation of effective antimicrobial therapy is the critical determinant of survival in human septic shock. Crit Care Med 2006;34(6):1589–96.
10. Lagier JC, Edouard S, Pagnier I, et al. Current and past strategies for bacterial culture in clinical microbiology. Clin Microbiol Rev 2015;28(1):208–36.
11. Tabak YP, Vankeepuram L, Ye G, et al. Blood culture turnaround time in U.S. acute care hospitals and implications for laboratory process optimization. J Clin Microbiol 2018;56(12).
12. MacVane SH, Oppermann N, Humphries RM. Time to result for pathogen identification and antimicrobial susceptibility testing of bronchoalveolar lavage and endotracheal aspirate specimens in U.S. acute care hospitals. J Clin Microbiol 2020;58(11):e01468.
13. Fernandes CM, Walker R, Price A, et al. Root cause analysis of laboratory delays to an emergency department. J Emerg Med 1997;15(5):735–9.
14. Srinivasan R, Karaoz U, Volegova M, et al. Use of 16S rRNA gene for identification of a broad range of clinically relevant bacterial pathogens. PloS One 2015;10(2):e0117617.
15. Spencer RC. Epidemiology of infection in ICUs. Intensive Care Med 1994;20(Suppl 4):S2–6.
16. Koenig SM, Truwit JD. Ventilator-associated pneumonia: diagnosis, treatment, and prevention. Clin Microbiol Rev 2006;19(4):637–57.
17. Li G, Cook DJ, Thabane L, et al. Risk factors for mortality in patients admitted to intensive care units with pneumonia. Respir Res 2016;17(1):80.
18. Kalil AC, Metersky ML, Klompas M, et al. Executive summary: management of adults with hospital-acquired and ventilator-associated pneumonia: 2016 clinical practice guidelines by the infectious diseases society of America and the American thoracic society. Clin Infect Dis 2016;63(5):575–82.
19. Metlay JP, Waterer GW, Long AC, et al. Diagnosis and treatment of adults with community-acquired pneumonia. an official clinical practice guideline of

the American thoracic society and infectious diseases society of America. Am J Respir Crit Care Med 2019;200(7):e45–67.

20. Mahony JB. Detection of respiratory viruses by molecular methods. Clin Microbiol Rev 2008;21(4): 716–47.

21. Boonyaratanakornkit J, Vivek M, Xie H, et al. Predictive value of respiratory viral detection in the upper respiratory tract for infection of the lower respiratory tract with hematopoietic stem cell transplantation. J Infect Dis 2019;221(3):379–88.

22. Walter JM, Wunderink RG. Testing for respiratory viruses in adults with severe lower respiratory infection. Chest 2018;154(5):1213–22.

23. Luyt C-E. Virus diseases in ICU patients: a long time underestimated; but be aware of overestimation. Intensive Care Med 2006;32(7):968–70.

24. Legoff J, Zucman N, Lemiale V, et al. Clinical significance of upper airway virus detection in critically Ill hematology patients. Am J Respir Crit Care Med 2019;199(4):518–28.

25. Martino R, Porras RP, Rabella N, et al. Prospective study of the incidence, clinical features, and outcome of symptomatic upper and lower respiratory tract infections by respiratory viruses in adult recipients of hematopoietic stem cell transplants for hematologic malignancies. Biol Blood Marrow Transplant 2005;11(10):781–96.

26. Evans SE, Jennerich AL, Azar MM, et al. Nucleic acid-based testing for noninfluenza viral pathogens in adults with suspected community-acquired pneumonia. an official American thoracic society clinical practice guideline. Am J Respir Crit Care Med 2021;203(9):1070–87.

27. Choi SH, Hong SB, Ko GB, et al. Viral infection in patients with severe pneumonia requiring intensive care unit admission. Am J Respir Crit Care Med 2012;186(4):325–32.

28. Afzal Z, Minard CG, Stager CE, et al. Clinical diagnosis, viral PCR, and antibiotic utilization in community-acquired pneumonia. Am J Ther 2016; 23(3):e766–72.

29. Gelfer G, Leggett J, Myers J, et al. The clinical impact of the detection of potential etiologic pathogens of community-acquired pneumonia. Diagn Microbiol Infect Dis 2015;83(4):400–6.

30. Webber DM, Wallace MA, Burnham C-AD, et al. Evaluation of the biofire filmarray pneumonia panel for detection of viral and bacterial pathogens in lower respiratory tract specimens in the setting of a tertiary care academic medical center. J Clin Microbiol 2020;58(7):00320–e00343.

31. Klein M, Bacher J, Barth S, et al. Multicenter evaluation of the unyvero platform for testing bronchoalveolar lavage fluid. J Clin Microbiol 2021;59(3).

32. Buchan BW, Windham S, Balada-Llasat JM, et al. Practical comparison of the biofire filmarray pneumonia panel to routine diagnostic methods and potential impact on antimicrobial stewardship in adult hospitalized patients with lower respiratory tract infections. J Clin Microbiol 2020;58(7).

33. Pickens C, Wunderink RG, Qi C, et al. A multiplex polymerase chain reaction assay for antibiotic stewardship in suspected pneumonia. Diagn Microbiol Infect Dis 2020;98(4):115179.

34. Dangerfield B, Chung A, Webb B, et al. Predictive value of methicillin-resistant Staphylococcus aureus (MRSA) nasal swab PCR assay for MRSA pneumonia. Antimicrob Agents Chemother 2014;58(2): 859–64.

35. Paonessa JR, Shah RD, Pickens CI, et al. Rapid detection of methicillin-resistant staphylococcus aureus in BAL: a pilot randomized controlled trial. Chest 2019;155(5):999–1007.

36. Pickens CI, Qi C, Postelnick M, et al. Association between a rapid diagnostic test to detect methicillin-resistant Staphylococcus Aureus pneumonia and decreased vancomycin use in a medical intensive care unit over a 30-month period. Infect Control Hosp Epidemiol 2021;42(11):1–3.

37. Sarikonda KV, Micek ST, Doherty JA, et al. Methicillin-resistant Staphylococcus aureus nasal colonization is a poor predictor of intensive care unit-acquired methicillin-resistant Staphylococcus aureus infections requiring antibiotic treatment. Crit Care Med 2010;38(10):1991–5.

38. Bush K, Fisher JF. Epidemiological expansion, structural studies, and clinical challenges of new β-lactamases from gram-negative bacteria. Annu Rev Microbiol 2011;65(1):455–78.

39. Bassetti M, Righi E, Carnelutti A. Bloodstream infections in the intensive care unit. Virulence 2016;7(3): 267–79.

40. Barnett AG, Page K, Campbell M, et al. The increased risks of death and extra lengths of hospital and ICU stay from hospital-acquired bloodstream infections: a case–control study. BMJ Open 2013; 3(10):e003587.

41. Laupland KB, Zygun DA, Davies HD, et al. Population-based assessment of intensive care unit-acquired bloodstream infections in adults: incidence, risk factors, and associated mortality rate. Crit Care Med 2002;30(11):2462–7.

42. Kaye KS, Marchaim D, Chen T-Y, et al. Effect of nosocomial bloodstream infections on mortality, length of stay, and hospital costs in older adults. J Am Geriatr Soc 2014;62(2):306–11.

43. Shafazand S, Weinacker AB. Blood cultures in the critical care unit: improving utilization and yield. Chest 2002;122(5):1727–36.

44. Tuma RSP. MALDI-TOF mass spectrometry: getting a feel for how it works. Oncol Times 2003;25(19):26.

45. French K, Evans J, Tanner H, et al. The clinical impact of rapid, direct MALDI-ToF identification of

bacteria from positive blood cultures. PLoS One 2016;11(12):e0169332.

46. Faron ML, Buchan BW, Samra H, et al. Evaluation of WASPLab software to automatically read chromID CPS elite agar for reporting of urine cultures. J Clin Microbiol 2019;58(1).

47. Ferreira L, Sánchez-Juanes F, Porras-Guerra I, et al. Microorganisms direct identification from blood culture by matrix-assisted laser desorption/ionization time-of-flight mass spectrometry. Clin Microbiol Infect 2011;17(4):546–51.

48. Vlek AL, Bonten MJ, Boel CH. Direct matrix-assisted laser desorption ionization time-of-flight mass spectrometry improves appropriateness of antibiotic treatment of bacteremia. PLoS One 2012;7(3): e32589.

49. Tan KE, Ellis BC, Lee R, et al. Prospective evaluation of a matrix-assisted laser desorption ionization-time of flight mass spectrometry system in a hospital clinical microbiology laboratory for identification of bacteria and yeasts: a bench-by-bench study for assessing the impact on time to identification and cost-effectiveness. J Clin Microbiol 2012;50(10): 3301–8.

50. Charnot-Katsikas A, Tesic V, Love N, et al. Use of the accelerate pheno system for identification and antimicrobial susceptibility testing of pathogens in positive blood cultures and impact on time to results and workflow. J Clin Microbiol 2018;56(1):e01166.

51. Humphries R, Di Martino T. Effective implementation of the Accelerate Pheno™ system for positive blood cultures. J Antimicrob Chemother 2019; 74(Supplement_1):i40–3.

52. Banerjee R, Teng CB, Cunningham SA, et al. Randomized trial of rapid multiplex polymerase chain reaction-based blood culture identification and susceptibility testing. Clin Infect Dis 2015;61(7): 1071–80.

53. Friedrich AK, Cahan M. Intraabdominal infections in the intensive care unit. J Intensive Care Med 2014; 29(5):247–54.

54. Bagdasarian N, Rao K, Malani PN. Diagnosis and treatment of Clostridium difficile in adults: a systematic review. JAMA 2015;313(4):398–408.

55. Riddle DJ, Dubberke ER. Clostridium difficile infection in the intensive care unit. Infect Dis Clin North America 2009;23(3):727–43.

56. Spina A, Kerr KG, Cormican M, et al. Spectrum of enteropathogens detected by the FilmArray GI Panel in a multicentre study of community-acquired gastroenteritis. Clin Microbiol Infect 2015; 21(8):719–28.

57. Debast SB, Bauer MP, Kuijper EJ. European Society of Clinical Microbiology and Infectious Diseases: update of the treatment guidance document for Clostridium difficile infection. Clin Microbiol Infect 2014; 20(Suppl 2):1–26.

58. Barbut F, Surgers L, Eckert C, et al. Does a rapid diagnosis of Clostridium difficile infection impact on quality of patient management? Clin Microbiol Infect 2014;20(2):136–44.

59. Marcos MA, Martínez E, Almela M, et al. New rapid antigen test for diagnosis of pneumococcal meningitis. Lancet 2001;357(9267):1499–500.

60. Moïsi JC, Saha SK, Falade AG, et al. Enhanced diagnosis of pneumococcal meningitis with use of the binax NOW immunochromatographic test of streptococcus pneumoniae antigen: a multisite study. Clin Infect Dis 2009;48(Supplement_2): S49–56.

61. Leber AL, Everhart K, Balada-Llasat JM, et al. Multicenter evaluation of biofire filmarray meningitis/encephalitis panel for detection of bacteria, viruses, and yeast in cerebrospinal fluid specimens. J Clin Microbiol 2016;54(9):2251–61.

62. Fleischer E, Aronson PL. Rapid diagnostic tests for meningitis and encephalitis—biofire. Pediatr Emerg Care 2020;36(8):397–401.

63. Poplin V, Boulware DR, Bahr NC. Methods for rapid diagnosis of meningitis etiology in adults. Biomark Med 2020;14(6):459–79.

64. Domingues RB, Santos MVd, Leite FBVdM, et al. FilmArray Meningitis/Encephalitis (ME) panel in the diagnosis of bacterial meningitis. Braz J Infect Dis 2019;23(6):468–70.

65. Laupland KB, Bagshaw SM, Gregson DB, et al. Intensive care unit-acquired urinary tract infections in a regional critical care system. Crit Care 2005; 9(2):R60–5.

66. Xu R, Deebel N, Casals R, et al. A new gold rush: a review of current and developing diagnostic tools for urinary tract infections. Diagnostics (Basel) 2021; 11(3).

67. García LT, Cristancho LM, Vera EP, et al. A new multiplex-PCR for urinary tract pathogen detection using primer design based on an evolutionary computation method. J Microbiol Biotechnol 2015; 25(10):1714–27.

Pharmacologic Management of Delirium in the Intensive Care Unit

Perry J. Tiberio, MD, PhD[a], Niall T. Prendergast, MD[a],
Timothy D. Girard, MD, MSCI[b],*

KEYWORDS

• Delirium • Intensive care • Mechanical ventilation • Treatment • Prevention

KEY POINTS

• Delirium in the ICU is common and contributes to significant morbidity and mortality.
• Approaches to reducing delirium in the ICU focus on prevention and treatment.
• The choice and quantity of sedative drugs influence the risk of delirium.
• Haloperidol did not prevent or treat delirium in the ICU in large, randomized, placebo-controlled trials.
• Dexmedetomidine may prevent and treat delirium in select ICU patients.

INTRODUCTION
What is Delirium?

Delirium is a common medical condition characterized by acute and fluctuating disturbances in attention, awareness, and cognition. There are many triggers and risk factors for delirium, including acute illness, substance withdrawal or intoxication, and medical therapies. Because of the severity of the illnesses and the treatments required to manage these illnesses, critically ill intensive care unit (ICU) patients are typically exposed to numerous delirium risk factors. It is therefore not surprising that delirium is common in the ICU. Without the use of validated assessments, delirium in the ICU is easily underdiagnosed.[1] A meta-analysis of 42 studies published in 2015 found that 32% (5280 of 16,595) of patients (mechanically ventilated and nonventilated) admitted to the ICU developed delirium.[2] Various studies have reported 50% to 80% of patients who require mechanical ventilation during critical illness develop delirium.[3–6] Moderate to heavy sedation, which is often used to manage mechanically ventilated ICU patients, is a delirium risk factor, with the strongest evidence linking exposure to benzodiazepines with increased risk of delirium.[7]

When faced with delirium in an ICU patient, clinicians should first seek to identify and mitigate delirium risk factors. We present an overview of the predisposing risk factors and precipitating triggers associated with delirium in **Fig. 1**. Although not amenable to modification, predisposing risk factors should be recognized, including advancing age, preexisting cognitive impairment, comorbid disease (particularly respiratory disease), and vision or hearing impairment.[8] Precipitating risk factors, however, can often be addressed and include severity of illness; emergent or major

The authors have nothing to disclose.
[a] Division of Pulmonary, Allergy, and Critical Care Medicine, Department of Medicine, University of Pittsburgh, NW 628 UPMC Montefiore, 3459 Fifth Avenue, Pittsburgh, PA 15213, USA; [b] Department of Critical Care Medicine, The Clinical Research, Investigation, and Systems Modeling of Acute Illness (CRISMA) Center, University of Pittsburgh, 3520 Fifth Avenue, 101 Keystone Building, Pittsburgh, PA, 15213, USA
* Corresponding author. 3520 Fifth Avenue, 101 Keystone Building, Pittsburgh, PA 15213.
E-mail address: timothy.girard@pitt.edu
Twitter: @timothygirard (T.D.G.)

Clin Chest Med 43 (2022) 411–424
https://doi.org/10.1016/j.ccm.2022.04.004
0272-5231/22/© 2022 Elsevier Inc. All rights reserved.

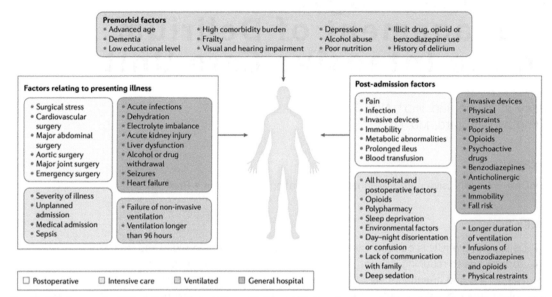

Fig. 1. Risk factors for ICU delirium. From Wilson JE, Mart MF, Cunningham C, Shehabi Y, Girard TD, MacLullich AMJ, Slooter AJC, Ely EW. Delirium. *Nat Rev Dis Primers* 2020; 6: 90.

surgery; organ failure; metabolic disturbance; sepsis; substance withdrawal; mechanical ventilation; and the use of sedatives, especially benzodiazepines.[8]

How is Delirium Evaluated?

Delirium is often underrecognized and undiagnosed during critical illness when a validated tool is not used to detect delirium. Evidence-based clinical practice guidelines, therefore, recommend the routine use of validated assessment tools to detect delirium early, facilitating the reversal of modifiable risk factors.[9] Two tools are recommended based on extensive validation research: the Confusion Assessment Method for the ICU (CAM-ICU)[10] and the Intensive Care Delirium Screening Checklist (ICDSC).[11] Both are easy to implement into clinical practice and may effect patient outcomes; a prospective cohort found that adherence to delirium screening was associated with reduced in-hospital mortality.[12] Whereas each tool has high sensitivity when used by trained clinicians, ICDSC is less specific,[10,11] and a prospective study comparing CAM-ICU and ICDSC found that CAM-ICU more accurately diagnosed delirium.[13] A secondary analysis of a prospective study found the level of sedation (based on the Richmond Agitation-Sedation Scale [RASS]) influenced outcomes of delirium assessments: at RASS of −3, CAM-ICU led to higher rates of delirium, but at RASS of 0, CAM-ICU led to lower rates of delirium.[14] Newer tools, such as CHART-

DEL-ICU and CAM-ICU-7, might aid in evaluating patients at risk of delirium,[15,16] but more evidence is needed before these tools are recommended for widespread use.

What is the Pathophysiology of Delirium?

Despite identifying numerous etiologies, the pathophysiology of delirium is not fully understood. Although a full discussion of the mechanisms thought to underlie delirium during critical illness is beyond the scope of this article, we summarize several important points here:

- Certain patients are predisposed to delirium because of preexisting cognitive dysfunction or advancing age.[17] Host vulnerability, whether at the blood-brain barrier or in the neuroinflammatory response to critical illness, likely contributes to the development of delirium.[18,19]
- Hypoxia was initially described as a cause for delirium in 1959,[20] with a more recent study demonstrating that early cerebral hypoxia in critical illness is associated with delirium.[21]
- Critical illness alters energy metabolism, resulting in relative insulin resistance, mitochondrial dysfunction, and other metabolic derangements that may contribute to delirium.[22]
- System inflammation is often increased during critical illness and can lead to changes in the permeability of the blood-brain barrier,

resulting in central nervous system (CNS) inflammation and the development of delirium.[23,24]

- Dysregulation occurs in neurotransmitter homeostasis during critical illness, and disruption in pathways of acetylcholine and dopamine,[25] adrenaline,[26] and γ-aminobutyric acid (GABA)[27] signaling likely contribute to delirium.

Why Care About Delirium?

Delirium in the ICU is associated with important short- and long-term adverse outcomes. In the short-term, delirium can lead to patient interference in medical care (eg, physical therapy, respiratory therapy), accidental removal of life-sustaining equipment (eg, central venous catheters, endotracheal tube), longer times on the ventilator, and extended ICU and hospital length of stays.[3,28,29] A recent retrospective analysis of 5936 propensity-matched critically ill adults with and without delirium found that delirium was associated with increased 30-day post-hospital discharge mortality (hazard ratio, 1.44; 95% confidence interval [CI], 1.08–1.92).[28] The duration of ICU delirium has also been associated with increased mortality,[30] re-emphasizing the importance of using validated identification tools in daily clinical practice for the early identification of delirium. In addition, delirium is associated with short-term[3] and long-term cognitive dysfunction up to 12 months after discharge.[4,5] This cognitive impairment contributes to difficulties with daily living, including employment.[31,32] It is therefore important that delirium is identified early and effectively addressed.

Summary of Introduction

In summary, delirium is a prevalent condition in the ICU with an unclear pathophysiology and several predisposing risk factors and precipitating triggers. Clinicians should use validated assessment tools to identify delirious patients early to reduce short- and long-term morbidity and mortality. For the remainder of the review, we focus on evidence regarding the pharmacologic prevention and treatment of delirium in the ICU and conclude by highlighting emerging, but unproven, therapies.

MANAGEMENT OF DELIRIUM IN THE INTENSIVE CARE UNIT

Many patients are already delirious when they are admitted to the ICU, whereas others develop it during their ICU stay. Given the profound short- and long-term consequences of delirium, it is crucial that clinicians have successful means for its prevention and treatment. The literature on delirium prevention and treatment varies in its methodologies, creating challenges when deciding what to incorporate into clinical practice. Strategies used to prevent delirium frequently overlap those used to treat delirium in the ICU; for instance, dexmedetomidine may be used as an alternative to benzodiazepines and other deliriogenic sedatives to reduce the risk of delirium or to treat existing delirium. Many clinical trials recruited patients with and without delirium, therefore, examining a medication's efficacy for delirium treatment and prevention. We use the remainder of this review to discuss pharmacologic strategies for preventing and treating delirium in the ICU, describing drug classes, mechanisms of action, existing evidence, and current recommendations (**Table 1**).

Prevention of Delirium in the Intensive Care Unit

Early studies of the prevention and treatment of delirium focused on sedative classes and depth of sedation. Numerous trials demonstrated that less sedation improves patient outcomes. In the Awakening and Breathing Controlled (ABC) trial,[33] a protocol that paired daily spontaneous awakening trials with spontaneous breathing trials reduced oversedation and time on the ventilator and improved mortality. In a more recent prospective multicenter international cohort, critically ill ventilated patients who received lighter sedation experienced less delirium, more ventilator-free days, and lower mortality than those who received heavy sedation.[34] These and other studies led the 2018 Society of Critical Care Medicine (SCCM) guidelines to make a conditional recommendation to use light sedation in critically ill, mechanically ventilated adults[9]; there is no consensus on what defines light, moderate, and heavy sedation. Further research is needed to clarify the effects of deep sedation on posthospital patient-centered outcomes, such as cognition and physical rehabilitation.

Propofol

Propofol is a short-acting general anesthetic that acts through agonism at $GABA_A$ receptors with possible glutamatergic activity through N-methyl-D-aspartic acid (NMDA) receptor blockade. A large number of critical care trials compared propofol with benzodiazepines. Whereas multiple studies found that sedation with propofol rather than benzodiazepines was associated with improved mortality,[35] lighter sedation, and shorter time to extubation,[36] the studies that compared propofol

Table 1
Major trials of pharmacologic prevention and treatment of delirium in the ICU

Trial	Year	Study Design	Number	Treatment	Results
Trials evaluating both prevention and treatment of ICU delirium					
MENDS	2007	Multicenter, double-blind RCT	106 ventilated patients	Dexmedetomidine vs lorazepam for sedation	Significant increase in delirium- and coma-free days in the dexmedetomidine group
SEDCOM	2009	Multicenter, double-blind RCT	375 ventilated patients	Dexmedetomidine vs midazolam for sedation	Significant reduction in delirium and increase in delirium-free days in the dexmedetomidine group
HOPE-ICU	2013	Single-center, double-blinded RCT	142 ventilated patients	Haloperidol vs placebo	No significant difference in incidence or duration of delirium
SAILS	2016	Multicenter, double-blind RCT	272 ventilated patients	Rosuvastatin vs placebo	No significant difference in incidence of delirium
MoDUS	2017	Multicenter, double-blind RCT	142 ventilated patients	Simvastatin vs placebo	No significant difference in incidence of delirium or in delirium- and coma-free days
DESIRE	2017	Multicenter, open-label RCT	201 ventilated patients	Dexmedetomidine + fentanyl vs usual care	No significant difference in prevalence of delirium
Perbet et al,[45] 2018	2018	Single-center, double-blind RCT	162 ventilated patients	Ketamine vs placebo for sedation	Significant reduction in delirium and increase in delirium-free days in ketamine group
Nishikimi et al,[60] 2018	2018	Single-center, double-blind RCT	92 ICU patients	Ramelteon vs placebo	Lower prevalence and shorter duration of delirium in the ramelteon group
Skrobik et al,[49] 2018	2018	Two-center, double-blinded RCT	100 patients without delirium	Low-dose nocturnal dexmedetomidine vs placebo	Significant reduction in incidence of delirium, more delirium-free days

Trial	Year	Study design	Population	Intervention	Outcome
REDUCE	2018	Multicenter, double-blind RCT	1796 nondelirious patients	Haloperidol vs placebo	No significant difference in incidence or duration of delirium
SPICE-III	2019	Global, double-blind RCT	4000 ventilated patients	Dexmedetomidine vs usual care	Significant increase in delirium- and coma-free days in the dexmedetomidine group but no difference in mortality
Gandolfi et al,[61] 2020	2020	Multicenter, double-blind RCT	203 ICU patients	Melatonin vs placebo	Significant improvement in sleep quality without a significant difference in incidence of delirium
MENDS2	2021	Multicenter, double-blind RCT	422 ventilated patients with sepsis	Dexmedetomidine vs propofol	No significant difference in delirium- and coma-free days
Trials evaluating treatment of preexisting ICU delirium					
van Eijk et al,[65] 2010	2010	Multicenter, double-blind RCT	104 delirious ICU patients	Rivastigmine vs placebo	Trial halted because of higher mortality and longer duration of delirium in the rivastigmine group
DahLIA	2016	Multicenter RCT	71 patients with agitated delirium	Dexmedetomidine vs placebo	Significant increase in median ventilator-free hours, faster resolution of delirium, shorter duration of delirium
MIND-USA	2018	Multicenter, double-blind RCT	566 ventilated delirious patients	Haloperidol vs ziprasidone vs placebo	No difference in delirium- and coma-free days for either intervention group

Abbreviation: RCT, randomized controlled trial.

with benzodiazepines did not specifically examine delirium as an outcome measure. Nevertheless, because of the other adverse outcomes (eg, over-sedation and delayed liberation from mechanical ventilation) that result from sedation with benzodiazepines, the 2018 guidelines made a conditional recommendation to favor the use of propofol over benzodiazepines.

Opioids

Opioids are a class of medications that act through opioid receptors to induce analgesia and sedation. The opioid most often used in the ICU is fentanyl, a synthetic opioid that is 100 times more potent than morphine. It is used as an analgesic and sedative in the ICU (inducing so-called analgosedation) and is delivered as a continuous infusion or via intermittent intravenous (IV) injections.

The relationship between opioids and delirium in the ICU is complex. Untreated pain is a trigger for delirium; therefore, pain must be treated appropriately. In of study of patients admitted to the surgical ICU or trauma ICU, the use of morphine was associated with decreased delirium.[37] Alternatively, two prospective studies found that critically ill ventilated patients who received benzodiazepines and/or opioids had longer duration of delirium in the ICU[38] or a higher likelihood of developing delirium.[39] More recently a large retrospective analysis of 4075 adults admitted to the ICU demonstrated that exposure to any dose of opioid was associated with subsequent delirium (odds ratio [OR], 1.45; 95% CI, 1.24–1.69) and every 10 mg of IV morphine equivalent was associated with a 2.4% increase in next-day delirium.[40] Unexpectedly, the study also found an inverse association between the presence of severe pain and risk of transitioning to delirium (OR, 0.72; 95% CI, 0.53–0.97). A randomized controlled trial further clarifying the relationships between opioid exposure, pain, and development of delirium in the ICU is needed.

Benzodiazepines

Benzodiazepines are a class of drugs that cause sedation by stimulating $GABA_A$ receptors; benzodiazepines also act as anxiolytics, anticonvulsants, and hypnotics. There is significant evidence linking benzodiazepines to delirium. In a prospective study of 1112 critically ill patients, continuous IV benzodiazepines, but not intermittent IV benzodiazepines, were associated with delirium.[41] However, numerous other studies of ICU patients found that the association between benzodiazepines and delirium is dose-dependent rather than related to the route or timing of delivery. Additionally, an open-label trial

published in 2006 randomized ventilated patients requiring high doses of lorazepam to either receive intermittent boluses of lorazepam or a continuous infusion of propofol.[42] Although delirium was not assessed as an outcome in this trial, the propofol arm had significantly fewer median ventilator days compared with the intermittent lorazepam group (5.8 days vs 8.4 days; $P = .04$). The 2018 SCCM guidelines recommend choosing propofol or dexmedetomidine as sedatives over benzodiazepines.[9]

Ketamine

Ketamine is a general dissociative anesthetic, which functions as a noncompetitive NMDA receptor antagonist. Initial studies among cardiac surgery patients receiving a single perioperative dose of ketamine showed promise in reducing rates of delirium[43]; however, a larger follow-up trial did not find that ketamine reduced delirium in this patient population.[44] Few studies have evaluated delirium in patients receiving continuous infusions of ketamine for sedation in the ICU. One single-center, double-blind randomized trial found lower rates and duration of delirium in patients receiving continuous ketamine compared with placebo.[45] Ongoing trials, such as the ATTAINMENT trial,[46] will further elucidate the relationship between ketamine and delirium. Guidelines recommend against the use of ketamine as a treatment of delirium but do not make recommendations for its use for sedation.

Dexmedetomidine

Dexmedetomidine is a centrally acting α_2-agonist that leads to light sedation and provides some degree of analgesia. Several trials have evaluated delirium in patients receiving dexmedetomidine as a primary sedative drug (see **Table 1**). Note that some trials that evaluated delirium prevention also simultaneously evaluated delirium treatment. Two early trials, MENDS and SEDCOM, demonstrated reduced rates of delirium in patients sedated with dexmedetomidine. In the MENDS study, critically ill ventilated patients who were randomized to receive dexmedetomidine spent more days without delirium or coma (median days, 7.0 vs 3.0; $P = .01$) and were less likely to be comatose (63% vs 92%; $P < .001$) than patients who received midazolam.[47] In the SEDCOM study, 375 ventilated patients were randomized to receive either dexmedetomidine or midazolam for sedation, and those who received dexmedetomidine had lower incidence of delirium.[48]

Examining a different strategy, Skrobik and colleagues[49] published trial results in 2018 that evaluated the addition of low-dose dexmedetomidine at night to preexisting sedation (dosages were reduced by 50%). Patients who received nocturnal dexmedetomidine had a lower incidence of delirium (20% vs 46%; $P = .006$) with a relative risk of 0.44 (95% CI, 0.23–0.88; $P = .006$).

Two recent trials, the 2019 SPICE III study and the 2021 MENDS 2 study, compared sedation with dexmedetomidine with propofol rather than benzodiazepine-based sedation. In the open-label SPICE III trial, 4000 ventilated patients were randomized to receive dexmedetomidine or usual care (primarily propofol) as a primary sedative.[50] The dexmedetomidine group experienced 1 more day free of delirium and coma and 1 more ventilator-free day compared with the usual care group, but there was no significant difference in the primary outcome of 90-day mortality. In the MENDS 2 study, 432 patients with sepsis were randomized to either dexmedetomidine or propofol as a primary sedative[51] and there was no significant difference in the primary outcome of days alive without delirium or coma. In SPICE III and MENDS 2, patients sedated with dexmedetomidine had more adverse events, including bradycardia, hypotension, and self-extubation, than did those in the control groups. Given the adverse events seen in these trials, it might be favorable to prioritize propofol over dexmedetomidine as a first-line sedative agent.

Antipsychotics
The first-generation, or typical, antipsychotics work primarily by inhibiting D_2-dopaminergic receptors, but they also inhibit α-adrenergic, M_1-muscarinic, and H_1 histamine receptors. Haloperidol is the most used typical antipsychotic when treating agitation and delirium in the ICU. In the 2013 HOPE-ICU single-center, randomized trial of 142 ventilated patients, patients treated with haloperidol demonstrated no difference in the incidence or duration of delirium compared with placebo.[52] Similar findings were reported in 2018 from the larger multicenter REDUCE trial that examined whether haloperidol prevented delirium among 1796 critically ill adults who were not delirious at the time of recruitment.[53] The 2018 SCCM guidelines recommend against using haloperidol to prevent delirium in critically ill adults.

The second-generation, or atypical, antipsychotics work primarily to inhibit D_2- and D_3-dopaminergic receptors, but they also inhibit α_1-adrenergic receptors and are a partial agonist to $5HT_{1A}$ serotonergic receptors. The most commonly used atypical antipsychotics in the ICU are olanzapine, risperidone, and quetiapine. However, no placebo-controlled trials have examined whether these medications can prevent

delirium during critical illness. The multicenter, placebo-controlled, MIND study randomized high-risk ICU patients to receive haloperidol, ziprasidone (an atypical antipsychotic), or placebo, and found no evidence of prevention of delirium.[54] Atypical antipsychotics are not recommended for prevention of delirium in the 2018 SCCM guidelines.

Statins
HMG-CoA reductase inhibitors, or statins, are a class of medications that reduce cholesterol levels and improve cardiovascular outcomes. Their anti-inflammatory properties led investigators to hypothesize that reducing neuroinflammation with statins would reduce delirium during critical illness.[55] Preliminary studies suggested that statin use in critically ill patients may reduce the incidence of delirium,[56,57] but two large randomized, controlled trials did not find a benefit. In a secondary analysis of the 2016 ARDSNet SAILS trial evaluating the role of rosuvastatin on mortality in acute respiratory distress syndrome, no difference between the rosuvastatin group and placebo in days of delirium was found (34% in rosuvastatin group vs 30% in placebo group; $P = .22$).[58] In 2017, the Modifying Delirium Using Simvastatin (MoDUS) trial randomized ventilated patients to receive simvastatin or placebo; there was no difference in the primary outcome of days free of delirium and coma (mean of 5.7 in the simvastatin group vs 6.1 in the placebo group; $P = .66$).[59] Without compelling evidence from randomized controlled trials, guidelines do not recommend that statins be used to prevent delirium in critically ill patients.

Melatonin agonists
Melatonin is produced by the body to maintain the circadian rhythm and is used to help patients with shift work sleep disorder. Ramelteon is a drug that acts as a potent agonist of the MT_1 and MT_2 melatonin receptors and aids in syncing the sleep-wake cycle. Because sleep disruption is a potentially modifiable risk factor for delirium in the ICU, a single-center trial randomized 92 ICU patients to receive ramelteon or placebo.[60] Patients in the ramelteon group had significantly lower rates of delirium and more delirium-free days compared with those in the placebo group. In contrast, a multicenter trial in 2020 randomized 203 critically ill patients to receive melatonin or placebo and found that the quality of sleep improved, but the rate of delirium was not significantly different. Further research is necessary before melatonin or ramelteon are recommended as standard management for critically ill adults.[61]

Nonpharmacologic methods

Although outside the scope of this review, it should be noted that the 2018 SCCM guidelines recommend using a multicomponent, nonpharmacologic approach to reduce risk factors (see **Fig. 1**) and improve sleep, hearing, vision, and mobility.[9] An example of this approach includes the awakening and breathing coordination, delirium monitoring/management, early exercise/mobility, and family engagement (ABCDEF) bundle, which has been associated with significantly lower delirium rates in multiple large quality improvement projects.[62,63] Alternatively, a randomized controlled trial in 2016 demonstrated that continuous light therapy did not reduce the incidence or duration of delirium in critically ill adults.[64]

Treatment of Delirium in the Intensive Care Unit

Medications have been used to treat delirium for decades, but recent evidence suggests that most pharmacologic approaches lack efficacy (see **Table 1**). Most clinical trials evaluated the effects of medications on the prevention and treatment of delirium. Three major trials, however, evaluated the treatment of delirium in critically ill patients that was present at the time of recruitment: a 2010 trial evaluating rivastigmine,[65] the 2016 Dexmedetomidine to Lessen ICU Agitation (DahLIA) trial,[66] and the 2018 Modifying the Impact of ICU-Associated Neurologic Dysfunction-USA (MIND-USA) trial.[67]

Rivastigmine

Rivastigmine is an acetylcholinesterase inhibitor used primarily to treat Alzheimer disease by increasing acetylcholine in the CNS. In 2010, a multicenter, placebo-controlled, randomized trial randomized critically ill adults with delirium to receive rivastigmine or placebo as an adjunct to haloperidol for treatment of delirium.[65] Although the planned enrollment was 440 patients, the trial was halted early after 104 patients were enrolled because of increased mortality in patients receiving rivastigmine compared with those who received placebo (22% vs 8%; $P = .07$). The trial also found a nonsignificant trend toward longer duration of delirium in the rivastigmine group (5 days vs 3 days; $P = .06$). As such, rivastigmine is not recommended as a treatment of delirium in the ICU.

Dexmedetomidine

Dexmedetomidine has been studied extensively to reduce the incidence and duration of delirium in the ICU. In 2016, DahLIA, a multicenter, double-blind, placebo-controlled randomized trial, evaluated the role of low-dose dexmedetomidine in improving ability to extubate 71 agitated, delirious, mechanically ventilated patients.[66] The investigators found a significant increase in the primary outcome of median ventilator-free hours at 7 days (144.8 vs 127.5 hours; $P = .01$). There was also a significant reduction in the median hours to first resolution of delirium (23.3 vs 40 hours; $P = .01$) and fewer hours in the presence of delirium (36 vs 62 hours; $P = .009$). Although this trial suggests a role for dexmedetomidine among ventilated patients with agitated delirium, confirmatory trials are needed to determine if delirious mechanically ventilated patients benefit from dexmedetomidine given specifically during the weaning phase.

Antipsychotics

For decades, practitioners have used antipsychotics, such as haloperidol, to treat agitation and delirium in the ICU. The largest trial to examine antipsychotics as treatment of preexisting delirium in critical illness was the 2018 MIND-USA study.[67] In this multicenter, double-blind, placebo-controlled trial, 566 delirious ICU patients with respiratory failure and/or shock were randomized to receive haloperidol, ziprasidone, or placebo. The trial found no difference in the primary outcome of number of days alive without delirium and coma during the 14-day study period (8.5 days in placebo vs 7.9 days in haloperidol group vs 8.7 days in ziprasidone group; $P = .26$). Guidelines therefore recommend against using haloperidol or atypical antipsychotics to treat delirium in the ICU. A small randomized trial in 2010, however, suggested some benefit when quetiapine, an atypical antipsychotic, was used to treat delirium in critically ill patients already treated with as-needed haloperidol.[68] Further research is needed, therefore, to determine if quetiapine effectively treats delirium in larger trials.

In summary, the 2018 SCCM guidelines do not recommend treatment with haloperidol. They do recommend the use of dexmedetomidine when agitation interferes with ventilator weaning.[9]

EMERGING AND POSSIBLE FUTURE TREATMENTS

Without solid evidence supporting pharmacologic prevention and treatment of delirium in the ICU, ongoing research in emerging treatments is vital. Several observational studies and a few randomized trials have evaluated different pharmacologic approaches to reduce delirium (eg, adjunctive analgesia to reduce opioid consumption). Whereas some of this research is specific to the ICU, other studies were conducted in surgical

Table 2
Emerging treatments

Drug	Mechanism of Action	Evidence
Acetaminophen	Nonopioid analgesic that activates serotonergic inhibitory pathways	DEXACET: single-center RCT of 120 patients undergoing CT surgery found that postoperative scheduled IV acetaminophen combined with propofol or dexmedetomidine reduced in-hospital delirium.[72] PANDORA: multicenter RCT currently enrolling.[73]
Valproic acid	Enhances GABA neurotransmission, blocks voltage-dependent sodium channels	Case series in which 13/16 critically ill patients treated with VPA had resolution of hyperactive delirium.[69] Retrospective cohort of 80 ICU patients with resolution of delirium in patients receiving VPA alone compared with VPA + antipsychotic.[70] Retrospective of 47 ICU patients treated with VPA showed improvement in delirium with additional sedative drug-sparing effects.[71]
Gabapentin	Influences GABA neurotransmission, binds to voltage-gated calcium channels	A 2017 RCT evaluated gabapentin in noncardiac surgery patients and found an increase in incidence of postoperative delirium in patients treated with gabapentin.[74]
Pregabalin	Similar to gabapentin, binds to voltage-gated calcium channels	Evidence limited to post hoc analysis of an RCT evaluating perioperative pregabalin with inconclusive results because of overall low incidence of delirium.[75]
Clonidine	α_2-adrenergic agonist, reducing sympathetic tone in the CNS	Single-center RCT of patients undergoing surgical repair of aortic dissection found lower incidence of delirium with IV clonidine compared with placebo.[76] RCT in 2019 was halted because of slow enrollment; the trial did not find clonidine reduced delirium.[79] A prospective observational study found that delirious ICU patients treated with clonidine had a lower likelihood of delirium resolution.[77]
Baclofen	Inhibits reflexes at the spinal cord level and induces muscle relaxation	No evidence to support an effect on delirium. A multicenter RCT found that ventilated patients with unhealthy alcohol use had fewer agitation-related events compared with placebo, but at the expense of more patients experiencing delayed awakening.[78]

Abbreviations: CT, cardiothoracic; RCT, randomized controlled trial; VPA, valproic acid.

and/or geriatric populations. A brief overview of emerging treatments from the growing body of literature is discussed here (**Table 2**).

- Valproic acid: Valproic acid is an anticonvulsant that primarily enhances GABA neurotransmission and secondarily blocks voltage-dependent sodium channels. The medication may also have anti-inflammatory properties and block glutamatergic and NMDA receptors, which has led to recent interest in valproic acid as a treatment of delirium in the ICU.[69–71] One retrospective analysis found that agitation and delirium resolved more often in patients treated with valproic acid monotherapy than in patients receiving valproic acid plus antipsychotics.[70] Given that such analyses are confounded by selection bias, valproic acid's role as a delirium treatment should be evaluated in a placebo-controlled randomized trial before the medication is incorporated into practice.
- Acetaminophen: Acetaminophen is a nonopioid analgesic that has the potential benefit of reducing opioid use during critical illness. The IV form of acetaminophen was approved in 2011 by the Food and Drug Administration; it has excellent bioavailability and strong anti-inflammatory properties. The 2019 Dexmedetomidine and IV acetaminophen for the prevention of postoperative delirium following cardiac surgery (DEXACET) trial randomized 120 cardiac surgery patients to receive IV acetaminophen or placebo paired with dexmedetomidine or propofol.[72] The trial found a significant reduction in the primary outcome of in-hospital delirium in patients who received IV acetaminophen (10% vs 28% with placebo; difference, −18% [95% CI, −32% to −5%]; P = .01; hazard ratio, 2.8 [95% CI, 1.1–7.8]). Further research is necessary to determine if DEXACET's results are replicated and generalizable. PANDORA, a larger trial with plans to include 900 older cardiac surgery patients, is currently enrolling.[73]
- Gabapentin: Gabapentin is an anticonvulsant that influences GABA neurotransmission and secondarily binds to voltage-gated calcium channels, which may affect the release of excitatory neurotransmitters. A single-center, randomized trial evaluated the role of perioperative gabapentin in reducing postoperative delirium for 697 patients undergoing noncardiac surgery.[74] Although gabapentin reduced postoperative opioid consumption, no evidence of an effect on delirium was found (24.0% in the gabapentin arm vs 20.8% in

the placebo arm; P = .30). No studies have evaluated the role of gabapentin in the ICU.
- Pregabalin: Pregabalin is an anticonvulsant related to gabapentin and GABA that acts on voltage-gated calcium channels in the CNS and inhibits the release of glutamate, norepinephrine, serotonin, and dopamine. A post hoc analysis of a randomized trial of surgical patients receiving perioperative pregabalin is the only published study and was inconclusive because of an overall low prevalence of delirium.[75]
- Clonidine: Clonidine is an α_2-adrenergic agonist, like dexmedetomidine, that reduces sympathetic tone in the CNS and provides some analgesia. A pilot placebo-controlled randomized trial found that patients undergoing surgical repair of acute aortic dissection had lower postoperative delirium (measured by the Delirium Detection Score, which was created by modifying the Clinical Withdrawal Assessment for Alcohol) in the clonidine arm.[76] In contrast, a large prospective observational study of 3614 critically ill delirious patients found that the delirium was less likely to resolve in patients who received clonidine (OR, 0.78; 95% CI, 0.63–0.97) than in those who did not.[77] A larger randomized trial evaluating the role of clonidine is needed.
- Baclofen: Baclofen is a skeletal muscle relaxant that inhibits reflexes at the spinal cord level through $GABA_B$ agonism. Although there is no evidence to support its role in preventing or treating delirium, there is some evidence that receipt of baclofen reduces agitation in mechanically ventilated patients with unhealthy alcohol use in the ICU. A multicenter trial that randomized 314 ventilated patients with unhealthy alcohol use to either baclofen or placebo found a significant decrease in number of agitation-related events in the baclofen group compared with placebo (19.7% vs 29.7%; adjusted OR, 0.59; 95% CI, 0.35–0.99).[78] However, more patients in the baclofen group had the adverse effect of delayed awakening, and therefore more research is needed to determine its role in agitation and specifically evaluating its role in potentially reducing delirium.

SUMMARY

Delirium, often underdiagnosed in the ICU, is a common complication of critical illness that contributes to significant morbidity and mortality. Validated assessment tools, such as the CAM-ICU and ICDSC, can reliably identify delirium in this population. Clinicians should be aware of common risk factors and triggers and should work to mitigate these as much as possible to reduce the occurrence of delirium.

Because of the highly variable disease course, delirium prevention and treatment often overlap. Most clinical trials focused on delirium examined strategies designed to prevent and treat delirium in the ICU, although some trials specifically evaluated treatment of delirium. When sedating ICU patients, clinicians should avoid benzodiazepines and target light rather than heavy sedation. It is unclear if opioids in the ICU lead to delirium, and ongoing studies should elucidate the relationships between opioids, ketamine, and delirium. Dexmedetomidine as a primary sedative does not improve mortality compared with modern standards of care, but the medication may have a role in treating hyperactive delirious patients in the weaning phase of mechanical ventilation. Several clinical trials showed that most antipsychotics do not affect delirium during critical illness, but several potentially promising treatments require further investigation.

CLINICS CARE POINTS

- Delirium affects up to 50% to 80% of critically ill patients.

- Two validated assessment tools can reliably identify delirium in critically ill patients: the CAM-ICU and ICDSC.

- Delirium is associated with numerous adverse short- and long-term outcomes, including long-term cognitive impairment in survivors of critical illness.

- Benzodiazepines are a common and modifiable risk factor for delirium during critical illness.

- Antipsychotics did not reduce delirium in large randomized, placebo-controlled trials.

- Dexmedetomidine may be beneficial when treating agitation and delirium in mechanically ventilated patients who are close to extubation.

- Promising therapies, such as acetaminophen and clonidine, are being evaluated for the treatment of delirium.

DISCLOSURE

Dr. Girard receives research funding from Ceribell, Inc., served previously as a consultant for Haisco Pharmaceutical Group Co., Ltd., and is on an advisory board for Lungpacer Medical Inc. The other authors have nothing to disclose.

REFERENCES

1. Devlin JW, Marquis F, Riker RR, et al. Combined didactic and scenario-based education improves the ability of intensive care unit staff to recognize delirium at the bedside. Crit Care 2008;12:R19.

2. Salluh JI, Wang H, Schneider EB, et al. Outcome of delirium in critically ill patients: systematic review and meta-analysis. BMJ 2015;350:h2538.

3. Ely EW, Shintani A, Truman B, et al. Delirium as a predictor of mortality in mechanically ventilated patients in the intensive care unit. JAMA 2004;291:1753–62.

4. Girard TD, Thompson JL, Pandharipande PP, et al. Clinical phenotypes of delirium during critical illness and severity of subsequent long-term cognitive impairment: a prospective cohort study. Lancet Respir Med 2018;6:213–22.

5. Pandharipande PP, Girard TD, Jackson JC, et al. Long-term cognitive impairment after critical illness. N Engl J Med 2013;369:1306–16.

6. Ely EW, Gautam S, Margolin R, et al. The impact of delirium in the intensive care unit on hospital length of stay. Intensive Care Med 2001;27:1892–900.

7. Pandharipande P, Shintani A, Peterson J, et al. Lorazepam is an independent risk factor for transitioning to delirium in intensive care unit patients. Anesthesiology 2006;104:21–6.

8. Wilson JE, Mart MF, Cunningham C, et al. Delirium. Nat Rev Dis Primers 2020;6:90.

9. Devlin JW, Skrobik Y, Gelinas C, et al. Clinical practice guidelines for the prevention and management of pain, agitation/sedation, delirium, immobility, and sleep disruption in adult patients in the ICU. Crit Care Med 2018;46:e825–73.

10. Ely EW, Inouye SK, Bernard GR, et al. Delirium in mechanically ventilated patients: validity and reliability of the confusion assessment method for the intensive care unit (CAM-ICU). JAMA 2001;286:2703–10.

11. Bergeron N, Dubois MJ, Dumont M, et al. Intensive care delirium screening checklist: evaluation of a new screening tool. Intensive Care Med 2001;27:859–64.

12. Luetz A, Weiss B, Boettcher S, et al. Routine delirium monitoring is independently associated with a reduction of hospital mortality in critically ill surgical patients: a prospective, observational cohort study. J Crit Care 2016;35:168–73.

13. Tomasi CD, Grandi C, Salluh J, et al. Comparison of CAM-ICU and ICDSC for the detection of delirium in critically ill patients focusing on relevant clinical outcomes. J Crit Care 2012;27:212–7.

14. van den Boogaard M, Wassenaar A, van Haren FMP, et al. Influence of sedation on delirium recognition in critically ill patients: a multinational cohort study. Aust Crit Care 2020;33:420–5.

15. Krewulak KD, Hiploylee C, Ely EW, et al. Adaptation and validation of a chart-based delirium detection tool for the ICU (CHART-DEL-ICU). J Am Geriatr Soc 2021;69:1027–34.

16. Khan BA, Perkins AJ, Gao S, et al. The confusion assessment method for the ICU-7 delirium severity scale: a novel delirium severity instrument for use in the ICU. Crit Care Med 2017;45:851–7.

17. Persico I, Cesari M, Morandi A, et al. Frailty and delirium in older adults: a systematic review and meta-analysis of the literature. J Am Geriatr Soc 2018;66:2022–30.

18. Sweeney MD, Kisler K, Montagne A, et al. The role of brain vasculature in neurodegenerative disorders. Nat Neurosci 2018;21:1318–31.

19. Hasel P, Dando O, Jiwaji Z, et al. Neurons and neuronal activity control gene expression in astrocytes to regulate their development and metabolism. Nat Commun 2017;8:15132.

20. Engel GL, Romano J. Delirium, a syndrome of cerebral insufficiency. J Chronic Dis 1959;9:260–77.

21. Wood MD, Maslove DM, Muscedere JG, et al. Low brain tissue oxygenation contributes to the development of delirium in critically ill patients: a prospective observational study. J Crit Care 2017;41:289–95.

22. Sejling AS, Kjaer TW, Pedersen-Bjergaard U, et al. Hypoglycemia-associated changes in the electroencephalogram in patients with type 1 diabetes and normal hypoglycemia awareness or unawareness. Diabetes 2015;64:1760–9.

23. Munster BC, Aronica E, Zwinderman AH, et al. Neuroinflammation in delirium: a postmortem case-control study. Rejuvenation Res 2011;14:615–22.

24. Varatharaj A, Galea I. The blood-brain barrier in systemic inflammation. Brain Behav Immun 2017;60:1–12.

25. Gainetdinov RR, Jones SR, Caron MG. Functional hyperdopaminergia in dopamine transporter knock-out mice. Biol Psychiatry 1999;46:303–11.

26. Deiner S, Lin HM, Bodansky D, et al. Do stress markers and anesthetic technique predict delirium in the elderly? Dement Geriatr Cogn Disord 2014;38:366–74.

27. Sanders RD. Hypothesis for the pathophysiology of delirium: role of baseline brain network connectivity and changes in inhibitory tone. Med Hypotheses 2011;77:140–3.

28. Fiest KM, Soo A, Hee Lee C, et al. Long-term outcomes in intensive care unit patients with delirium: a population-based cohort study. Am J Respir Crit Care Med 2021;204(4):412–20.

29. Ouimet S, Kavanagh BP, Gottfried SB, et al. Incidence, risk factors and consequences of ICU delirium. Intensive Care Med 2007;33:66–73.

30. Pisani MA, Kong SY, Kasl SV, et al. Days of delirium are associated with 1-year mortality in an older intensive care unit population. Am J Respir Crit Care Med 2009;180:1092–7.

31. Brummel NE, Jackson JC, Pandharipande PP, et al. Delirium in the ICU and subsequent long-term disability among survivors of mechanical ventilation. Crit Care Med 2014;42:369–77.

32. Norman BC, Jackson JC, Graves JA, et al. Employment outcomes after critical illness: an analysis of the bringing to light the risk factors and incidence of neuropsychological dysfunction in ICU survivors cohort. Crit Care Med 2016;44:2003–9.

33. Girard TD, Kress JP, Fuchs BD, et al. Efficacy and safety of a paired sedation and ventilator weaning protocol for mechanically ventilated patients in intensive care (Awakening and Breathing Controlled trial): a randomised controlled trial. Lancet 2008;371:126–34.

34. Shehabi Y, Bellomo R, Kadiman S, et al. Sedation practice in intensive care evaluation study I, the A, New Zealand Intensive Care Society Clinical Trials G. Sedation intensity in the first 48 hours of mechanical ventilation and 180-day mortality: a multinational prospective longitudinal cohort study. Crit Care Med 2018;46:850–9.

35. Lonardo NW, Mone MC, Nirula R, et al. Propofol is associated with favorable outcomes compared with benzodiazepines in ventilated intensive care unit patients. Am J Respir Crit Care Med 2014;189:1383–94.

36. Zhou Y, Jin X, Kang Y, et al. Midazolam and propofol used alone or sequentially for long-term sedation in critically ill, mechanically ventilated patients: a prospective, randomized study. Crit Care 2014;18:R122.

37. Pandharipande P, Cotton BA, Shintani A, et al. Prevalence and risk factors for development of delirium in surgical and trauma intensive care unit patients. J Trauma 2008;65:34–41.

38. Pisani MA, Murphy TE, Araujo KL, et al. Benzodiazepine and opioid use and the duration of intensive care unit delirium in an older population. Crit Care Med 2009;37:177–83.

39. Kamdar BB, Niessen T, Colantuoni E, et al. Delirium transitions in the medical ICU: exploring the role of sleep quality and other factors. Crit Care Med 2015;43:135–41.

40. Duprey MS, Dijkstra-Kersten SMA, Zaal IJ, et al. Opioid use increases the risk of delirium in critically ill adults independently of pain. Am J Respir Crit Care Med 2021;204(5):566–72.

41. Zaal IJ, Devlin JW, Hazelbag M, et al. Benzodiazepine-associated delirium in critically ill adults. Intensive Care Med 2015;41:2130–7.

42. Carson SS, Kress JP, Rodgers JE, et al. A randomized trial of intermittent lorazepam versus propofol with daily interruption in mechanically ventilated patients. Crit Care Med 2006;34:1326–32.

43. Hudetz JA, Iqbal Z, Gandhi SD, et al. Ketamine attenuates post-operative cognitive dysfunction after cardiac surgery. Acta Anaesthesiol Scand 2009;53: 864–72.

44. Avidan MS, Maybrier HR, Abdallah AB, et al. Intraoperative ketamine for prevention of postoperative delirium or pain after major surgery in older adults: an international, multicentre, double-blind, randomised clinical trial. Lancet 2017;390:267–75.

45. Perbet S, Verdonk F, Godet T, et al. Low doses of ketamine reduce delirium but not opiate consumption in mechanically ventilated and sedated ICU patients: a randomised double-blind control trial. Anaesth Crit Care Pain Med 2018;37:589–95.

46. Bawazeer M, Amer M, Maghrabi K, et al. Adjunct low-dose ketamine infusion vs standard of care in mechanically ventilated critically ill patients at a Tertiary Saudi Hospital (ATTAINMENT Trial): study protocol for a randomized, prospective, pilot, feasibility trial. Trials 2020;21:288.

47. Pandharipande PP, Pun BT, Herr DL, et al. Effect of sedation with dexmedetomidine vs lorazepam on acute brain dysfunction in mechanically ventilated patients: the MENDS randomized controlled trial. JAMA 2007;298:2644–53.

48. Riker RR, Shehabi Y, Bokesch PM, et al. Dexmedetomidine vs midazolam for sedation of critically ill patients: a randomized trial. JAMA 2009;301:489–99.

49. Skrobik Y, Duprey MS, Hill NS, et al. Low-dose nocturnal dexmedetomidine prevents ICU delirium. A randomized, placebo-controlled trial. Am J Respir Crit Care Med 2018;197:1147–56.

50. Shehabi Y, Howe BD, Bellomo R, et al. Early sedation with dexmedetomidine in critically ill patients. N Engl J Med 2019;380:2506–17.

51. Hughes CG, Mailloux PT, Devlin JW, et al. Dexmedetomidine or propofol for sedation in mechanically ventilated adults with sepsis. N Engl J Med 2021; 384:1424–36.

52. Page VJ, Ely EW, Gates S, et al. Effect of intravenous haloperidol on the duration of delirium and coma in critically ill patients (Hope-ICU): a randomised, double-blind, placebo-controlled trial. Lancet Respir Med 2013;1:515–23.

53. van den Boogaard M, Slooter AJC, Bruggemann RJM, et al. Effect of haloperidol on survival among critically ill adults with a high risk of delirium: the REDUCE randomized clinical trial. JAMA 2018;319:680–90.

54. Girard TD, Pandharipande PP, Carson SS, et al. Feasibility, efficacy, and safety of antipsychotics for intensive care unit delirium: the MIND randomized, placebo-controlled trial. Crit Care Med 2010;38:428–37.

55. Morandi A, Hughes CG, Girard TD, et al. Statins and brain dysfunction: a hypothesis to reduce the burden of cognitive impairment in patients who are critically ill. Chest 2011;140:580–5.

56. Page VJ, Davis D, Zhao XB, et al. Statin use and risk of delirium in the critically ill. Am J Respir Crit Care Med 2014;189:666–73.

57. Mather JF, Corradi JP, Waszynski C, et al. Statin and its association with delirium in the medical ICU. Crit Care Med 2017;45:1515–22.

58. Needham DM, Colantuoni E, Dinglas VD, et al. Rosuvastatin versus placebo for delirium in intensive care and subsequent cognitive impairment in patients with sepsis-associated acute respiratory distress syndrome: an ancillary study to a randomised controlled trial. Lancet Respir Med 2016;4: 203–12.

59. Page VJ, Casarin A, Ely EW, et al. Evaluation of early administration of simvastatin in the prevention and treatment of delirium in critically ill patients undergoing mechanical ventilation (MoDUS): a randomised, double-blind, placebo-controlled trial. Lancet Respir Med 2017;5:727–37.

60. Nishikimi M, Numaguchi A, Takahashi K, et al. Effect of administration of ramelteon, a melatonin receptor agonist, on the duration of stay in the ICU: a single-center randomized placebo-controlled trial. Crit Care Med 2018;46:1099–105.

61. Gandolfi JV, Di Bernardo APA, Chanes DAV, et al. The effects of melatonin supplementation on sleep quality and assessment of the serum melatonin in ICU patients: a randomized controlled trial. Crit Care Med 2020;48:e1286–93.

62. Balas MC, Burke WJ, Gannon D, et al. Implementing the awakening and breathing coordination, delirium monitoring/management, and early exercise/mobility bundle into everyday care: opportunities, challenges, and lessons learned for implementing the ICU Pain, Agitation, and Delirium Guidelines. Crit Care Med 2013;41:S116–27.

63. Pun BT, Balas MC, Barnes-Daly MA, et al. Caring for critically ill patients with the ABCDEF bundle: results of the ICU liberation collaborative in over 15,000 adults. Crit Care Med 2019;47:3–14.

64. Simons KS, Laheij RJ, van den Boogaard M, et al. Dynamic light application therapy to reduce the incidence and duration of delirium in intensive-care patients: a randomised controlled trial. Lancet Respir Med 2016;4:194–202.

65. van Eijk MM, Roes KC, Honing ML, et al. Effect of rivastigmine as an adjunct to usual care with haloperidol on duration of delirium and mortality in critically ill patients: a multicentre, double-blind, placebo-controlled randomised trial. Lancet 2010;376: 1829–37.

66. Reade MC, Eastwood GM, Bellomo R, et al. Australian, New Zealand Intensive Care Society Clinical

Trials G. Effect of dexmedetomidine added to standard care on ventilator-free time in patients with agitated delirium: a randomized clinical trial. JAMA 2016;315:1460–8.

67. Girard TD, Exline MC, Carson SS, et al. Haloperidol and ziprasidone for treatment of delirium in critical illness. N Engl J Med 2018;379:2506–16.

68. Devlin JW, Roberts RJ, Fong JJ, et al. Efficacy and safety of quetiapine in critically ill patients with delirium: a prospective, multicenter, randomized, double-blind, placebo-controlled pilot study. Crit Care Med 2010;38:419–27.

69. Sher Y, Miller AC, Lolak S, et al. Adjunctive valproic acid in management-refractory hyperactive delirium: a case series and rationale. J Neuropsychiatry Clin Neurosci 2015;27:365–70.

70. Quinn NJ, Hohlfelder B, Wanek MR, et al. Prescribing practices of valproic acid for agitation and delirium in the intensive care unit. Ann Pharmacother 2021;55:311–7.

71. Crowley KE, Urben L, Hacobian G, et al. Valproic acid for the management of agitation and delirium in the intensive care setting: a retrospective analysis. Clin Ther 2020;42:e65–73.

72. Subramaniam B, Shankar P, Shaefi S, et al. Effect of intravenous acetaminophen vs placebo combined with propofol or dexmedetomidine on postoperative delirium among older patients following cardiac surgery: the DEXACET randomized clinical trial. JAMA 2019;321:686–96.

73. Khera T, Mathur PA, Banner-Goodspeed VM, et al. Scheduled prophylactic 6-hourly IV AcetaminopheN

to prevent postoperative delirium in older CaRdiac SurgicAl patients (PANDORA): protocol for a multicentre randomised controlled trial. BMJ Open 2021;11:e044346.

74. Leung JM, Sands LP, Chen N, et al. Perioperative gabapentin does not reduce postoperative delirium in older surgical patients: a randomized clinical trial. Anesthesiology 2017;127:633–44.

75. Farlinger C, Clarke H, Wong CL. Perioperative pregabalin and delirium following total hip arthroplasty: a post hoc analysis of a double-blind randomized placebo-controlled trial. Can J Anaesth 2018;65:1269–70.

76. Rubino AS, Onorati F, Caroleo S, et al. Impact of clonidine administration on delirium and related respiratory weaning after surgical correction of acute type-A aortic dissection: results of a pilot study. Interact Cardiovasc Thorac Surg 2010;10:58–62.

77. Smit L, Dijkstra-Kersten SMA, Zaal IJ, et al. Haloperidol, clonidine and resolution of delirium in critically ill patients: a prospective cohort study. Intensive Care Med 2021;47:316–24.

78. Vourc'h M, Garret C, Gacouin A, et al. Effect of high-dose baclofen on agitation-related events among patients with unhealthy alcohol use receiving mechanical ventilation: a randomized clinical trial. JAMA 2021;325:732–41.

79. Hov KR, Neerland BE, Undseth O, et al. The Oslo study of clonidine in elderly patients with delirium; LUCID: a randomised placebo-controlled trial. Int J Geriatr Psychiatry 2019;34:974–81.

Management of the Critically Ill Patient with Pulmonary Arterial Hypertension and Right Heart Failure

John Granton, MD, FRCPC[a],*, Ricardo Teijeiro-Paradis, MD[b]

KEYWORDS

- Pulmonary hypertension • Right ventricle • Echocardiography • Extracorporeal support
- Heart failure

KEY POINTS

- Right ventricular failure is a common cause of death and morbidity in patients with pulmonary arterial hypertension.
- An approach needs to be developed based on physiologic principles.
- Echocardiography can complement a physiologic approach and guide treatment decisions.
- Extracorporeal support is a useful strategy in selected patients as a bridge to transplant or recovery.

INTRODUCTION

Pulmonary hypertension (PH) is characterized by an increase in right ventricular (RV) afterload that results in an increase in pulmonary arterial pressure. PH is defined as a mean pulmonary arterial pressure greater than 20 mm Hg.[1] PH is further classified into 5 groups. Group 1, pulmonary arterial hypertension (PAH) represents a distinct phenotype characterized by a pulmonary vasculopathy, leading to an effective reduction in the cross-sectional area of the pulmonary vasculature. PAH may be idiopathic or occur secondary to connective tissue diseases, congenital heart disease/ left to right shunts, portal hypertension, human immunodeficiency virus, or drugs. Several genes have been implicated in the development of heritable and sporadic disease. Group II disease relates to PH in the context of left-sided heart/valvular disease, group III disease from underlying structural lung disease or hypoxic pulmonary conditions, and group IV from chronic thromboembolic disease. Group V PH is due to miscellaneous conditions including hemoglobinopathies (most commonly sickle cell disease).

Although this review focuses on RV failure in the context of PAH, all forms of PH can be characterized by RV dysfunction. Therefore, many of the principles in management of RV failure presented may apply while also considering treatment of the underlying condition (eg, left heart disease, lung disease). Although there are many studies addressing the treatment of PAH, there are no systematic studies informing the best strategy to manage the failing RV. Our goal is to help the reader understand some of the physiologic principles that can be used as a guide to a strategy for managing these patients. We will highlight the use of echocardiography in management.

[a] University of Toronto, Pulmonary and Critical Care Medicine, University Health Network, 9-9023 MARS Building, 585 University Avenue, Toronto, Ontario M5G 2N2, Canada; [b] Interdepartmental Division of Critical Care, University of Toronto, University Health Network, 585 University Avenue, Toronto, Ontario M5G 2N2, Canada
* Corresponding author.
E-mail address: John.granton@uhn.ca

Clin Chest Med 43 (2022) 425–439
https://doi.org/10.1016/j.ccm.2022.04.005
0272-5231/22/© 2022 Elsevier Inc. All rights reserved.

Normal Right Ventricular Physiology

After the first breath of life our RV begins to morph into the adult phenotype—a thin-walled, crescent-shaped structure that ejects into a low-resistance, high-compliance, low-impedance circuit.[2] Although the adult RV is less muscular than the LV, it ejects the same amount of blood per cycle under lower pressure, making it energetically more efficient. Much of the ejection may in fact be passive, as the absence of the RV (eg, Fontan circuit) can be tolerated in so far as venous pressure exceeds mean pulmonary pressure to sustain pulmonary perfusion. In addition, left ventricular (LV) ejection aids in RV ejection through contraction of the intraventricular septum. To function efficiently in case of elevation of pulmonary vascular resistance (PVR), the RV will initially adapt and couple its elastance—end systolic pressure divided by end systolic volume—to match the elastance of the arterial system.[3]

In the acute care setting, rapid noninvasive assessment of cardiac function during critical illness has been adopted as standard of practice at some centers. Echocardiography is a reliable, safe, and useful modality in the management of unselected critically ill patients.[4] We will emphasize its role in managing patients with RV failure, as it may provide prognostic information and be a valuable tool to guide and monitor therapeutic interventions.[4,5]

Sonographically, the RV is identified by a more apical insertion of the tricuspid valve, by the presence of the moderator band, extensive trabeculations, a greater number of papillary muscles, and by the disposition and lack of fibrous continuity between the inflow and outflow tract (Fig. 1).[6] The RV is typically described as having a conical shape. This particular shape makes the sonographic assessment of the RV, in particular its volumetric components, challenging.[6,7]

Assessment of the RV has 3 major components: size, function, and ventricular interdependence. Because of its shape, the plane of imaging is critical. Foreshortening (imaging off plane) can significantly alter the reliability of the measurements. Semiquantitative assessment of size is recommended in the setting of point-of-care imaging. An approximation of the end-diastolic area ratio of RV and LV in the apical 4-chamber view is the simplest semiquantitative parameter to determine if the RV is dilated. When the RV end-diastolic area is close to or equal to the LV area (RV/LV ratio 0.6–1), the RV is moderately dilated. If the RV area exceeds the end-diastolic area of the LV (RV/LV ratio >1), the RV is severely dilated. One important caveat is that the ratio depends on the size of both ventricles. In instances where the size of the LV is abnormal, the approximation of the RV size will be imprecise. Other qualitative signs of RV dilatation are loss of its triangular shape, visualization of the moderator band, and a predominantly RV constituted cardiac apex. Quantitative measurements of RV size are provided in Fig. 2.

Systolic function of the RV is more difficult to assess than that of the LV. Its shape, sequential contraction (peristalsis-like), and the significant contribution of the interventricular septum in RV ejection render parameters such as ejection fraction by disc summation (Simpson method) unreliable.[6] Assessing RV systolic function begins by visually comparing its contractility with that of the LV (benchmark). Quantitative parameters measure the approximation of the tricuspid annulus to the apex (longitudinal contraction) and the RV free wall to the septum (area of change).[5] Pressure gradients derived from Doppler velocities aid in estimating pressures in the cardiac chambers. Parameters used to characterize the RV systolic function and their thresholds are listed in Fig. 3. Novel technologies including speckle tracking and multiplane imaging have made RV strain and RV 3-dimensional (3D) imaging available at the bedside, further expanding the capabilities of assessing RV function.

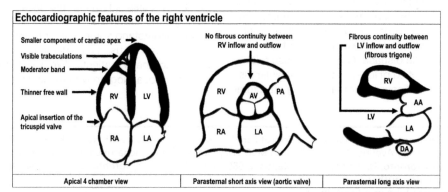

Fig. 1. Echocardiographic features of the right ventricle. AA, ascending aorta; AV, aortic valve; DA, descending aorta; LA, left atrium; LV, left ventricle; RA, right atrium; RV, right ventricle; PA, pulmonary artery.

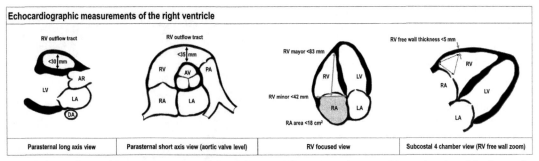

Fig. 2. Echocardiographic measurements of the right ventricle. AR, aortic root; AV, aortic valve; DA, descending aorta; LA, left atrium; LV, left ventricle; PA, pulmonary artery; RA, right atrium; RV, right ventricle.

Echocardiographic assessment of RV systolic function

	Parameter	Example/Tracings	Values	Caveats

LV benchmark	Apical 4 chamber view		• Visual comparison of systolic function
			• RV end-diastolic volume (50-100 mL)
			• LV end-diastolic volume (40-90 mL)
			• Same stroke volume
			• Normal ejection fraction:
			  • RV 45-50%
			  • LV 55-70%
				• RV systolic function may be overestimated in the setting of LV systolic dysfunction
				• LV systolic function is always overestimated in in the setting of RV failure (poor LV preload, high contractility)

TAPSE – M mode	Tricuspid valve lateral annulus excursion / RV focused view / M mode cursor	Measure the height of the excursion, not the slope of the excursion	• Tricuspid annulus plane systolic excursion (TAPSE) • Normal values: 25-35 mm • Abnormal systolic function: ≤16 mm • Established prognostic value • Validated against estimation of ejection fraction by other modalities • Inter-observer variability: 1.9 mm • Meaningful change from baseline: >1.9mm	• Assessment limited to longitudinal contraction • No utility for grading severity • Unreliable measurement if the angle of excursion is different to the angle of interrogation (M-mode) • Overestimates systolic function in severe tricuspid regurgitation • Underestimates systolic function post-pericardiotomy • Unreliable measurement if the heart is swinging (pericardial effusion)
S' velocity – tissue doppler	Tricuspid valve lateral annulus excursion / RV focused view / PW cursor	Systole / Diastole	• S' (systolic) velocity of the tricuspid annulus (Pulsed wave Doppler) with tissue Doppler imaging • Abnormal value: <9.5 cm/s • Established prognostic value • Inter-observer variability: 1.6 m/sec • Meaningful change from baseline: >1.6m/sec	• Same caveats as TAPSE • Limited to longitudinal contraction

Fractional area of change (FAC)	RV end-diastolic area / RV end-systolic area / RV focused view		• Fractional area of change (FAC)
			• FAC= End-diastolic area - End-systolic area / End-diastolic area
			• Normal value: >35%
			• Abnormal values:
			  • 35% - 26% mild dysfunction
			  • 25% - 17% moderate dysfunction
			  • <17% severe dysfunction
			• Established prognostic value
			• Assessment of longitudinal and radial contraction of the RV
			• Inter-observer variability: 10%
			• Meaningful change from baseline: 10%
				• Moderator band and trabeculations must be included in area tracing
				• Off-plane scanning will give unreliable values
				• Moderate inter-observer variability
				• Obviates the contribution of the outflow tract to contraction

Fig. 3. Echocardiographic assessment of RV systolic function. LA, left atrium; LV, left ventricle; PW, pulsed wave; RA, right atrium; RV, right ventricle.

Pathophysiology of Right Ventricular Failure in Pulmonary Arterial Hypertension

Although capable of handling acute changes in preload, the adult RV phenotype is unable to accommodate sudden increases in RV afterload. Following an acute increase in afterload, heightened contractility may overcome the increase in afterload, end-systolic volume, and diastolic volumes, thus maintaining adequate coupling of the RV to the pulmonary circuit. Sustained or excessive increases in afterload will lead to uncoupling with further RV dilation, increased wall stress, and decreased stroke volume. With chronic increase in PVR, RV hypertrophy is the main compensatory mechanism to reduce wall tension. If the increase in afterload is too severe, the RV will no longer be able to eject—generally the naïve RV is unable to generate pressures greater than 60 mm Hg. Chronic increases in RV afterload, either through an increase in PVR (as in the case of PAH) or from an increase in left atrial (LA) pressure (as in the case of mitral valve disease or chronic systolic or diastolic LV disease), stimulate adaptive remodeling. However, if the afterload continues to increase, remodeling may no longer be adaptive with abnormalities in metabolism, oxidative stress, capillary rarefaction, inflammation, and neurohormonal activation characterizing the decompensated state.[8]

The dilated, dysfunctional RV creates several challenges. First the increase in RV afterload may reduce stroke volume and LV preload. Initially the heart can compensate for this reduction in stroke volume through an increase in heart rate. At some point the reduction in stroke volume may become limiting. In a constrained space the dilated RV will lead to deviation of both the intraatrial and intraventricular septum (**Fig. 4**). Therefore, in addition to a reduction in forward flow to the LV (series effect), there is a superimposed parallel effect that can also impair LA and LV filling. Dilation also leads to an increase in RV wall stress, essentially an increase in RV afterload. Rising myocardial oxygen consumption (MVO_2) joins with coexisting adverse influence of wall tension on coronary perfusion to produce acute or chronic ischemia. This mismatch between coronary perfusion and MVO_2 can be compounded by systemic hypotension, further impairing RV contractility. This eventually becomes a vicious cycle, leading to progressive circulatory failure.

Causes for Decompensation

It is important to consider and treat conditions or complications that may lead to destabilization of the RV (**Table 1**). These conditions are associated by one or more of increased cardiac demand, reduced systemic blood pressure (with falling

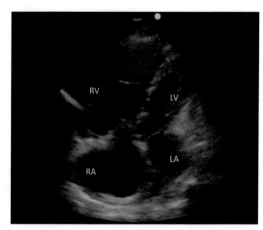

Fig. 4. Parasternal long axis view of a heart in a patient with advanced right ventricle failure. This image demonstrates the influence of a dilated right ventricle (RV) and right atrium (RA) on left ventricle (LV) and left atrial (LA) filling.

coronary perfusion), increased myocardial oxygen consumption (increased heart rate or RV wall tension), increased RV afterload, or reduced contractility. Atrial arrhythmias are often poorly tolerated owing to a loss of atrial contribution to ventricular filling as well as higher heart rates that reduce ventricular filling and increase MVO_2. Arrhythmias are also ominous signs, indicating advanced PAH and RV failure. As such they should prompt reconsideration of treatment options and referral for lung transplantation if eligible.

Special Circumstances

Pregnancy

Although outcomes have improved with PAH-targeted treatments and advances in high-risk pregnancy care, the risk of maternal mortality or need for urgent extracorporeal support and lung transplant remains high: 12% to 20%.[9] The risk primarily relates to the increase in plasma volume, cardiac demands from the fetal/placental circuit, and hormonal changes as nicely summarized in a review by Sanghavi and colleagues.[10] Plasma volume expansion begins early in the first trimester, increases steeply in the second trimester, and is around 50% greater than prepregnancy values by the third trimester.[10] This increase in plasma volume exceeds the 20% to 30% increase in red cell mass, resulting in a physiologic dilutional anemia with normal hemoglobin levels as low as 105 g/L (10.5 g/dL) in the second and third trimesters. The sharp increase of cardiac output (CO) in the first trimester is followed by a more gradual increase to peak values 30% to 50% greater than the prepregnancy baseline[11]; this is mediated by

Table 1
Causes and conditions that may contribute to right ventricular decompensation in a patient with pulmonary arterial hypertension

Stressor	Examples
Increase in RV preload	Pregnancy Acute volume resuscitation Acute kidney injury Noncompliance or ineffective diuretics
Increase in RV afterload	Mechanical ventilation (increase in alveolar pressure) Embolism in pulmonary artery (clot, fat) Noncompliance with PAH medications Progression of vasculopathy (PVR)
Worsening RV function	Myocardial ischemia Sepsis Progression of PAH Arrhythmia
Increase in cardiac demand	Sepsis Pregnancy Surgery

an early increase in stroke volume of up to 35% by the end of the second trimester, in conjunction with a progressive increase in heart rate of 10 to 20 bpm throughout the pregnancy.[12] Oxygen consumption increases by 20%.

Although LV and RV ejection fractions remain unchanged, there is an increase in LV and RV end-diastolic volumes. LV and RV mass increase by 40% to 50%.[13] Systemic vascular resistance (SVR) decreases by up to 40%, mediated by the vasodilatory effects of progesterone and estrogen, in addition to the development of the high-flow, low-resistance uteroplacental circulation.[10] The net effect of changes in cardiac output and SVR is a slight decrease in systemic blood pressure with a nadir at 22 to 24 weeks of gestation.[14]

Abrupt and physiologically demanding changes in the cardiovascular system occur during labor and delivery, affecting RV preload and afterload. Increased respiratory efforts and Valsalva maneuvers lead to intrathoracic pressure swings that cause fluctuations in central venous and pulmonary arterial pressures. In addition, blood volume increases via autotransfusion of 300 to 500 mL of blood into the systemic circulation after each uterine contraction. Intermittent inferior vena cava compression and release further contributes to volume shifts.[10]

Patients with PAH have markedly impaired compensatory mechanisms to adapt to the hemodynamic changes of pregnancy.[15,16] The inability to modulate PVR to accommodate an increase in pulmonary blood flow leads to higher pulmonary pressures and an increase in RV afterload and RV work. In addition to an increase in RV preload,

this leads to RV dilation and an increase in RV wall tension and MVO_2. In the face of a lower systemic pressure and reduced coronary perfusion (due to low systemic blood pressure and high RV wall tension), this may lead to RV ischemia and decreased RV contractility. Tricuspid regurgitation may also be aggravated, further increasing venous pressure and worsening peripheral oedema and hepatic congestion. Cardiac output is compromised from a combination of reduced pulmonary blood flow and ventricular/atrial interdependence, where the dilated, pressurized right atrial (RA) and RV lead to shift of the intraatrial and intraventricular septum, impairing LV filling. Systemic hypotension ensues, further impairing myocardial perfusion and exacerbating RV ischemia, thus setting up a perilous spiral into cardiogenic shock.[9,17] Impaired oxygen delivery is further compounded by increased peripheral oxygen consumption.

The risk of deterioration and death from RV failure is most pronounced at gestational weeks 20 to 24, during labor and delivery, and in the postpartum period[9,18]; these represent the time points during which large and rapid changes in hemodynamics and volume status occur. Venous thromboembolism is an added risk and may contribute to RV failure and circulatory collapse in the peripartum period. For the fetus, most deaths are secondary to antepartum maternal death, whereas outcomes for live-born infants are much more favorable.[9,18]

Although guidelines continue to issue a strong recommendation to avoid pregnancy in patients with PAH,[16,19] women with PAH do become pregnant and, occasionally, PAH manifests de novo during pregnancy. The quoted risks of mortality have been based primarily on retrospective cohort series that may not reflect contemporaneous treatments nor be reflective of women who are on active therapy. In the 13 studies included in a recent systematic review, only 48% of women received PAH-specific therapy.[9] Recent reports and our own experience favor a risk-based approach to guide couples in making an informed decision about their risks based on clinical, physiologic, and hemodynamic features while on full medical treatments (recognizing that this would necessarily exclude treatments that are potentially teratogenic).[20,21]

Surgery

Patients with PAH have worse outcomes after surgery.[22] The anesthetic approach (regional, general anesthesia) in addition to the type of surgery (thoracic, intraabdominal, peripheral) are important considerations in determining outcomes. The marginalized RV is unable to compensate for sudden hemodynamic changes or demands related to sepsis or rapid fluid shifts. Consequently, the physiologic state and RV reserve are important considerations in determining the optimum approach to surgical interventions, intraoperative management, and perioperative care.

A risk-based assessment that considers the patient's hemodynamics, RV function, RV reserve, and underlying comorbidities—particularly if the PAH is associated with systemic conditions such as autoimmune disease with inherent complexities related to other organ dysfunction or immune suppressants—is required.[23] Emergency surgeries are associated with the highest risk of perioperative morbidity and mortality.[22] A multidisciplinary team composed of the surgeon, anesthesiologist, nurse specialist, and intensivist needs to perform a risk assessment and map out a care plan. If possible, these patients should be transferred to a high-volume center with expertise in PAH care. The interdisciplinary team should first focus on the timing or need for surgery. Ideally, surgery should be deferred to allow for optimization of PAH and RV function. Once the decision is made to proceed with surgery, the anesthetic technique, mode of induction (for general anesthesia), interoperative management, and monitoring need to be considered.[24,25] Spinal or epidural approaches may not be successful in mitigating risks of a general anesthetic owing to adverse effects on systemic blood pressure.[24] Consideration includes method of induction, agents used for induction, maintenance of anesthesia, and mechanical ventilation.[26] The net effect of mechanical ventilation on RV function will depend on the balance between the effects of higher mean airway pressure (via use of higher levels of positive end-expiratory pressure (PEEP), tidal volumes, or pressure support) on venous return (typically decrease) and RV afterload (increase).

The surgical approach also needs to be considered. In general, laparoscopic surgery may not offer the same benefits in patients with PAH as in the general population. The Trendelenburg position and insufflation of the abdomen may lead to increases in venous return. Insufflation of the abdomen with CO_2 many also lead to systemic absorption that persists—even following surgery—increasing PVR.[27] Although dental, endoscopic, ophthalmologic, and peripheral surgeries may be at low risk for adverse events, specialized planning and care are essential during thoracic surgery—in particular single lung ventilation and lateral thoracotomy—as well as for upper abdominal surgical procedures, owing to the higher risk of postoperative atelectasis. Although use of traditional PAH therapies can be considered for other causes of PH in patients undergoing surgery, it needs to be understood that there is limited data in regard to safety or efficacy and that they are not being used for their approved indication. Indeed, some studies suggest that their use in these indications may be harmful and should caution us about using these treatments based on perceived benefit and biological plausibility.

Management of Right Ventricular Failure

Monitoring and setting goals

The monitoring of a patient with RV decompensation should consider the treatment goals outlined later. In our view, invasive monitoring of pulmonary arterial pressure, wedge pressure, or cardiac output is not routinely required. Central venous catheters will allow measurement of central venous saturations, reflective of effective oxygen delivery relative to utilization. It will also provide the opportunity to measure RA pressure—to guide efforts to optimize RV preload and net RV function—a reduction in RA pressures being the desired goal. It is difficult to assign a desired RA pressure—the optimum RA pressure being dependent on the degree of RV diastolic function, tricuspid regurgitation, and any influence of intrathoracic pressure. Heart rate is also an important parameter to consider. An increase in heart rate may be secondary to adrenergic agents to the detriment of the RV by increasing MVO_2 or reflect a deterioration in stroke volume.

Measurement of serum lactate and other favorable biochemical markers of organ perfusion/function are important goals. Quantification of tissue perfusion using the method adopted in the Andromeda trial (based on capillary refill time) is worthy of consideration, as it may provide a reliable and reproducible marker of tissue perfusion that can be followed at the bedside.[28]

Echocardiography has become an essential tool in the management of RV failure. Its growing availability in the intensive care unit allows for on-demand or even continuous hemodynamic monitoring, providing real-time guidance for clinicians.[4,7,29] As no evidence-based guidelines are available, the following sections provide examples of the utility of sonography in the management of these complex patients. They should be used in concert with the other parameters mentioned earlier to guide treatment decisions.

All parameters to assess RV systolic function have limitations. Tricuspid annular plane systolic excursion (TAPSE) may overestimate RV systolic function in cases of severe tricuspid regurgitation by conflating regurgitant volume and forward stroke volume. In the early postoperative period after cardiac surgery, TAPSE may be underestimated, as the pericardium limits movement of the RV free wall and tricuspid annulus.[6,30] The tissue Doppler–derived S′ velocity at the tricuspid annulus faces the same caveats as TAPSE.[6] Incorrect identification of myocardial borders and the exclusion of RV trabeculations can severely alter the reliability of the fractional area of change.

Pressure estimation based on velocity gradients across the tricuspid valve is reliable.[4,5,30] However, in severe, free-flowing tricuspid regurgitation, the pressure gradient across the valve is lost and the RV-RA pressures equalize rapidly in systolé, significantly underestimating RV systolic pressure (RVSP). When estimation of RVSP is unreliable, Doppler velocities across the RV outflow tract and pulmonary valve provide estimates of the mean and diastolic pulmonary artery pressures (**Fig. 5**). Novel technologies such as RV strain and RV 3D imaging provide a reliable automated assessment of RV systolic function; however, they depend on good endocardial border definition, which is at times impossible to obtain in the critical care setting. In addition, its intervendor variability has limited its widespread adoption.

Ventricular interdependence is identified by assessing the conformation of both ventricles in the parasternal short-axis view and by observing the displacement of the interventricular septum within the cardiac cycle. Changes in conformation due to RV dysfunction may lead to a D-shaped LV (**Fig. 6**). Septal displacement may be more difficult to observe and requires scrolling through the clip at a rate that allows seeing the point of maximum displacement. Maximum mid-diastolic displacement with normal mid-late systolic morphology indicates RV volume overload, whereas continuous flattening and greatest displacement at end-systole suggest pressure and volume overload. Establishing the degree of ventricular interdependence provides further understanding of the mechanism of RV failure (increased RV afterload vs normal RV afterload;(**Fig. 7**)) and may guide the clinician through adopted therapeutic interventions.

Simple findings can point toward chronic RV dysfunction. Although not specific, pericardial effusion is generally a marker of chronicity in RV failure and an ominous prognostic indicator. Similarly, RA dilatation and right ventricular free wall hypertrophy almost exclusively occur during chronic conditions. The degree of PH, or surrogates such as RVSP, also provide orientation. The right ventricle is not capable of overcoming acute increases in afterload; hence, high RVSP (>60 mm Hg) is an unlikely finding in the setting of isolated, acute RV failure, such as pulmonary embolism. For example, in acute pulmonary embolism, echocardiography shows an acutely dilated, thin-walled RV with poor systolic function and only mildly elevated pulmonary artery pressure (RVSP <60 mm Hg). Pulmonary acceleration time (see **Fig. 5**), using pulsed wave Doppler in the RV outflow tract, is a marker of increased pulmonary vascular resistance and is typically shortened; hence, the 60/60 rule for pulmonary embolism, RVSP less than 60 mmHg and pulmonary acceleration time less than 60 mSec. When pulmonary embolism becomes hemodynamically significant, enhanced ventricular interdependence becomes evident in the form of dynamic septal displacement and LV compression (see **Fig. 6**). Sonography can also identify clot in transit, further increasing the likelihood of pulmonary embolism driving RV failure.

Echocardiography can identify signs of left ventricular dysfunction or hemodynamically significant valvular abnormalities, which may drive RV dysfunction and failure. It is important to mention that ventricular interdependence affects both ventricles, and the LV is not exempted from functional abnormalities in isolated RV dysfunction or failure. Chronic underfilling of the LV in patients with chronic thromboembolic PH leads to LV atrophy.[31] These subclinical LV abnormalities become apparent after pulmonary endarterectomy, unmasking severe LV dysfunction.[31]

Echocardiography is a potentially valuable tool to follow dynamic changes from therapeutic intervention (**Fig. 8**).[32] The estimation of the pulmonary artery pressure by Doppler is simple and

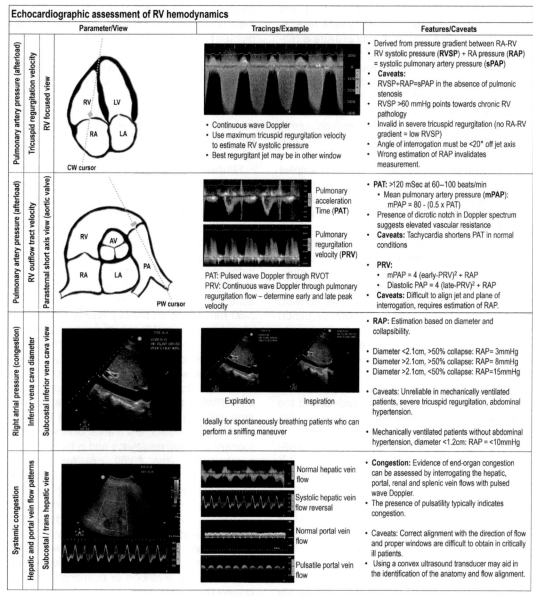

Fig. 5. Echocardiographic assessment of right ventricle hemodynamics. AV, aortic valve; CW, continuous wave; LA, left atrium; LV, left ventricle; RA, right atrium; RV, right ventricle; PA, pulmonary artery; PW, pulsed wave.

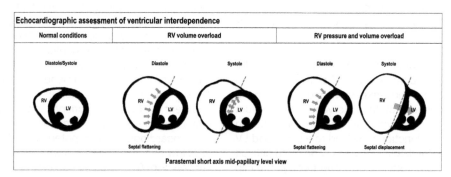

Fig. 6. Echocardiographic assessment of ventricular interdependence. LV, left ventricle; RV, right ventricle.

Ventricular interactions during right ventricular failure

Increased RV afterload	Normal RV afterload

Primary mechanism

↑Afterload

Normal afterload

↑RV workload

RV ischemia

Hemodynamic pathway

Systemic congestion

↑ Tricuspid regurgitation

↓ Venous return

↑Afterload

↓LV preload → ↓Cardiac output

↑ RV pressure overload

↓LV relaxation

↑ Interventricular Septal Shift

Systemic congestion

↑ RA pressure

↓ Venous return

↑ RV end-diastolic pressure

↓LV preload → ↓Cardiac output

↓ RV contractility

Ventricular interdependence

RV pressure and volume overload
Diastole — Systole

RV — LV
Septal flattening

RV — LV
Septal displacement

RV volume overload
Diastole — Systole

RV — LV
Septal flattening

RV — LV

Fig. 7. Ventricular interactions during right ventricular failure. LV, left ventricle; RA, right atrium; RV, right ventricle.

reliable.[4,5] However, the clinician needs to pay close attention to trends in pulmonary artery pressure in concert with other markers of RV function. A significant reduction in RVSP, considered in isolation, may not be a positive sign as it could signal worsening RV systolic function. The dynamic effects of diuresis and pulmonary vasodilators can be reliably tracked by monitoring the degree of RV dilatation, the magnitude and time of maximum septal displacement, and other markers of RV systolic function such as TAPSE and fractional area change (see **Fig. 8**).[7] When available, RV strain and 3D echo have shown potential to predict and detect subclinical RV dysfunction and failure, allowing for timely deployment of therapeutic interventions.[6,29]

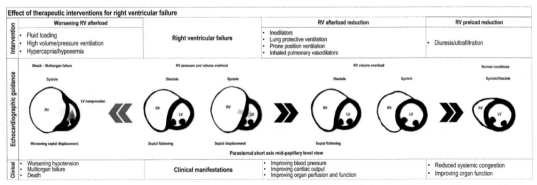

	Worsening RV afterload	Right ventricular failure	RV afterload reduction	RV preload reduction
Intervention	• Fluid loading • High volume/pressure ventilation • Hypercapnia/hypoxemia		• Inodilators • Lung protective ventilation • Prone position ventilation • Inhaled pulmonary vasodilators	• Diuresis/ultrafiltration

Effect of therapeutic interventions for right ventricular failure

Echocardiographic guidance:
Shock – Multiorgan failure (Systole) — RV pressure and volume overload (Diastole, Systole) — RV volume overload (Diastole, Systole) — Normal conditions (Systole/Diastole)

Worsening septal displacement — Septal flattening — Septal displacement — Septal flattening

Parasternal short axis mid-papillary level view

| **Clinical** | • Worsening hypotension
• Multiorgan failure
• Death | Clinical manifestations | • Improving blood pressure
• Improving cardiac output
• Improving organ perfusion and function | • Reduced systemic congestion
• Improving organ function |

Fig. 8. Effect of therapeutic interventions for right ventricular failure. LV, left ventricle; RV, right ventricle.

Echocardiography is also useful in diagnosing and guiding management of RV failure in patients with acute respiratory failure and mechanical ventilation. Mechanical ventilation can cause acute cor pulmonale and hemodynamic instability in patients with acute respiratory distress syndrome (ARDS) by increasing RV afterload and limiting preload (see **Fig. 7**).[7,29] Echocardiographic evidence of RV dilation and systemic congestion has been used as the diagnostic definition in research studies.[5,7,29,33] In practice, using the degree and timing of septal displacement may be a simpler and more reliable way to evidence the hemodynamic impact of the increased RV afterload.[7] In hypoxemic patients with borderline hemodynamics, the size of the RV and degree of septal displacement may help guide titration of ventilatory support by observing the effects of increasing or decreasing PEEP (see **Fig. 8**).[7]

Evidence of systemic congestion is generally determined using central venous pressure or echocardiographic surrogates of RA pressure,[29,34] in particular, inferior vena cava diameter and its respiratory variation. However, in critically ill patients on mechanical ventilation, estimation of systemic congestion using ultrasound of the inferior vena cava is imprecise.[7] Only extreme values of size and respiratory variation are helpful in the right patient and in the right context. Recently, indices of venous congestion, looking into pattern changes in pulsed wave Doppler in hepatic, portal, and renal veins, have been described.[35] These indices are relatively easy to obtain, provide tangible evidence of end-organ congestion, and can be helpful tracking the effectiveness of treatment, particularly fluid removal (see **Fig. 8**).

Principles of Managing the Failing Right Ventricle

A strategy to treat the failing RV must consider optimizing RV preload (to reduce RV wall tension and adverse influence of a dilated RV on LV filling), reducing RV afterload, and improving contractility while maintaining adequate systemic blood pressure (**Table 2**, see **Fig. 8**).[23,36,37]

Medical Management

Support systemic blood pressure

A successful strategy must preserve coronary perfusion by supporting systemic blood pressure; this is particularly important, as many therapies aimed at improving RV afterload and contractility may reduce systemic blood pressure. Although no systematic studies have been performed, noradrenaline and/or vasopressin are generally advocated. Vasopressin is particularly attractive, as it is not associated with tachycardia at therapeutic doses.[26]

Table 2
Goals and therapies to manage right ventricular decompensation in a patient with pulmonary arterial hypertension

Variable	Benefit	Intervention
Preserve systemic blood pressure	Preserve coronary perfusion	Alpha agonists (norepinephrine, phenylephrine) Vasopressin
Reduce ventricular volume	Reduce wall tension (improve coronary perfusion, reduce MVO2) Reduce adverse influence of RV on LV filling	Diuretics Ultrafiltration
Reduce RV afterload	Improve RV stroke volume	Pulmonary vasodilators (nitric oxide, prostanoids, PDE3 inhibitors) Reduce atelectasis Maintain oxygenation Avoid hypercapnia
Improve RV contractility	Improve RV stroke volume	PDE3 inhibitors PDE5 inhibitors? Beta agonists (adrenaline, dobutamine) Calcium sensitizers

Right Ventricular Preload

Optimization of RV preload is critical. In acute RV infarction, administration of fluids may be required to increase venous return and maintain pulmonary perfusion. However, overdistention of an ischemic RV may worsen cardiac function. Indeed, in patients with chronic PH, diuresis may be one of the most important treatment strategies in patients with decompensated and dilated RV. Reduced RV volume should lower RV wall tension, thereby reducing MVO_2 and improving coronary blood flow to the RV. In addition, diuresis may reduce tricuspid regurgitation and limit ventricular interdependence.[38] The resulting improvement in LV filling may lead to improved oxygen delivery and renal perfusion, even in patients with cardiorenal syndrome.

Reduce right ventricular afterload

PVR is conventionally considered to quantify the degree of RV afterload. However, pulmonary vascular compliance and impedance as well as LA pressure are other forces that constitute RV afterload.[39] Any event that reduces the cross-sectional area of the pulmonary vasculature (pulmonary embolism), provokes vasoconstriction (eg, hypoxemia, hypercapnia), or increases LA pressure will increase RV afterload. RV afterload may also be increased by atelectasis (via hypoxic pulmonary vasoconstriction). Therefore, mechanically ventilated patients with RV failure may benefit from judicious titration of PEEP. PEEP must be applied with caution, as alveolar overdistention may also load the RV by compressing or stretching the pulmonary capillaries.[40]

Pulmonary vasodilators may be beneficial in acute RV failure. The ideal pulmonary vasodilator has a rapid onset of action, short half-life, and selectivity for the pulmonary vasculature. In that regard the use of inhaled pulmonary vasodilators is attractive. Nitric oxide, prostanoids, and phosphodiesterase 5 (PDE_5) inhibitors have been reported to improve RV afterload.[41] The use of systemic agents is limited by a longer half-life and off-target effects on the systemic vasculature as well as potentially increased intrapulmonary shunt by nonselective pulmonary vasodilation.

We consider using inhaled nitric oxide or PGI2 in conjunction with an oral or parenteral PDE_5 inhibitor. For naïve patients with World Health Organization group I PH (PAH), parenteral prostanoids should be considered, as they may salvage patients who present de novo with advanced PAH and RV failure.

Improve contractility

The agents to increase RV contractility are the same as those used to treat LV failure. Their effectiveness may be limited by 2 constraints. First, the RV is less muscular than the LV. Second, the ischemic, overloaded RV may have limited contractile reserve. Although PDE_3 inhibitors (eg, milrinone) and calcium channel sensitizers (eg, levosimendan) have been shown to improve RV function acutely, there are no large outcome-based studies to support one strategy over another.[42] The use of PDE_3 inhibitors may also be limited by systemic vasodilation and hypotension. Epinephrine may also be used; however, it can lead to an undesired tachycardia.

Heart rate

Tachycardia increases myocardial oxygen consumption and may reduce stroke volume by reducing diastolic filling time. The effects of tachycardia are compounded in the setting of RV overload when RV systolic duration increases relative to the LV, further impairing diastolic LV filling. Changes in heart rate should be monitored as a marker of progressive worsening or as a cautionary sign of unwanted effects of treatment (eg, beta-adrenergic agents).

Surgical/Device Management

It is important to recognize failure of medical treatments before multisystem organ dysfunction occurs.[43] Mechanical circulatory support should be considered if medical treatments are not improving tissue perfusion or not tolerated. Before embarking on these options, the team needs to consider exit strategies for the patient. For a naïve patient with PAH, this may include migration from extracorporeal life support (ECLS) to medical therapies such as parenteral prostanoids. More commonly, however, migration from ECLS to lung or heart-lung transplant is the only durable therapeutic option.[44] In our program we cannulate eligible patients as a bridge-to-transplant or, less commonly when they have not been formally evaluated, bridge-to-transplant decision. For patients who are not candidates for ECLS or transplant, discussions around goals of care and end-of-life treatments are warranted.

Several configurations for ECLS are possible.[43,45] In general, venoarterial support is required. **Table 3** summarizes the considerations for different forms of support listing the advantages and disadvantages of each approach. The ideal configuration is one that provides support of tissue oxygen delivery, offloads the failing RV, is durable, and allows the patient to participate in treatment decisions and physiotherapy. An

Table 3
Extracorporeal configurations to support the failing right ventricle. Advantages and limitations of each configuration are provided

Configuration	Advantages	Limitations
Venovenous		
Inflow and outflow using 2 separate venous cannulae	Relatively easy to establish Improves oxygenation Improves hypercapnia Reduced risk of arterial embolic events	Does not directly support RV function
Single cannulae—dual lumen (RA to PA) cannulae Dual lumen cannulae + atrial septostomy	Venous access May offload the right heart Reduced risk of arterial embolic events	May not fully offload the RV Limitations in flow rates Durability + creation of atrial septostomy
Veno-arterial		
Systemic venous inflow and retrograde systemic arterial return	Percutaneous Offloads RV	May not fully correct severe oxygenation failure Risk of systemic embolization Limb ischemia Desaturation across aortic arch—Harlequin syndrome
PA to LA configuration (eg, Novalung)	Pumpless configuration Offloads RV Allows for retraining of LV and adaptation/remodeling of RV Durable Allows ambulation without pump	Requires sternotomy Difficult to wean and migrate off configuration Risk of systemic embolization
Central venoarterial configuration	Not dependent on retrograde flow—offloads RV and LV	Requires operation or sternotomy Risk of systemic embolization Less durable

Abbreviations: LA, left atrium; LV, left ventricle; PA, Pulmonary artery.

important consideration is a strategy that allows for retraining of the chronically underfilled LV to potentially avoid the development of pulmonary edema after lung transplant—a well-described but mechanistically uncertain syndrome, presumed related to failure of the LV to adapt to an increase in preload.[46,47] In some centers, ECLS is continued in the perioperative period to mitigate the development of LV dysfunction and allow time for the RV to adapt to its new circuit.[48] Centers have reported lower rates of primary graft dysfunction using this approach. A systematic evaluation of this strategy has not been performed.

SUMMARY

RV failure is a recognized and formidable complication in patients with PAH. An approach based on physiologic principles is key to salvaging these patients. Early recognition and correction of reversible causes is an important consideration.

A multidisciplinary team including intensivists, anesthesiologist, surgeons, and allied health professionals, drawing on expertise from specialized centers, is important to ensure that all avenues are explored. Goals for management should include markers of tissue perfusion. Echocardiography can complement hemodynamic assessments and assist in treatment decisions. Treatment strategies should consider methods to optimize RV preload, contractility, and afterload. When appropriate, referral for mechanical circulatory support or lung transplantation should be considered when RV failure is refractory to medical therapies.

DISCLOSURE

Dr J. Granton has received support for research and education programs through unrestricted grants to his institution from Bayer and Janssen Pharmaceuticals.

CLINICS CARE POINTS

- Right ventricular failure is a recognized complication of acute and chronic pulmonary hypertension.
- Pregnancy and surgery impose unique challenges in patients with pulmonary hypertension.
- Management of right ventricular failure in pulmonary hypertension requires an interprofessional approach, and treatment based on robust physiological principles.
- Early recognition of the failure of medical therapies and implementation of mechanical circulatory support (if appropriate) may avoid irreversible shock and organ failure.

REFERENCES

1. Simonneau G, Montani D, Celermajer DS, et al. Haemodynamic definitions and updated clinical classification of pulmonary hypertension. Eur Respir J 2019;53(1). https://doi.org/10.1183/13993003.01913-2018.
2. Pinsky MR. The right ventricle: interaction with the pulmonary circulation. Crit Care 2016;20(1):266.
3. Vonk Noordegraaf A, Westerhof BE, Westerhof N. The relationship between the right ventricle and its load in pulmonary hypertension. J Am Coll Cardiol 2017;69(2):236–43.
4. Porter TR, Shillcutt SK, Adams MS, et al. Guidelines for the use of echocardiography as a monitor for therapeutic intervention in adults: a report from the American society of echocardiography. J Am Soc Echocardiogr 2015;28(1):40–56.
5. Harjola VP, Mebazaa A, Čelutkienė J, et al. Contemporary management of acute right ventricular failure: a statement from the heart failure association and the working group on pulmonary circulation and right ventricular function of the european society of cardiology. Eur J Heart Fail 2016;18(3):226–41.
6. Lang RM, Badano LP, Mor-Avi V, et al. Recommendations for cardiac chamber quantification by echocardiography in adults: an update from the American society of echocardiography and the European association of cardiovascular imaging. J Am Soc Echocardiogr 2015;28(1):1–39. e14.
7. Krishnan S, Schmidt GA. Acute right ventricular dysfunction: real-time management with echocardiography. Chest 2015;147(3):835–46.
8. Gomez-Arroyo J, Mizuno S, Szczepanek K, et al. Metabolic gene remodeling and mitochondrial dysfunction in failing right ventricular hypertrophy secondary to pulmonary arterial hypertension. Circ Heart Fail 2013;6(1):136–44.
9. Low TT, Guron N, Ducas R, et al. Pulmonary arterial hypertension in pregnancy-a systematic review of outcomes in the modern era. Pulm Circ 2021;11(2). 20458940211013671.
10. Sanghavi M, Rutherford JD. Cardiovascular physiology of pregnancy. Circulation 2014;130(12):1003–8.
11. Mahendru AA, Foo FL, McEniery CM, et al. Change in maternal cardiac output from preconception to mid-pregnancy is associated with birth weight in healthy pregnancies. Ultrasound Obstet Gynecol 2017;49(1):78–84.
12. Vartun A, Flo K, Wilsgaard T, et al. Maternal functional hemodynamics in the second half of pregnancy: a longitudinal study. PLoS One 2015;10(8): e0135300.
13. Ducas RA, Elliott JE, Melnyk SF, et al. Cardiovascular magnetic resonance in pregnancy: insights from the cardiac hemodynamic imaging and remodeling in pregnancy (CHIRP) study. J Cardiovasc Magn Reson 2014;16:1.
14. Grindheim G, Estensen ME, Langesaeter E, et al. Changes in blood pressure during healthy pregnancy: a longitudinal cohort study. J Hypertens 2012;30(2):342–50.
15. Bassily-Marcus AM, Yuan C, Oropello J, et al. Pulmonary hypertension in pregnancy: critical care management. Pulm Med 2012;2012:709407.
16. Hemnes AR, Kiely DG, Cockrill BA, et al. Statement on pregnancy in pulmonary hypertension from the pulmonary vascular research institute. Pulm Circ 2015;5(3):435–65.
17. Goland S, Tsai F, Habib M, et al. Favorable outcome of pregnancy with an elective use of epoprostenol and sildenafil in women with severe pulmonary hypertension. Cardiology 2010;115(3):205–8.
18. Jais X, Olsson KM, Barbera JA, et al. Pregnancy outcomes in pulmonary arterial hypertension in the modern management era. Eur Respir J 2012;40(4): 881–5.
19. Galie N, Humbert M, Vachiery JL, et al. 2015 ESC/ERS Guidelines for the diagnosis and treatment of pulmonary hypertension: the joint task force for the diagnosis and treatment of pulmonary hypertension of the european society of cardiology (ESC) and the european respiratory society (ers): endorsed by: association for european paediatric and congenital cardiology (AEPC), international society for heart and lung transplantation (ISHLT). Eur Heart J 2016; 37(1):67–119.

20. Kamp JC, von Kaisenberg C, Greve S, et al. Pregnancy in pulmonary arterial hypertension: midterm outcomes of mothers and offspring. J Heart Lung Transpl 2021;40(3):229–33.
21. Kiely DG, Condliffe R, Webster V, et al. Improved survival in pregnancy and pulmonary hypertension using a multiprofessional approach. BJOG 2010; 117(5):565–74.
22. Meyer S, McLaughlin VV, Seyfarth HJ, et al. Outcomes of noncardiac, nonobstetric surgery in patients with PAH: an international prospective survey. Eur Respir J 2013;41(6):1302–7.
23. Price LC, Martinez G, Brame A, et al. Perioperative management of patients with pulmonary hypertension undergoing non-cardiothoracic, non-obstetric surgery: a systematic review and expert consensus statement. Br J Anaesth 2021;126(4):774–90.
24. Caddigan S, Granlund B. Anesthesia for patients with pulmonary hypertension or right heart failure, . StatPearls (Internet). Treasure Island (FL): StatPearls Publishing; 2021. https://www.ncbi.nlm.nih.gov/books/NBK572071/. [Accessed July 2021].
25. Seyfarth HJ, Gille J, Sablotzki A, et al. Perioperative management of patients with severe pulmonary hypertension in major orthopedic surgery: experience-based recommendations. GMS Interdiscip Plast Reconstr Surg DGPW 2015;4:Doc03.
26. Reimer CGGJ. Pharmacology of the pulmonary circulation. In: Slinger P, editor. Principles and practice of anesthesia for thoracic surgery. 2nd edition. Springer; 2019.
27. Atkinson TM, Giraud GD, Togioka BM, et al. Cardiovascular and ventilatory consequences of laparoscopic surgery. Circulation 2017;135(7):700–10.
28. Zampieri FG, Damiani LP, Bakker J, et al. Effects of a resuscitation strategy targeting peripheral perfusion status versus serum lactate levels among patients with septic shock. a bayesian reanalysis of the ANDROMEDA-SHOCK Trial. Am J Respir Crit Care Med 2020;201(4):423–9.
29. Vieillard-Baron A, Naeije R, Haddad F, et al. Diagnostic workup, etiologies and management of acute right ventricle failure : a state-of-the-art paper. Intensive Care Med 2018;44(6):774–90.
30. Konstam MA, Kiernan MS, Bernstein D, et al. Evaluation and management of right-sided heart failure: a scientific statement from the american heart association. Circulation 2018;137(20):e578–622. Epub 2018 Apr 12.
31. Verbelen T, Van De Bruaene A, Cools B, et al. Postoperative left ventricular function in different types of pulmonary hypertension: a comparative study. Interactive CardioVascular Thorac Surg 2018;26(5):813–9.
32. Arrigo M, Huber LC, Winnik S, et al. Right ventricular failure: pathophysiology, diagnosis and treatment. Card Fail Rev 2019;5(3):140–6.
33. Repessé X, Charron C, Vieillard-Baron A. Acute respiratory distress syndrome: the heart side of the moon. Curr Opin Crit Care 2016;22(1):38–44.
34. Vieillard-Baron A, Prigent A, Repessé X, et al. Right ventricular failure in septic shock: characterization, incidence and impact on fluid responsiveness. Crit Care 2020;24(1):630.
35. Beaubien-Souligny W, Rola P, Haycock K, et al. Quantifying systemic congestion with Point-Of-Care ultrasound: development of the venous excess ultrasound grading system. Ultrasound J 2020;12(1):16.
36. Hoeper MM, Granton J. Intensive care unit management of patients with severe pulmonary hypertension and right heart failure. Am J Respir Crit Care Med 2011;184(10):1114–24.
37. Kaestner M, Schranz D, Warnecke G, et al. Pulmonary hypertension in the intensive care unit. expert consensus statement on the diagnosis and treatment of paediatric pulmonary hypertension. the european paediatric pulmonary vascular disease network, endorsed by ISHLT and DGPK. Heart 2016;102(Suppl 2):ii57–66.
38. Kasner M, Westermann D, Steendijk P, et al. Left ventricular dysfunction induced by nonsevere idiopathic pulmonary arterial hypertension: a pressure-volume relationship study. Am J Respir Crit Care Med 2012;186(2):181–9.
39. Tedford RJ. Determinants of right ventricular afterload (2013 Grover Conference series). Pulm Circ 2014;4(2):211–9.
40. Guerin C, Matthay MA. Acute cor pulmonale and the acute respiratory distress syndrome. Intensive Care Med 2016. https://doi.org/10.1007/s00134-015-4197-z.
41. McGinn K, Reichert M. A comparison of inhaled nitric oxide versus inhaled epoprostenol for acute pulmonary hypertension following cardiac surgery. comparative study. Ann Pharmacother 2016;50(1):22–6.
42. Papp Z, Agostoni P, Alvarez J, et al. Levosimendan efficacy and safety: 20 years of SIMDAX in clinical use. J Cardiovasc Pharmacol 2020;76(1):4–22.
43. Granton J, Mercier O, de Perrot M. Management of severe pulmonary arterial hypertension. Semin Respir Crit Care Med 2013;34(5):700–13.
44. Hoeper MM, Benza RL, Corris P, et al. Intensive care, right ventricular support and lung transplantation in patients with pulmonary hypertension. Eur Respir J 2019;53(1). https://doi.org/10.1183/13993003.01906-2018.

45. Machuca TN, de Perrot M. Mechanical support for the failing right ventricle in patients with precapillary pulmonary hypertension. Rev Circ 2015;132(6): 526–36.

46. Gupta S, Torres F, Bollineni S, et al. Left ventricular dysfunction after lung transplantation for pulmonary arterial hypertension. Transpl Proc 2015;47(9): 2732–6.

47. Avriel A, Klement AH, Johnson SR, et al. Impact of left ventricular diastolic dysfunction on lung transplantation outcome in patients with pulmonary arterial hypertension. Am J Transpl 2017;17(10): 2705–11.

48. Toyoda Y, Bhama JK, Shigemura N, et al. Efficacy of extracorporeal membrane oxygenation as a bridge to lung transplantation. J Thorac Cardiovasc Surg 2013;145(4):1065–70. discussion 1070-1.

Caring for the Critically Ill Patient with COVID-19

Matthew K. Hensley, MD, MPH[a],*, Hallie C. Prescott, MD, MSc[b,c]

KEYWORDS

- Critical care • COVID-19 • SARS-CoV-2 • Pandemic • Healthcare disparities • Resource allocation

KEY POINTS

- One in 4 patients hospitalized with COVID-19 become critically ill, with up to 80% of those requiring mechanical ventilation.
- In-hospital mortality varies but with appropriate resources and capacity, it can be as low as 12% in some cohorts.
- Long-term outcomes after COVID-19 remain poor, with 50% to 70% reporting persistent symptoms such as shortness of breath or fatigue.
- Acute respiratory failure from COVID-19 represents a similar spectrum of disease to other historical cohorts of viral acute respiratory distress syndrome (ARDS).
- Corticosteroids remain the mainstay of treatment of COVID-19, though optimal dosing and duration remain unknown.

INTRODUCTION

Since its identification in late 2019, severe acute respiratory syndrome coronavirus 2 (SARS-CoV-2) leading to COVID-19 illness has become a global pandemic, with nearly 182,101,209 cases and 3,950,876 deaths worldwide as of July 2, 2021.[1] Best practices for critical care, including intensive care unit (ICU) bed capacity and staffing,[2,3] respiratory support,[4] and therapeutics,[5] evolved rapidly during the course of the pandemic as our understanding of transmission,[6] virus variants,[7] and outcomes matured. SARS-CoV-2 fueled debates about the most basic aspects of supportive critical care, including the methods and timing of endotracheal intubation,[8] personal protective equipment, timing of prone positioning,[9,10] and oxygen saturation goals.[11] Furthermore, the global spread of COVID-19 has highlighted disparities in care not only between ethnic and racial minorities[12] but also between countries.[13] Special populations, including

patients with hematologic malignancy, have demonstrated unique host factors contributing to higher mortality[14] and delayed viral clearance,[15] leading to persistent infectivity and need for further study on isolation precautions. Considering together, critical illness related to COVID-19 has proven to be the biggest challenge of our generation, causing us to reimagine research design and methods, develop innovative ways to expand critical care capacity, and adapt our communication strategies with patients, families, and providers (**Fig. 1**).

EPIDEMIOLOGY, OUTCOMES, RESOURCE UTILIZATION, AND DISPARITIES
Asia

Early in the pandemic, case series and cohort studies from China described the early epidemiology and outcomes of COVID-19.[16–20] Of 1099 patients hospitalized in China with COVID-19 during December 2019 and January 2020, 55 (5.0%)

[a] Department of Internal Medicine, Division of Pulmonary and Critical Care, University of Pittsburgh Medical Center, 5200 Centre Avenue, Suite 610, Pittsburgh, PA 15232, USA; [b] Department of Internal Medicine, University of Michigan, NCRC Building 16, Room 341E / 2800 Plymouth Road, Ann Arbor, MI 48109-2800, USA; [c] VA Center for Clinical Management Research, HSR&D Center of Innovation, Ann Arbor, MI, USA
* Corresponding author.
E-mail address: hensleymk2@upmc.edu
Twitter: @HalliePrescott (H.C.P.)

Clin Chest Med 43 (2022) 441–456
https://doi.org/10.1016/j.ccm.2022.04.006
0272-5231/22/© 2022 Elsevier Inc. All rights reserved.

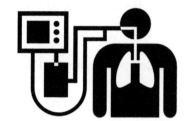

COVID-19 Critical Illness Outcomes

Critical Care Resource Allocation   Healthcare Disparities

ARDS and Ventilator Management   Sedation practices

Prone positioning   Timing of Intubation

Therapeutics in COVID-19

Fig. 1. Comprehensive care of the critically ill patient with COVID-19.

were admitted to the ICU, 25 (2.3%) underwent mechanical ventilation, and 2 (1.4%) died.[19] In a similar cohort of 191 adults hospitalized with COVID-19 in China, 53 (28%) required ICU admission, of whom 42 (78%) ultimately died of multiorgan failure.[16] Among 32 patients treated with mechanical ventilation, 10 (31%) developed ventilator-associated pneumonia and 31 (97%) died after a median 8 days of ICU care (interquartile ratio (IQR) 4.0–12.0 days)[16] (**Table 1**). Half of the decedents (27/54) experienced a secondary infection.[16] Although these studies provided important early data on COVID-19 outcomes, caution was needed when interpreting such early reports because 613 patients (76.2% of the entire cohort) were still hospitalized at the time of publication and excluded from the original analysis.[16] Therefore, true rates of mortality, mechanical ventilation, and other outcomes were uncertain.

Europe

Outside Asia, Italy was among the first countries to experience a surge of COVID-19. Among 17,713 laboratory-confirmed cases in Italy through March 18, 2020, 1593 (9%) were admitted to tier 3 ICUs (highest level of care) and included in an early case series.[21] This critically ill cohort was a majority male (82%), median age of 63 years (IQR 56–70), and most had at least one comorbidity (N = 709, 68%).[21] Among 1300 with available treatment data, 1150 (88%) received mechanical ventilation and 137 (11%) received noninvasive ventilation (NIV); median positive end expiratory pressure (PEEP) was 14 cm H_2O (IQR 12–16), and median P/F ratio was 160 (IQR 114–220).[21] In a subgroup of the first 1715 patients, as of May 30 2020,[22] 865 (50.4%) were discharged

from the ICU, 836 (48.7%) died, and 14 (0.8%) were still in the ICU.[22] Risk factors for mortality included older age (HR 1.75 [95%CI: 1.60–1.92]) and male gender (HR 1.57 [95%CI: 1.31–1.88]), whereas higher P/F ratio on ICU admission (HR 0.8 per 100 units [95%CI: 0.74–0.87]) was protective.[22]

North America

By March 2020, COVID-19 was spreading rapidly within the United States. Small, early case series from Seattle, Washington highlighted the severity of illness,[23,24] with nearly 70% of patients receiving mechanical ventilation, and in-hospital mortality ranging from 50% to 67%.[23,24] Half of all patients received vasopressors, and median durations of ICU and mechanical ventilation were 14 and 10 days, respectively.[23] By late March 2020, New York city became the epicenter of COVID-19 in the United States, yielding larger cohort studies.[25–27] Of 1150 adults hospitalized with COVID-19 in New York city through April 1, 2020, 257 (22%) were critically ill.[27] Of these 257, 203 (79%) received mechanical ventilation for a median of 18 days (IQR 9–28), 170 (66%) received vasopressors, and 79 (31%) received renal replacement therapy.[27] In a larger cohort of 2741 patients hospitalized from March through April 2020 in New York city, 647 (23.6%) received mechanical ventilation but was lacking in data in terms of duration, vasopressor use, or renal replacement therapy.[26] In a subsequent cohort of 5700 adults hospitalized during March and April 2020, 373 (14.2%), who had either died or were discharged from the hospital, required intensive care.[25] Of the 373 critically ill patients, 320 (85.8%) received mechanical ventilation, and 81

Table 1
Epidemiologic studies of critically ill patients with COVID-19

Author(s)	Population	Mechanical Ventilation (N, %)	Duration of Mechanical Ventilation (Median, IQR)	Prone Positioning (N, %)	PEEP (Median, IQR)	P/F Ratio (Median, IQR)	Compliance (Median, IQR)	Outcomes
Guan et al,[19] 2020	1099 hospitalized patients with COVID-19 across China	25 (2.3%)	-	-	-	-	-	In-hospital mortality, 2 (1.4%)
Zhou et al,[16] 2020	191 patients hospitalized with COVID-19 who were either discharged or died by Jan 31, 2020	32 (16.8%)	-	-	-	-	-	31/32 (97%) of mechanically ventilated patients died
Grasselli et al,[21] 2020	1591 critically ill patients with COVID-19 in Italy	1150 (88%)	-	240 (27%)	14 (12–16)	160 (114–220)	-	405 (26%) died, 920 (58%) still admitted
Richardson et al,[25] 2020	373 critically ill patients with COVID-19 in United States	320 (85.8%)	-	-	-	-	-	282/320 (88.1%) mortality for mechanically ventilated patients
Petrilli et al,[26] 2020	990 critically ill patients with COVID-19 in United States	647 (65.4%)	-	-	-	-	-	57% mortality among all ICU or ventilated patients
Cummings et al,[27] 2020	257 critically ill patients with COVID-19 in United States	203 (79%)	18 d (9–28)	35 (17%)	15 (12–18)	129 (80–203)	27 (22–36)	41% mortality for mechanically ventilated patients
Ziehr et al,[62] 2020	66 mechanically ventilated patients with COVID-19	66 (100%)	16 d (10–21)	31 (47%)	10 (8–12)	182 (135–245)	35 (30–43)	16.7% mortality, 62% successfully extubated, 21% underwent tracheostomy

(21.7%) were received renal replacement therapy. As of April 4, 2020, 1151 (20.2%) patients requiring mechanical ventilation, 38 (3.3%) were discharged alive, 282 (24.5%) died while admitted, and 831 (72.2%) remained in the hospital.[25] Pulmonary dysfunction was a key driver of mortality, accounting for 56.1% of COVID-related hospital deaths compared with just 21.6% of deaths in recent cohorts of decedents with acute hypoxemia respiratory failure.[28]

Hospital Mortality

Estimates of hospital mortality have varied markedly across studies and over time, likely reflecting differences in completeness of COVID case ascertainment, patient case-mix, hospital resource availability, prevalence of different SARS-CoV-2 strains, COVID treatments, and overall volume of patients. In a study of 8516 patients admitted to 88 US Veterans Affairs hospitals, Bravata and colleagues showed that in-hospital mortality varied by month (22.9% in March 2020, 25% in April, 15.5% in May, 13.6% in June, 12.5% in July, and 12.8% in August) and was strongly associated ICU demand.[29] In particular, when COVID-19 ICU demand was more than 75% to 100% of baseline ICU demand, risk of mortality increased markedly [HR 1.94 (95%CI: 1.46–2.59)].[29] A meta-analysis across the United States, Europe, and Asia included 10,150 patients admitted to the ICU with COVID-19, assessing outcomes for those who were discharged from the ICU or died.[30] Reported mortality across studies varied widely from 0% to 84%. In studies with complete ICU disposition data (ie, death or discharge), combined ICU mortality was 41.6% (95% CI: 34.0%–49.7%).[30] The meta-analysis did not account for patients still admitted to the ICU; therefore, interpretation and generalizability are limited. Other studies have similarly shown that mortality rates have waxed and waned in conjunction with hospital demand.

Resource Allocation and Availability

Critical care requires trained clinicians, supplies, and space. Early in the pandemic, there was widespread fear that a shortage of ventilators[31–33] would contribute to excess mortality. With roughly 62,000 working ventilators in the United States before the pandemic,[34] the feasibility of ventilator sharing was considered. In one New York hospital, 3 pairs of critically ill patients (N = 6) were placed on one mechanical ventilator, using volume control mode.[32] Deep sedation and continuous paralysis were used to avoid ventilator dyssynchrony. Although the authors concluded that ventilator sharing may be safe and feasible for short periods of time, multiple professional societies published a consensus statement advising against ventilator sharing due to the risk for causing more harm than good.[35] Ultimately, industry partners (eg, Ford, General Motors, Dyson) helped to manufacture ventilator equipment[34] and expand the US supply of ventilators to nearly 120,000 by August 2020, alleviating concerns of ventilator shortage.[34]

Despite the early focus on ventilator availability, it quickly became evident that having trained clinicians, adequate space, and basic supplies were more important than ventilators. In particular, the availability of nurses,[36] respiratory therapists,[37] acute care providers,[38] and well-ventilated space[29] proved to be the most important scare resources. Many hospitals had to rapidly expand ICU bed capacity with critical care trained and noncritical care trained staff.[3] Using a tiered system, the most experienced critical care provider can safely supervise midlevel or noncritically-care trained providers to care for up to 24 patients at some institutions with appropriate bed capacity and resources.[3] Alternatively, telemedicine services where an off-site hospital provides critical care expertise serves as another method for expanding capacity in resource-constrained areas.[39] To expand physical ICU space, some hospital repurposed floor rooms to serve as ICU beds with negative pressure capabilities, whereas other countries such as China rapidly built new ICUs.[40] Personal protective equipment was sanitized and reused to maintain supply. Incentive programs were developed to hire traveling nurses in areas of shortage, or to have a back-up supply of staff in the event of health-care workers contracting COVID-19. Nevertheless, shortages of key resources required organizations to develop triage committees, if critical care demand would far exceed available resources.[41]

Long-Term Outcomes

Data on longer-term outcomes from COVID-19 continue to accrue but existing evidence indicates not only high in-hospital mortality but also a high burden of subsequent morbidity among hospital survivors.[42,43] Among 1648 patients hospitalized with COVID-19 at 38 Michigan hospitals, 398 (24.2%) died in-hospital, and an additional 84 (5.1% of the cohort, 6.7% of hospital survivors) died within 60 days of discharge. Total mortality by 60 days postdischarge was 29.2% (482/1648) but was much higher among ICU-treated patients (257/405, 63.5%).[42] Among 488 who completed 60-day postdischarge telephone follow-up, 159 (32.6%) reported at least one new or worsened cardiopulmonary symptom, 188 (39%) were not yet back to their normal activities, 78 (40% of previously employed) were not yet back to work, 124 (25%) were at least moderately emotionally impacted, and 124 (25%) were at least moderately financially impacted as a result of COVID.[42]

Subsequent studies have examined outcomes at 4 to 6 months posthospitalization and similarly shown persistent morbidity in a large subset of patients. Among 478 adult survivors of COVID-19 in France who completed 4-month telephone follow-up after being hospitalized between March 1, 2020 and May 20, 2020, 244 (51%) reported at least 1 new symptom including fatigue (31%), cognitive symptoms (21%), and new onset dyspnea (16%).[43] Among 2469 patients hospitalized with COVID-19 in China and discharged between Jan 7, 2020 and May 20, 2020, 1733 were followed to 6 months.[44] Among patients seen at 6-month follow-up, 63% (1038 of 1655) endorsed fatigue or muscle weakness, 26% (437 of 1655) endorsed sleeping difficulties, and 23% (367 of 1617) endorsed anxiety or depression.[44] Among 116 who were critically ill at the time of hospitalization, 29% (34 of 116) had a 6-minute walk test result below the lower limit of normal, 56% (48 of 86) had reduced diffusion on pulmonary function testing, and 45% (41 of 92) had persistent ground glass opacities seen on chest CT imaging.[44] Furthermore, a recent systematic review of 9751 COVID-19 survivors found that 72.5% (IQR 55%–80%) reported at least 1 persistent symptom, including dyspnea in 36% (IQR 27.6%–50.0%), fatigue in 40% (IQR 31%–57%), and sleep difficulties in 29.4% (IQR 24.4%–33.0%), although there was significant heterogeneity of symptom onset, follow-up, and patient care settings among studies included.[45]

In a cohort study of 2354 patients hospitalized with critical COVID-19 in Sweden during March through June 2020, 90-day mortality was 26.9%. In multivariable models, male sex [HR 1.28 (95% CI: 1.06–1.55)], malignancy [HR 1.81 (95%CI: 1.19–2.74)], and morbid obesity [HR 1.46 (95% CI: 1.05–1.99)] were identified as risk factors for 90-day mortality.

Disparities

Disparities in health outcomes by race and ethnicity have been on stark display during the COVID-19 pandemic.[46] COVID incidence and outcomes have differed by race and ethnicity, driven by inequalities in risk of SARS-CoV-2 exposure and chronic health status that are perpetuated by structures and policy that perpetuate inequality.[47] People of color are more likely to live in densely populated or polluted areas, be unable to do their job remotely (or in a physically distanced manner), and experience a disproportionate burden of comorbid illnesses,[46] all of which increase the risk of exposure to SARS-CoV2 and worse outcomes from COVID-19.[48] Poverty alone prevents access to critical care resources, with 49% of low-income areas having no ICU beds compared with just 3% of high-income communities.[49]

Of 94,683 patients with COVID-19 who presented to emergency departments at 87 US Health Systems between December 1, 2019 and September 30, 2020, Black people accounted for 26.7% and Hispanic 33.6%,[50] far more than their corresponding US population percentages of 13.4% and 18.5%, respectively.[51] Of the 29,687 patients who were admitted with COVID-19 through the emergency department, admission rates were similar across racial and ethnic groups, although in-hospital mortality was greater in Black (RR 1.18, 95%CI: 1.06–1.31) and Hispanic patients (RR 1.28, 95%CI: 1.13–1.44) compared with White patients.[50]

Similarly, of 1551 patients who tested positive for COVID-19 in Houston, Texas, between March 5, 2020 and May 31, 2020, 22% (N = 341) were Black and 18% (N = 279) were Hispanic.[52] The authors postulated that population density contributed to the disparities in infection rates, with non-Hispanic-Black (OR 2.23, 95% CI: 1.90–2.60) and Hispanic (OR 1.95, 95%CI: 1.72–2.20) residents having a higher likelihood of infection compared with White residents of Houston.

MANAGEMENT

Because of infection precautions and high patient volume, many ICU practices changed during the COVID-19 pandemic, including delirium assessment, sedation practices, family involvement, and end-of-life care. Meanwhile, clinicians debated the optimal approach to respiratory support, including the threshold for initiation and approach to mechanical ventilation. Finally, therapeutics were controversial and evolved rapidly as clinical trial data emerged.

Supportive Care: ABCDEF Bundle

The ABCDEF bundle[53] is a collection of 6 evidence-based practices (pain assessment and treatment, spontaneous awakening and breathing trials, choice of sedation, delirium assessment, early mobility, and family engagement) that serve as the cornerstone for supportive care in the ICU. In a 2-day point prevalence study of ABCDEF bundle implementation in 212 ICUs in 38 countries on June 3, 2020 and July 1, 2020, there was low implementation of all elements, including pain assessment (45%), spontaneous breathing trials (28%), sedation assessment (52%), delirium assessment (35%), early mobility (47%), and family engagement (16%).[54] The study did not assess reasons for low compliance but hypothesized reasons include high patient census, scarcity of personnel, drug shortages, and time needed to don/doff PPE.

Sedation practices have differed during the pandemic as well. In a multinational study of 2088 critically ill patients, across 69 ICUs (January 20, 2020 through April 28, 2020), 1337 (64%) were sedated with benzodiazepine infusions for a median of 7 days (IQR 4-12 days).[55] As would be expected, benzodiazepine infusion (OR 1.59 [95% CI: 1.33–1.91]) was associated risk of acute brain dysfunction.[55] Despite guidelines[56] recommending against benzodiazepine infusions, their use have increased during the pandemic due to drug shortages, need for multiple sedating medications to prevent self-extubation, and high patient-to-nurse ratios limiting the ability to reorient and calm patients.

Family visitation, goals of care discussions, and end-of-life care were substantially impacted during COVID-19, changing a key element of critical care and the ABCDEF bundle. Of 89 hospitals across the state of Michigan, 49 (55%) responded to surveys conducted between April 6, 2020 and May 8, 2020.[57] One hospital (2%) indicated that visitation was still allowed, whereas all others (98%) had a "no visitation" policy during early months in the pandemic, with 29 (59%) making exceptions in certain situations such as end-of-life.[57] Of the 49 hospitals surveyed, 40 (82%) endorsed changes in communication strategies either through video conferencing or telephone. Patient and family communication was similarly altered, with 34 hospitals (69%) encouraging video communication through tablets or smart phones. Similarly, a single center case series found that family or friends were present in only one-third of deaths.[28]

Respiratory Support: Phenotypes, Intubation, Self-Proning, Ventilator Management, Fluid Resuscitation

From the early days of the pandemic, there has been ongoing debate over the extent to which the pathophysiology of COVID-19-related respiratory failure is similar (or not) to other causes of acute hypoxic respiratory failure, and, following along this line, whether we should treat patients with COVID-19-related respiratory failure as we would treat patients with non-COVID-related acute respiratory distress syndrome.

There was much debate about the pathophysiology of acute hypoxic respiratory failure due to COVID-19. Some believed the primary cause was due to endothelial dysfunction and hypoxic vasoconstriction with increased compliance relative to historical cohorts.[58–60] This led to the theoretic subphenotypes of COVID-19 respiratory failure: (1) "L" phenotype with low elastance, normal compliance and (2) "H" phenotype with high elastance and low compliance.[61] Investigators further postulated a need for differing ventilation strategies in each group, with the "L" phenotype requiring liberalized tidal volume with lower PEEP and the "H" phenotype requiring typical ventilation strategies including higher PEEP and low tidal volume ventilation.[58] As further evidence emerged, significant heterogeneity of disease was observed, with varying compliance consistent with prior cohorts of patients with ARDS.[62,63] This resulted in a call to study the disease further before changing decades of critical care practice and continuing to advocate for lung protective low tidal volume ventilation.[64] In a study comparing 130 critically ill mechanically ventilated patients with COVID-19 ARDS to 382 non-COVID ARDS mechanically ventilated patients, there was no difference in time-to-breathing unassisted at 28 days or 28-day mortality.[65] Other studies have similarly found similar outcomes when comparing COVID-19 ARDS to other viral ARDS cohorts.[66] Further investigation using semiquantitative methods found the "L" and "H" phenotypes were not mutually exclusive and likely represent a spectrum of disease.[67] Furthermore, historical investigation of personalized mechanical ventilation techniques have not improved outcomes in ARDS patients when compared with typical lung-protective ventilation techniques.[68] In summary, there is not enough evidence to suggest acute hypoxic respiratory failure from COVID-19 is different from historical ARDS cohorts, or that mechanical ventilation strategies should deviate from current best practice guidelines.

When Should the Hypoxic Patient with COVID-19 Be Intubated?

Early in the pandemic, there was widespread concern that heated high-flow nasal cannula (HHFNC) and NIV may increase the risk for aerosolization of SARS-CoV-2, and thereby drive the transmission of COVID-19 to health-care workers. This concern led many clinicians to electively intubate patients and initiate mechanical ventilation once oxygenation saturation could not be maintained with low levels of nasal cannula oxygen. However, subsequent studies have not borne out this early concern. Humans are highly effective at generating aerosols via coughing but HHFNC and NIV do not cause meaningful increases in the aerosol generation over and beyond what is produced by patients on room air.[69]

Even after HHFNC and NIV were shown safe from the aerosol-generation standpoint, there remained equipoise regarding the optimal threshold for the initiation of invasive mechanical ventilation.[70] Some clinicians opt for earlier intubation, recognizing the added time associated with intubation under airborne precautions. Other clinicians delay intubation as long as possible, recognizing that some patients may be able to avoid invasive mechanical ventilation altogether.

Several observational studies have examined outcomes by timing of intubation. In a study of 47 patients with hypoxic respiratory failure in Korea (February 17, 2020 through April 23, 2020), 23 (48.9%) were intubated on the first day meeting ARDS criteria (P/F ≤ 300 with bilateral infiltrates not fully explained by heart failure), whereas 24 (51.1%) were intubated on a subsequent day, more than 24 hours after suspected ARDS diagnosis.[71] In-hospital mortality was numerically higher (56.5% vs 43.8%, $P = .43$), whereas ventilator free days were lower in the early intubation group (median 9 days vs 28 days, $P = .008$).[71]

In a study of 231 patients with hypoxic respiratory failure in Georgia (March 6, 2020 through May 7, 2020),[63] 109 (47.2%) were treated with high-flow nasal cannula, whereas 97 (42.0%) were intubated directly without preceding high-flow nasal cannula. Ultimately, 78 (71.6%) in the high-flow group required intubation.[63] In-hospital mortality was similar across subgroups defined by timing of intubation: 8 hours or less (38.2%), between 8 and 24 hours (31.6%), and ≥24 hours (38.1%), $P = .7$.

In a study of 245 patients with hypoxic respiratory failure in 11 ICUs in France (February 15, 2020 through May 1, 2020), 117 (47.8%) received early mechanical ventilation, 85 (34.6%) high-flow nasal cannula, 18 (7.4%) CPAP, 16 (6.6%) nasal cannula, and 9 noninvasive positive pressure ventilation (3.6%).[72] The 60-day mortality was higher among patients treated with early mechanical ventilation versus noninvasive oxygen therapy (42.7% vs 21.9%, $P<.01$), and similar among patients who were intubated earlier (within 2 days) versus later (42.2% vs 42.7%).

In a study of 75 mechanically ventilated patients with COVID-19 at Temple University (February 2020 through May 2020), respiratory mechanics were compared by timing of intubation (before or after the median time of intubation, 1.27 days).[73] Patients in the late intubation group (>1.27 days)

had higher P/F ratios (160 vs 205, $P = .46$), higher PEEP (11 vs 9, $P = .27$), and higher plateau pressure (26 vs 22, $P = .02$), with similar compliance (35 vs 41, $P = .13$) at the time of intubation.[73] The late intubation group had longer ICU length of stay (median 12.3 vs 7.4 days, $P = .001$) and duration of mechanical ventilation. This observational design, however, does not account for patients receiving alternative respiratory support such as HHFNC and never require intubation.

A recent meta-analysis included 8944 critically ill patients with COVID-19 across 12 studies, assessing the impact of early intubation, within 24 hours of ICU admission, versus later.[74] Interestingly, early versus late intubation did not affect all-cause mortality (45.4% vs 39.1%; RR 1.07, 95% CI: 0.99–1.15) or duration of mechanical ventilation (mean difference −0.58 days, 95% CI: −3.06–1.89). Secondary outcomes including ICU length of stay and need for renal replacement therapy were similar between groups.[74] One significant limitation, however, is that observational data may have residual confounding by indication. Patients with higher illness severity may be intubated sooner while also having higher risk of mortality, thereby introducing bias, and limiting our overall interpretation of these studies.

Considering together, observational data suggests later intubation is associated with worse respiratory mechanics,[73] although mortality among invasive mechanically ventilated patients may be the same regardless of timing of intubation.[63,72,74] Noninvasive support modalities (HHFNC, NIV) seem safe, although it is unclear whether they reduce mortality and may prolong the length of stay.[63,72] Bias associated with observational data limits interpretation of whether patients should be intubated early or late in their course, and randomized trials are not available presently.

Is Proning the Nonintubated Patient with COVID-19 Safe and Does It Prevent Intubation?

Given the benefits seen in historical groups of ARDS patients placed in the prone position,[75] providers began proning the awake nonintubated patient with respiratory failure from COVID-19 (self-proning), hoping to prevent intubation and utilization of scarce resources. New York city emergency medicine providers enrolled 50 consecutive patients with respiratory failure from COVID-19 between March 1, 2020 and April 1, 2020, excluding those with limited code status, those requiring NIV, and including those who remained hypoxic (saturation <94% with supplemental oxygen).[76] Of the 50 patients who self-proned, 13 (24%) were intubated within 24 hours of arrival to the emergency room.[76] Of the remaining 37 patients admitted to the hospital, 5 (13.5%) were intubated during their hospital stay and 36% in total requiring intubation. Notably, 7 (14%) patients required intubation within 1 hour of proning.[76] Lack of a control group limits interpretation.

A separate case series of 24 awake nonintubated spontaneously breathing French patients with respiratory failure due to COVID-19 between March 27, 2020 and April 8, 2020 examined tolerance of prone positioning and outcomes.[10] Of the 24 patients enrolled, 4 (17%) did not tolerate prone positioning for more than 1 hour, 5 (21%) tolerated it for 1 to 3 hours, and 15 (63%) tolerated it for more than 3 hours. Of the 24 patients, 6 (25%) were considered responders defined as a PaO_2 increase 20% or greater during proning, with half of those nonsustained after resupination.[10] Lack of control group and lack of outcomes data are limiting factors.

An Italian series of 15 non-ICU patients with respiratory failure due to COVID-19 demonstrated that continuous positive airway pressure (CPAP) administration outside the ICU (10 cm H_2O and FiO_2 0.6), whereas prone was feasible.[77] Of the 15 patients who were proned for 3 hours with CPAP, all patients had reduction in respiratory rate, and improved p/f ratio while proned ($P<.001$). At 14-day follow-up, 9 (60%) were discharged home, 1 (6%) improved and stopped proning but remained hospitalized, 3 (20%) continued proning, 1 (6%) patient was intubated, and 1 (6%) patient died.[77] Of 29 patients enrolled in a New York city hospital with respiratory failure from COVID-19 between April 6, 2020 and April 14, 2020, 25 completed at least 1 hour of self-proning.[78] All patients had improvement in oxyhemoglobin saturation with a median improvement of 7% (range 1%–34%). Of the 25 patients, 12 (48%) required intubation and 5 (20%) after the initial hour of proning.[78]

Although self-proning seems feasible with improvement in oxygenation for some patients, it is difficult to draw conclusions with the lack of comparison groups, randomization, and long-term outcomes.[4] The time of prone positioning was relatively brief in most case series and difficult to tell if patients had sustained improvements, or whether intubations were simply delayed. Randomized trials are needed to answer this question with confidence.

Should Shock Be Treated Differently in Patients with COVID-19?

To date, there are no well-controlled trials randomizing patients to various hemodynamic treatment strategies. Extrapolation from septic shock studies has guided authors to recommend assessing for fluid responsiveness,[79] giving balanced crystalloids over colloids,[80] and using norepinephrine as a first-line vasopressor targeting a mean arterial pressure of 60 to 65 mm Hg.[79,80] Similarly, the use of stress dose steroids is a clinical decision and no different in patients with COVID-19 and distributive shock.[80] There are several opinions on how much volume should be given,[81] but there is a paucity of data presently to make conclusions. Similar to historical cohorts of septic shock, the resuscitation volume and type will likely be an ongoing debate. Once shock has resolved, there is a question of the utility of diuresis with loop diuretics, which has been shown to reduce duration of mechanical ventilation in non-COVID-19 ARDS trials.[82] Investigation regarding the utility of nebulized furosemide in respiratory failure from COVID-19 is ongoing.[83]

Pharmacologic Therapies

The COVID-19 pandemic brought about rapid investigation in therapeutics. Early reports of hydroxychloroquine, a medication used to treat autoimmune diseases, showed promise in small noncontrolled studies. However, large observational[84] and randomized[85,86] trials demonstrated no benefit with hydroxychloroquine. Since that time, numerous other agents have failed to show benefit, including Zinc and Vitamin C,[87] convalescent plasma,[88] sarilumab,[89] lopinavir,[86] interferon,[86] canakinumab,[90] and acalabrutinib.[91] However, others have shown promise for reducing duration of illness, as well as mortality.

Corticosteroids were the first agents shown to reduce mortality from COVID-19. Of 6425 patients hospitalized with COVID-19 in the United Kingdom, dexamethasone 6 mg daily versus usual care for up to 10 days reduced 28-day mortality among those receiving mechanical ventilation (29.3% vs 41.4%, rate ratio 0.64 95% CI: 0.51–0.81) and those receiving oxygen without mechanical ventilation (23.3% vs 26.2%, rate ratio 0.82 95% CI: 0.72–0.94)[92] (**Table 2**). Furthermore, a recent meta-analysis including 73 studies and 21, 350 patients hospitalized with COVID-19 found corticosteroids were used with increasing frequency in mechanically ventilated patients (35%), ICU patients (51.3%), and severely ill patients (40%), demonstrating an overall mortality benefit (OR 0.65; 95%CI: 0.51–0.83).[93] Notably, steroids were not found to prolong viral shedding but interpretations are somewhat limited due to heterogeneity of study methodologies and reporting. As a result, the World Health Organization (WHO)

Table 2
Therapeutics in critically ill patients with COVID-19

Author(s)	Population	Intervention	Outcome	Adverse Events
Horby et al,[92]	Hospitalized patients with COVID-19	Oral or intravenous dexamethasone 6 mg daily (N = 2104) vs usual care (N = 4321)	28-d mortality improved with dexamethasone in pts receiving oxygen without MV (23.3% vs 26.2%) and pts receiving MV (29.3% vs 41.4%)	4 in dexamethasone group (2 hyperglycemia, 1 GI hemorrhage, 1 psychosis)
Angus et al,[108] 2020	Critically ill patients with COVID-19, Bayesian randomized adaptive platform (REMAP)	50 mg or 100 mg hydrocortisone for 7-d (N = 143), shock dependent steroid course (N = 152), or no steroids (N = 108)	93% and 80% probability of superiority with regards to organ-failure free days	9 in steroid groups (neuropathy, fungemia, pneumonia, pulmonary embolism, elevated troponin, postop hemorrhage, intracranial hemorrhage)
Tomazini et al,[109] 2020	Hospitalized patients with COVID-19 ARDS	20 mg dexamethasone daily for 5 d, 10 mg daily for 5 d (N = 151) vs usual care (N = 148)	Increased number of ventilator-free days (6.6 vs 4.0, P = .04), no difference in 28-d mortality	No difference between groups for hyperglycemia or secondary infections
Beigel et al,[96] 2020	Hospitalized patients with COVID-19 and lower respiratory tract infection	200 mg remdesivir once, then 100 mg daily for 4 more doses (N = 541) vs placebo (N = 521)	No difference in survival. Improved median recovery time (10 vs 15 d, P<.001) for those requiring supplemental oxygen not requiring mechanical ventilation	No difference in adverse events between groups
Pan et al,[86] 2021	Hospitalized patients with COVID-19	Remdesivir (N = 2750) vs no trial drug (N = 4088)	No difference in overall mortality (10.9% vs 11.2%) or need for mechanical ventilation (10.8% vs 10.5%)	Not reported

(continued on next page)

Table 2
(continued)

Author(s)	Population	Intervention	Outcome	Adverse Events
Rosas et al,[98] 2021	Hospitalized patients with COVID-19 pneumonia	Tocilizumab 8 mg/kg for 1 or 2 doses (N = 294) vs placebo (N = 144)	No difference in 28-d mortality (19.7% vs 19.4%) or clinical status improvement (between group difference −1.0, 95% CI: −2.5–0)	No difference in serious adverse events
Gordon et al,[99] 2021	Critically ill patients with COVID-19, Bayesian randomized adaptive platform (REMAP)	Tocilizumab (N = 353) vs control (N = 402)	99.9% posterior probability of improved survival, HR 1.61 (95%CI: 1.25–2.08)	No difference in serious adverse events (9 occurred including one secondary bacterial infection)

recommends dexamethasone 6 mg daily or 50 mg hydrocortisone every 8 hours for 7 to 10 days in severely or critically ill patients with COVID-19.[94] The optimal dose and duration of corticosteroids are not yet fully known.[95]

Remdesivir, an inhibitor of RNA-polymerase, was the next drug to show promise against the COVID-19 pandemic. Across 13 countries, 1062 patients hospitalized with COVID-19 from February 21, 2020 through April 19, 2020 were randomized to remdesivir versus placebo.[96] Although remdesivir did not confer survival benefit at 28 days (HR 0.73; 95% CI: 0.52–1.03), median recovery time (defined as time to neither being hospitalized nor hospitalized without supplemental oxygen requirement and no longer requiring medical care) was shorter with remdesivir (10 vs15 days; $P<.001$).[96] A larger randomized trial conducted by the WHO enrolled 2750 patients hospitalized with COVID-19, randomizing them to receive remdesivir and 4088 to no trial drug in 405 hospitals across 30 countries.[86] Authors concluded that remdesivir conferred no mortality benefit (RR 0.95; 95% CI: 0.81–1.11) or reducing need for mechanical ventilation, even when stratified by age and respiratory support at trial entry.[86] The Food and Drug Administration has approved remdesivir for use in patients hospitalized with respiratory failure from COVID-19, although not for those requiring mechanical ventilation.[97] Similarly, use beyond 10 days of symptoms is not recommended.

Tocilizumab, a monoclonal antibody targeting IL-6, was initially developed for the treatment of autoimmune diseases and cytokine release syndrome for chimeric antigen receptor therapy in patients with hematologic malignancy. Early investigations found no survival benefit with the use of tocilizumab in COVID-19.[98] Of 452 hospitalized patients with COVID-19 across 62 hospitals in 9 countries, treatment with tocilizumab versus placebo resulted in no difference in 28-day mortality (19.7% vs 19.4%, $P = .94$).[98] Similarly, tocilizumab treatment did not result in clinical status improvement, defined as being discharged home or hospitalized without supplemental oxygen need at 28-days from enrollment (ordinal clinical status score 1.0 vs 2.0, $P = .31$).[98] Later investigation using an adaptive platform randomized trial (randomizing to multiple domains allowing patients to be on multiple treatments) enrolled 353 patients treated with tocilizumab.[99] Interestingly, tocilizumab treatment resulted in more organ-failure-free days (10 versus 0 [OR 1.64; 95% CI: 1.25–2.14]) and improved 90-day survival (HR 1.61, 95% CI: 1.25–2.08) when compared with placebo.[99] Given the conflicting results, current recommendations are to consider adding tocilizumab to dexamethasone treatment when a patient has rapidly increasing oxygen requirements early in their illness with elevated C-reactive protein levels of 75 mg/L or greater (BIIa).[97]

Early observational data demonstrated a high incidence of venous thromboembolic disease in patients with COVID-19.[100] Further examination of autopsy investigations found up to 58% incidence of pulmonary emboli.[101] The American Society of Hematologists recommends using prophylactic dose anticoagulants over intermediate dose[102] based on randomized trial results.[103] The question of whether full dose anticoagulation should be used in the absence of clinically detected venous thromboembolism remains unknown. Early observations found improved in-hospital mortality with full-dose anticoagulation,[104] although increased rates of mechanical ventilation, raising questions of whether empiric full-dose should be used in all patients hospitalized with COVID-19. As a result, several ongoing trials are investigating full-dose anticoagulation effects on organ-failure free days and need for mechanical ventilation, although preliminary nonpeer-reviewed results suggests harm in the critically ill population but potential benefits in moderately ill patients with COVID-19 not requiring ICU level care or organ support (heated high flow, NIV, mechanical ventilation).[105]

The most effective treatment of COVID-19 is preventing infection from occurring. Among 43,548 participants aged 16 years and older across 152 sites around the world, 21,720 people received a 2-vaccine regimen 21-days apart, resulting in 95% efficacy in prevention of disease.[106] Preliminary nonpeer-reviewed work demonstrates a profound reduction in ICU admissions and deaths since vaccinations became available, by 65.6% (95%CI: 62.2%–68.6%) and 69.3% (95% CI: 65.5%–73.1%), respectively.[107]

DISCUSSION

COVID-19 not only changed the way we practice critical care but also forced us to reconsider resource allocation, staffing, and nonconventional strategies such as self-proning the awake patient in hopes of reducing the need for mechanical ventilation. Furthermore, the changing epidemiology and transmission forced critical care and researchers to rethink trial design, with a new adaptive platform trial not routinely performed before the COVID-19 pandemic.

However, some things do remain consistent over time. Respiratory failure due to COVID-19 seems to be consistent with prior cohorts of viral ARDS, with respect to mortality as well as ventilator management. Lung-protective ventilation remains the mainstay of critical care and should not change based on the current available evidence. Sedation practices, similarly, deviated from clinical practice guidelines with benzodiazepine infusions leading to increased risk of delirium. Remembering the basics of critical care is important for improving outcomes, even in times of a global pandemic.

Pharmacologic therapies have rapidly evolved over time reducing morbidity and mortality for patients with respiratory failure from COVID-19. First and foremost, vaccinations have drastically reduced transmission and severity of illness. Corticosteroids have consistently demonstrated benefit with regards to mortality, whereas other medications such as remdesivir and tocilizumab have conflicting results but may reduce severity of illness.

The pandemic has taken a global toll, both from a health perspective and from an economic standpoint. Because vaccinations have become widespread in certain parts of the world, restrictions will be lifted, and life will begin to normalize for many. However, we cannot forget the lessons learned from this global pandemic. We need to maintain a public health infrastructure capable of responding rapidly with resources, train and maintain staff to respond with appropriate bed capacity, understand the importance of isolation precautions for infection prevention, and use research techniques such as randomized, embedded, multifactorial, adaptive platform (REMAP) to rapidly assess therapeutics to improve care and outcomes for our patients.

CLINICS CARE POINTS

- One in 4 patients hospitalized with COVID-19 become critically ill, with up to 80% of those requiring mechanical ventilation.
- In-hospital mortality varies, but with appropriate resources and capacity, can be as low as 12% in some cohorts.
- Long-term outcomes after COVID-19 remain poor, with 50% to 70% reporting persistent symptoms such as shortness of breath or fatigue.
- Acute respiratory failure from COVID-19 represents a similar spectrum of disease to other historical cohorts of viral ARDS.
- Corticosteroids remain the mainstay of treatment of COVID-19, although optimal dosing and duration remain unknown.

DISCLOSURE

This article is the result of work supported with resources and use of facilities at the Ann Arbor VA Medical Center. The views expressed in this article are those of the authors and do not necessarily reflect the position or policy of the Department of Veterans Affairs or the US government.

REFERENCES

1. WHO coronavirus (COVID-19) Dashboard. Available at: https://covid19.who.int. Accessed July 2, 2021.
2. Grasselli G, Pesenti A, Cecconi M. Critical care utilization for the COVID-19 outbreak in Lombardy, Italy: early experience and Forecast during an emergency Response. JAMA 2020;323(16):1545–6.
3. Harris GH, Baldisseri MR, Reynolds BR, et al. Design for implementation of a system-level ICU pandemic surge staffing plan. Crit Care Explor 2020;2(6):e0136.
4. Alhazzani W, Møller MH, Arabi YM, et al. Surviving Sepsis Campaign: guidelines on the management of critically ill adults with Coronavirus Disease 2019 (COVID-19). Intensive Care Med 2020;46(5):854–87.
5. Del Rio C, Malani PN. COVID-19-New Insights on a rapidly changing epidemic. JAMA 2020;323(14):1339–40.
6. Modes of transmission of virus causing COVID-19: implications for IPC precaution recommendations. Available at: https://www.who.int/news-room/commentaries/detail/modes-of-transmission-of-virus-causing-covid-19-implications-for-ipc-precaution-recommendations. Accessed April 21, 2021.
7. CDC. COVID-19 and Your health. Centers for Disease Control and Prevention; 2020. Available at: https://www.cdc.gov/coronavirus/2019-ncov/long-term-effects.html. Accessed February 25, 2021.
8. Meng L, Qiu H, Wan L, et al. Intubation and ventilation amid the COVID-19 outbreak: Wuhan's experience. Anesthesiology 2020;132(6):1317–32.
9. Sarma A, Calfee CS. Prone positioning in awake, nonintubated patients with COVID-19: necessity is the Mother of Invention. JAMA Intern Med 2020. https://doi.org/10.1001/jamainternmed.2020.3027.
10. Elharrar X, Trigui Y, Dols A-M, et al. Use of prone positioning in nonintubated patients with COVID-19 and hypoxemic acute respiratory failure. JAMA 2020;323(22):2336–8.
11. Oxygenation and ventilation. COVID-19 treatment guidelines. Available at: https://www.covid19treatmentguidelines.nih.gov/critical-care/oxygenation-and-ventilation/. Accessed April 21, 2021.

12. CDC. Community, work, and School. Centers for disease control and prevention. 2020. Available at: https://www.cdc.gov/coronavirus/2019-ncov/community/health-equity/racial-ethnic-disparities/disparities-illness.html. Accessed April 21, 2021.

13. Sorci G, Faivre B, Morand S. Explaining among-country variation in COVID-19 case fatality rate. Sci Rep 2020;10(1):18909.

14. Malard F, Genthon A, Brissot E, et al. COVID-19 outcomes in patients with hematologic disease. Bone Marrow Transplant 2020. https://doi.org/10.1038/s41409-020-0931-4.

15. Hensley MK, Bain WG, Jacobs J, et al. Intractable coronavirus disease 2019 (COVID-19) and prolonged severe acute respiratory syndrome coronavirus 2 (SARS-CoV-2) Replication in a chimeric antigen receptor-Modified T-Cell therapy Recipient: a case study. Clin Infect Dis 2021. https://doi.org/10.1093/cid/ciab072.

16. Zhou F, Yu T, Du R, et al. Clinical course and risk factors for mortality of adult inpatients with COVID-19 in Wuhan, China: a retrospective cohort study. Lancet 2020;395(10229):1054–62.

17. Wu C, Chen X, Cai Y, et al. Risk factors associated with acute respiratory distress syndrome and death in patients with coronavirus disease 2019 pneumonia in Wuhan, China. JAMA Intern Med 2020; 180(7):934–43.

18. Chen N, Zhou M, Dong X, et al. Epidemiological and clinical characteristics of 99 cases of 2019 novel coronavirus pneumonia in Wuhan, China: a descriptive study. Lancet 2020;395(10223):507–13.

19. Guan W, Ni Z, Hu Y, et al. Clinical characteristics of coronavirus disease 2019 in China. N Engl J Med 2020;382(18):1708–20.

20. Yang X, Yu Y, Xu J, et al. Clinical course and outcomes of critically ill patients with SARS-CoV-2 pneumonia in Wuhan, China: a single-centered, retrospective, observational study. Lancet Respir Med 2020. https://doi.org/10.1016/S2213-2600(20)30079-5.

21. Grasselli G, Zangrillo A, Zanella A, et al. Baseline characteristics and outcomes of 1591 patients infected with SARS-CoV-2 admitted to ICUs of the Lombardy region, Italy. JAMA 2020. https://doi.org/10.1001/jama.2020.5394.

22. Grasselli G, Greco M, Zanella A, et al. Risk factors associated with mortality among patients with COVID-19 in intensive care Units in Lombardy, Italy. JAMA Intern Med 2020;180(10):1345–55.

23. Bhatraju PK, Ghassemieh BJ, Nichols M, et al. Covid-19 in critically ill patients in the Seattle region - case series. N Engl J Med 2020. https://doi.org/10.1056/NEJMoa2004500.

24. Arentz M, Yim E, Klaff L, et al. Characteristics and outcomes of 21 critically ill patients with COVID-19 in Washington state. JAMA 2020;323(16):1612–4.

25. Richardson S, Hirsch JS, Narasimhan M, et al. Presenting characteristics, Comorbidities, and outcomes among 5700 patients hospitalized with COVID-19 in the New York city area. JAMA 2020. https://doi.org/10.1001/jama.2020.6775.

26. Petrilli CM, Jones SA, Yang J, et al. Factors associated with hospital admission and critical illness among 5279 people with coronavirus disease 2019 in New York City: prospective cohort study. BMJ 2020;369:m1966.

27. Cummings MJ, Baldwin MR, Abrams D, et al. Epidemiology, clinical course, and outcomes of critically ill adults with COVID-19 in New York City: a prospective cohort study. Lancet 2020; 395(10239):1763–70.

28. Ketcham SW, Bolig T, Molling DJ, et al. Causes and Circumstances of death among patients hospitalized with COVID-19: a retrospective cohort study. Ann ATS 2020. https://doi.org/10.1513/AnnalsATS.202011-1381RL. AnnalsATS.202011-1381RL.

29. Bravata DM, Perkins AJ, Myers LJ, et al. Association of intensive care Unit patient Load and demand with mortality rates in US department of Veterans Affairs hospitals during the COVID-19 pandemic. JAMA Netw Open 2021;4(1): e2034266.

30. Armstrong RA, Kane AD, Cook TM. Outcomes from intensive care in patients with COVID-19: a systematic review and meta-analysis of observational studies. Anaesthesia 2020. https://doi.org/10.1111/anae.15201.

31. Ranney ML, Griffeth V, Jha AK. Critical supply shortages — the need for ventilators and personal protective equipment during the Covid-19 pandemic. N Engl J Med 2020;382(18):e41.

32. Beitler JR, Mittel AM, Kallet R, et al. Ventilator sharing during an acute shortage caused by the COVID-19 pandemic. Am J Respir Crit Care Med 2020;202(4):600–4.

33. Tonetti T, Zanella A, Pizzilli G, et al. One ventilator for two patients: feasibility and considerations of a last resort solution in case of equipment shortage. Thorax 2020;75(6):517–9.

34. Kobokovich A. Ventilator Stockpiling and availability in the US. 2020. Available at: https://www.centerforhealthsecurity.org/resources/COVID-19/COVID-19-fact-sheets/200214-VentilatorAvailability-factsheet.pdf. Accessed April 30, 2021.

35. SCCM | consensus statement on multiple patients per ventilator. Society of critical care medicine (SCCM). Available at: https://sccm.org/Clinical-Resources/Disaster/COVID19/Advocacy/Joint-Statement-on-Multiple-Patients-Per-Ventilato. Accessed June 29, 2021.

36. Arabi YM, Azoulay E, Al-Dorzi HM, et al. How the COVID-19 pandemic will change the future of critical care. Intensive Care Med 2021;47(3):282–91.

37. Hester TB, Cartwright JD, DiGiovine DG, et al. Training and Deployment of medical Students as respiratory therapist Extenders during COVID-19. ATS Scholar 2020;1(2):145–51.

38. Martin L. Shortage of ICU Providers Who Operate Ventilators Would Severely LImit Care During COVID-19 Outbreak. Society of critical care medicine (SCCM). Available at: https://sccm.org/getattachment/About-SCCM/Media-Relations/Final-Covid19-Press-Release.pdf?lang=en-US. Accessed June 20, 2021.

39. Williams D, Lawrence J, Hong Y, et al. Tele-ICUs for COVID-19: a Look at national prevalence and characteristics of hospitals providing Teleintensive care. J Rural Health 2020. https://doi.org/10.1111/jrh.12524.

40. Phua J, Weng L, Ling L, et al. Intensive care management of coronavirus disease 2019 (COVID-19): challenges and recommendations. Lancet Respir Med 2020;8(5):506–17.

41. Supady A, Curtis JR, Abrams D, et al. Allocating scarce intensive care resources during the COVID-19 pandemic: practical challenges to theoretical frameworks. Lancet Respir Med 2021;9(4):430–4.

42. Chopra V, Flanders SA, O'Malley M, et al. Sixty-day outcomes among patients hospitalized with COVID-19. Ann Intern Med 2020. https://doi.org/10.7326/M20-5661.

43. Writing Committee for the COMEBAC Study Group, Morin L, Savale L, et al. Four-month clinical status of a cohort of patients after hospitalization for COVID-19. JAMA 2021;325(15):1525–34.

44. Huang C, Huang L, Wang Y, et al. 6-month consequences of COVID-19 in patients discharged from hospital: a cohort study. Lancet 2021;397(10270):220–32.

45. Nasserie T, Hittle M, Goodman SN. Assessment of the frequency and variety of persistent symptoms among patients with COVID-19: a systematic review. JAMA Netw Open 2021;4(5):e2111417.

46. Webb Hooper M, Nápoles AM, Pérez-Stable EJ. COVID-19 and racial/ethnic disparities. JAMA 2020;323(24):2466–7.

47. Culture of Health Program. National Academy of medicine. Available at: https://nam.edu/programs/culture-of-health/. Accessed June 29, 2021.

48. Gross CP, Essien UR, Pasha S, et al. Racial and ethnic disparities in population-level Covid-19 mortality. J Gen Intern Med 2020;35(10):3097–9.

49. Kanter GP, Segal AG, Groeneveld PW. Income disparities in access to critical care services. Health Aff 2020;39(8):1362–7.

50. Wiley Z, Ross-Driscoll K, Wang Z, et al. Racial and ethnic differences and clinical outcomes of COVID-19 patients presenting to the emergency department. Clin Infect Dis 2021. https://doi.org/10.1093/cid/ciab290.

51. U.S. Census Bureau QuickFacts: United States. Available at: https://www.census.gov/quickfacts/fact/table/US/PST045219. Accessed May 14, 2021.

52. Vahidy FS, Nicolas JC, Meeks JR, et al. Racial and ethnic disparities in SARS-CoV-2 pandemic: analysis of a COVID-19 observational registry for a diverse US metropolitan population. BMJ Open 2020;10(8):e039849.

53. Marra A, Ely EW, Pandharipande PP, et al. The ABCDEF bundle in critical care. Crit Care Clin 2017;33(2):225–43.

54. Liu K, Nakamura K, Katsukawa H, et al. ABCDEF bundle and supportive ICU practices for patients with coronavirus disease 2019 infection: an International point prevalence study. Crit Care Explorations 2021;3(3):e0353.

55. Pun BT, Badenes R, Heras La Calle G, et al. Prevalence and risk factors for delirium in critically ill patients with COVID-19 (COVID-D): a multicentre cohort study. Lancet Respir Med 2021. https://doi.org/10.1016/S2213-2600(20)30552-X.

56. Barr J, Fraser GL, Puntillo K, et al. Clinical practice guidelines for the management of pain, agitation, and delirium in adult patients in the intensive care unit. Crit Care Med 2013;41(1):263–306.

57. Valley TS, Schutz A, Nagle MT, et al. Changes to visitation Policies and communication practices in Michigan ICUs during the COVID-19 pandemic. Am J Respir Crit Care Med 2020;202(6):883–5.

58. Gattinoni L, Coppola S, Cressoni M, et al. Covid-19 does not Lead to a "typical" acute respiratory distress syndrome. Am J Respir Crit Care Med 2020. https://doi.org/10.1164/rccm.202003-0817LE.

59. Marini JJ, Gattinoni L. Management of COVID-19 respiratory distress. JAMA 2020. https://doi.org/10.1001/jama.2020.6825.

60. Chiumello D, Busana M, Coppola S, et al. Physiological and quantitative CT-scan characterization of COVID-19 and typical ARDS: a matched cohort study. Intensive Care Med 2020;46(12):2187–96.

61. Gattinoni L, Chiumello D, Caironi P, et al. COVID-19 pneumonia: different respiratory treatments for different phenotypes? Intensive Care Med 2020;46(6):1099–102.

62. Ziehr DR, Alladina J, Petri CR, et al. Respiratory pathophysiology of mechanically ventilated patients with COVID-19: a cohort study. Am J Respir Crit Care Med 2020. https://doi.org/10.1164/rccm.202004-1163LE.

63. Hernandez-Romieu AC, Adelman MW, Hockstein MA, et al. Timing of intubation and mortality among critically ill coronavirus disease 2019 patients: a single-center cohort study. Crit Care

Med 2020. https://doi.org/10.1097/CCM.0000000 000004600.

64. Maley JH, Winkler T, Hardin CC. Heterogeneity of acute respiratory distress syndrome in COVID-19: "typical" or not? Am J Respir Crit Care Med 2020; 202(4):618–9.

65. Sjoding MW, Admon AJ, Saha AK, et al. Comparing clinical Features and outcomes in mechanically ventilated patients with COVID-19 and the acute respiratory distress syndrome. Ann Am Thorac Soc 2021. https://doi.org/10.1513/AnnalsATS. 202008-1076OC.

66. Bain W, Yang H, Shah FA, et al. COVID-19 versus non-COVID ARDS: comparison of Demographics, Physiologic Parameters, Inflammatory Biomarkers and clinical outcomes. Ann ATS 2021. https://doi. org/10.1513/AnnalsATS.202008-1026OC.

67. Bos LDJ, Paulus F, Vlaar APJ, et al. Subphenotyping acute respiratory distress syndrome in patients with COVID-19: consequences for ventilator management. Ann Am Thorac Soc 2020;17(9):1161–3.

68. Constantin J-M, Jabaudon M, Lefrant J-Y, et al. Personalised mechanical ventilation tailored to lung morphology versus low positive end-expiratory pressure for patients with acute respiratory distress syndrome in France (the LIVE study): a multicentre, single-blind, randomised controlled trial. Lancet Respir Med 2019;7(10):870–80.

69. Iwashyna TJ, Boehman A, Capecelatro J, et al. Variation in aerosol Production across oxygen Delivery Devices in spontaneously breathing Human Subjects. medRxiv 2020;2020. https://doi.org/10. 1101/2020.04.15.20066688. 04.15.20066688.

70. Nickson C, MD JI, Young P. "Silent hypoxaemia" and COVID-19 intubation. Life in the Fast Lane • LITFL. 2020. Available at: https://litfl.com/silent-hypoxaemia-and-covid-19-intubation/. Accessed July 9, 2021.

71. Lee YH, Choi K-J, Choi SH, et al. Clinical significance of timing of intubation in critically ill patients with COVID-19: a multi-center retrospective study. J Clin Med 2020;9(9). https://doi.org/10.3390/ jcm9092847.

72. Dupuis C, Bouadma L, de Montmollin E, et al. Association between early invasive mechanical ventilation and day-60 mortality in acute hypoxemic respiratory failure related to coronavirus disease-2019 pneumonia. Crit Care Explorations 2021; 3(1):e0329.

73. Pandya A, Kaur NA, Sacher D, et al. Ventilatory mechanics in early vs late intubation in a cohort of coronavirus disease 2019 patients with ARDS. Chest 2021;159(2):653–6.

74. Papoutsi E, Giannakoulis VG, Xourgia E, et al. Effect of timing of intubation on clinical outcomes of critically ill patients with COVID-19: a systematic

review and meta-analysis of non-randomized cohort studies. Crit Care 2021;25(1):121.

75. Guérin C, Reignier J, Richard J-C, et al. Prone positioning in severe acute respiratory distress syndrome. N Engl J Med 2013;368(23):2159–68.

76. Caputo ND, Strayer RJ, Levitan R. Early self-proning in awake, non-intubated patients in the emergency department: a single ED's experience during the COVID-19 pandemic. Acad Emerg Med 2020;27(5):375–8.

77. Sartini C, Tresoldi M, Scarpellini P, et al. Respiratory Parameters in patients with COVID-19 after using noninvasive ventilation in the prone position outside the intensive care Unit. JAMA 2020; 323(22):2338–40.

78. Thompson AE, Ranard BL, Wei Y, et al. Prone positioning in awake, nonintubated patients with COVID-19 hypoxemic respiratory failure. JAMA Intern Med 2020;180(11):1537–9.

79. Poston JT, Patel BK, Davis AM. Management of critically ill adults with COVID-19. JAMA 2020; 323(18):1839–41.

80. Hemodynamics. COVID-19 treatment guidelines. Available at: https://www.covid19treatment guidelines.nih.gov/critical-care/hemodynamics/. Accessed May 24, 2021.

81. Kazory A, Ronco C, McCullough PA. SARS-CoV-2 (COVID-19) and intravascular volume management strategies in the critically ill. Proc (Bayl Univ Med Cent) 2020;33(3):370–5.

82. Comparison of two fluid-management strategies in acute lung Injury | NEJM. Available at: https:// www.nejm.org/doi/full/10.1056/nejmoa062200. Accessed May 24, 2021.

83. Muscedere DJ. Nebulized Furosemide for pulmonary Inflammation in intubated patients with COVID-19 - a Phase 2/3 study. clinicaltrials.gov. 2021. Available at: https://clinicaltrials.gov/ct2/ show/NCT04588792. Accessed May 23, 2021.

84. Geleris J, Sun Y, Platt J, et al. Observational study of hydroxychloroquine in hospitalized patients with Covid-19. N Engl J Med 2020;382(25):2411–8.

85. Self WH, Semler MW, Leither LM, et al. Effect of hydroxychloroquine on clinical status at 14 Days in hospitalized patients with COVID-19: a randomized clinical trial. JAMA 2020;324(21):2165.

86. WHO Solidarity Trial Consortium, Pan H, Peto R, et al. Repurposed Antiviral drugs for Covid-19 - Interim WHO Solidarity trial results. N Engl J Med 2021;384(6):497–511.

87. Thomas S, Patel D, Bittel B, et al. Effect of high-dose Zinc and Ascorbic Acid Supplementation vs usual care on symptom length and reduction among Ambulatory patients with SARS-CoV-2 infection: the COVID A to Z randomized clinical trial. JAMA Netw Open 2021;4(2):e210369.

88. Simonovich VA, Burgos Pratx LD, Scibona P, et al. A randomized trial of convalescent plasma in Covid-19 severe pneumonia. N Engl J Med 2021; 384(7):619–29.

89. Sanofi. Regeneron shut down Kevzara trial in COVID-19 after finding no benefit for ventilated patients. FiercePharma. Available at: https://www. fiercepharma.com/pharma/sanofi-regeneron-s-kevzara-trial-covid-19-comes-to-a-screeching-halt-after-no-benefit-found. Accessed May 25, 2021.

90. Novartis provides update on CAN-COVID trial in hospitalized patients with COVID-19 pneumonia and cytokine release syndrome (CRS). Novartis. Available at: https://www.novartis.com/news/media-releases/novartis-provides-update-can-covid-trial-hospitalized-patients-covid-19-pneumonia-and-cytokine-release-syndrome-crs. Accessed May 25, 2021.

91. Update on CALAVI Phase II trials for Calquence in patients hospitalised with respiratory symptoms of COVID-19. Available at: https://www.astrazeneca. com/media-centre/press-releases/2020/update-on-calavi-phase-ii-trials-for-calquence-in-patients-hospitalised-with-respiratory-symptoms-of-covid-19.html. Accessed May 25, 2021.

92. Dexamethasone in hospitalized patients with Covid-19. N Engl J Med 2021;384(8):693–704.

93. Cano EJ, Fuentes XF, Campioli CC, et al. Impact of corticosteroids in coronavirus disease 2019 outcomes: systematic review and meta-analysis. CHEST 2021;159(3):1019–40.

94. Corticosteroids for COVID-19. Available at: https://www.who.int/publications-detail-redirect/WHO-2019-nCoV-Corticosteroids-2020.1. Accessed May 25, 2021.

95. Mishra GP, Mulani J. Corticosteroids for COVID-19: the search for an optimum duration of therapy. Lancet Respir Med 2021;9(1):e8.

96. Beigel JH, Tomashek KM, Dodd LE, et al. Remdesivir for the treatment of Covid-19 — Final report. N Engl J Med 2020;383(19):1813–26.

97. Therapeutic management. COVID-19 treatment guidelines. Available at: https://www. covid19treatmentguidelines.nih.gov/therapeutic-management/. Accessed May 26, 2021.

98. Rosas IO, Bräu N, Waters M, et al. Tocilizumab in hospitalized patients with severe Covid-19 pneumonia. N Engl J Med 2021;384(16):1503–16.

99. REMAP-CAP Investigators, Gordon AC, Mouncey PR, et al. Interleukin-6 receptor Antagonists in critically ill patients with Covid-19. N Engl J Med 2021;384(16):1491–502.

100. Bilaloglu S, Aphinyanaphongs Y, Jones S, et al. Thrombosis in hospitalized patients with COVID-19 in a New York city health system. JAMA 2020; 324(8):799–801.

101. Wichmann D, Sperhake J-P, Lütgehetmann M, et al. Autopsy Findings and venous thromboembolism in patients with COVID-19: a prospective cohort study. Ann Intern Med 2020;173(4):268–77.

102. ASH guidelines on Use of anticoagulation in patients with COVID-19 - Hematology.org. Available at: https://www.hematology.org:443/education/ clinicians/guidelines-and-quality-care/clinical-practice-guidelines/venous-thromboembolism-guidelines/ash-guidelines-on-use-of-anticoagulation-in-patients-with-covid-19. Accessed May 26, 2021.

103. INSPIRATION Investigators, Sadeghipour P, Talasaz AH, et al. Effect of intermediate-dose vs Standard-dose prophylactic anticoagulation on Thrombotic events, Extracorporeal Membrane oxygenation treatment, or mortality among patients with COVID-19 admitted to the intensive care Unit: the INSPIRATION randomized clinical trial. JAMA 2021;325(16):1620–30.

104. Paranjpe I, Fuster V, Lala A, et al. Association of treatment dose anticoagulation with in-hospital survival among hospitalized patients with COVID-19. J Am Coll Cardiol 2020;76(1):122–4.

105. Interim Presentation of ATTACC, ACTIV-4a & REMAP-CAP. ATTACC. https://www.attacc.org/ presentations. [Accessed 26 May 2021]. Accessed.

106. Polack FP, Thomas SJ, Kitchin N, et al. Safety and efficacy of the BNT162b2 mRNA Covid-19 vaccine. N Engl J Med 2020. https://doi.org/10.1056/ NEJMoa2034577.

107. Moghadas SM, Vilches TN, Zhang K, et al. The impact of vaccination on COVID-19 outbreaks in the United States. medRxiv 2021. https://doi.org/ 10.1101/2020.11.27.20240051.

108. Angus DC, Derde L, Al-Beidh F, et al. Effect of hydrocortisone on mortality and organ support in patients with severe COVID-19: the REMAP-CAP COVID-19 corticosteroid domain randomized clinical trial. JAMA 2020;324(13):1317–29.

109. Tomazini BM, Maia IS, Cavalcanti AB, et al. Effect of dexamethasone on Days alive and ventilator-free in patients with moderate or severe acute respiratory distress syndrome and COVID-19: the CoDEX randomized clinical trial. JAMA 2020; 324(13):1307–16.

Critical Care of the Lung Transplant Patient

Alyssa A. Perez, MD, MEd*, Rupal J. Shah, MD, MSCE

KEYWORDS

- Lung transplant Candidacy • The prelung transplant Patient in the ICU
- The immediate postlung transplant Patient in the ICU • Long-term complications of lung transplant
- Transplant and COVID-19

KEY POINTS

- Mechanical ventilation and extracorporeal membrane oxygenation (ECMO) support are no longer absolute contraindications for lung transplantation in carefully selected patients
- Some candidates are bridged to transplant using mechanical ventilation or ECMO, especially when these facilitate mobilization
- The immediate posttransplant intensive care unit (ICU) course is characterized by lung-protective ventilation, immunosuppression, and surveillance for primary graft dysfunction, daily bronchoscopy, and early rehabilitation
- Long-term complications of lung transplant include infection, drug toxicity, and chronic lung allograft dysfunction of obstructive and restrictive types
- COVID-19 has challenged lung transplant teams to define who are the best candidates for transplantation

INTRODUCTION TO LUNG TRANSPLANT

Lung transplantation is frequently the only therapeutic option for patients with end-stage lung disease. In the appropriate patient, lung transplant extends life, improves the quality of life, and reduces disability.[1] Between 1995 and 2018, more than 60,000 lung transplants were performed worldwide with the number of lung transplantations increasing each year.[2,3] The most common diagnoses leading to lung transplantation include chronic obstructive pulmonary disease (COPD), idiopathic pulmonary fibrosis (IPF), cystic fibrosis (CF), and non-IPF interstitial lung disease,[2] with fibrotic lung disease being the most common indication.[2] The age of lung transplant candidates has steadily increased over time with 32% of the waiting list candidates in 2018 more than age 65.[3–5] Survival after lung transplantation is improving over time, to a median survival of 6.7 years.[2,6]

Lung Transplant Candidacy

Lung transplantation should be considered for patients with end-stage lung disease who have both a high risk of death from their underlying lung disease (>50% in 1 year) as well as a high likelihood of survival after lung transplantation.[7] Absolute contraindications to lung transplantation include active malignancy, coronary artery disease without the ability to revascularize, significant extrapulmonary organ dysfunction, active tobacco or substance abuse, active infection with highly virulent organisms such as tuberculosis, morbid obesity, and lack of psychosocial support.[7] Relative contraindications vary based on transplant center. There is variability between centers on whether critical illness, mechanical ventilation (MV), and extracorporeal membrane oxygenation (ECMO) support are contraindications to transplant. The upper age limit for lung transplantation

Division of Pulmonary and Critical Care Medicine, University of California San Francisco, 400 Parnassus Street, 5th Floor, San Francisco, CA 94143, USA
* Corresponding author.
E-mail address: alyssa.perez@ucsf.edu

Clin Chest Med 43 (2022) 457–470
https://doi.org/10.1016/j.ccm.2022.04.007

also varies by center but generally is between 70 and 75 years of age.[7]

The Lung Allocation Score

In 2005, organ allocation for lung transplantation in the United States shifted from a time accrual system to the lung allocation score (LAS) in response to high wait list mortality.[8,9] The LAS ranges between 0 and 100, with higher scores prioritizing patients with an increased risk of waiting list mortality and a high probability of 1-year survival.[9,10] These clinical factors include the indication for lung transplantation, patient age, lung function, oxygen requirement, use of mechanical ventilation, and other factors developed to represent the acuity of the patient. Wait list mortality initially decreased with the introduction of the LAS; however, the shortage of available and acceptable donor organs remains a significant limitation to lung transplantation. Wait list mortality remains high, in 2019 being 14.6%.[9,11,12] Higher wait list mortality also reflects the simultaneous increase in the listing and transplantation of sicker and older patients.[3,9,12-16]

CARE OF THE PRELUNG TRANSPLANT PATIENT IN THE INTENSIVE CARE UNIT

Patients listed for lung transplantation ideally wait at home and come into the hospital at the time of donor offer. Factors contributing to prolonged wait time include low LAS, blood type, allosensitization, and recipient size.[17,18] A significant number of patients will outstrip oxygen or noninvasive positive pressure ventilation (NIPPV) needs necessitating hospital admission before the availability of a donor organ. In 2018, 25% of lung transplant wait list candidates were hospitalized before transplantation and 13.6% required intensive care unit level care before transplant.[3] Eight percent of all lung transplant recipients required ECMO and/or mechanical ventilation (MV).[3] As advanced lung disease progresses, ICU admission may be indicated for escalating oxygen requirements, prolonged periods of NIPPV, and bridge to transplant using MV and ECMO. In the absence of absolute, nonmodifiable contraindications to lung transplantation, acute exacerbations of ILD should prompt immediate referral to a transplant center for evaluation for lung transplantation.

Mechanical Ventilation as a Bridge to Lung Transplant

The use of MV was historically considered to be a contraindication to lung transplant because of the association with increased morbidity and mortality before and after lung transplant.[19–21] Early registry studies demonstrated increased mortality in the first year after lung transplant in patients who require MV as bridge.[5,22] An early study examining outcomes in patients with CF found the use of pretransplant MV was associated with prolonged MV after transplant, early graft dysfunction, and increased 1-year mortality.[23] Another early study using UNOS data found the pretransplant use of MV and ECMO correlated with worsened survival.[21,24]

Recent data confer more favorable outcomes after lung transplantation in patients who require bridge with MV. A single-center, retrospective cohort study evaluated outcomes of lung transplant recipients bridged with MV versus MV + ECMO versus no respiratory support; 11.7% (n = 97) of patients required MV before transplantation.[21] They found that MV and MV + ECMO resulted in longer hospital stays but the use of MV did not negatively impact survival.[21] Interestingly, the use of MV + ECMO compared with MV conferred greater survival after 1 year and exceeded survival compared with those who required MV only or no respiratory support pretransplant.[21]

Another larger study using UNOS registry data looked at outcomes of lung transplant recipients bridged with MV versus ECMO versus none between 2005 and 2017.[19] Patients in the bridged groups had greater risk for 1-year mortality compared with the no-bridge group although mortality did not differ between the MV- and ECMO-bridged groups.[19] Five-year mortality was also higher in the bridged groups versus the non-bridged groups, however, did not differ between the MV- and ECMO-bridged groups.[19]

The increasing use of MV as a bridge to lung transplant represents a shifting paradigm reflecting the listing of sicker patients with higher LAS coupled with the ongoing donor shortage and more recent data providing some reassurance that outcomes are acceptable.

Use of Pulmonary Vasodilators

Pulmonary vasodilators such as inhaled nitric oxide are frequently used in the management of refractory hypoxemia in the ICU; however, their use is controversial. While it may transiently improve oxygenation, it has not been found to improve outcomes and may risk acute kidney injury.[25] More than half of the patients awaiting lung transplant have or develop pulmonary hypertension (WHO group I or Group III pulmonary hypertension).[26] The use of pulmonary vasodilators in patients with WHO group III pulmonary hypertension is not well-studied and has not been shown to improve mortality.[27–30] In practice, inhaled pulmonary vasodilators are sometimes used as a bridge to transplant in candidates with worsening hypoxemia and evidence of right ventricular dysfunction or pulmonary hypertension.

Considerations For Mechanical Ventilation In Patients With Advanced Lung Disease

While MV before transplant may confer increased mortality after transplant, outcomes after the utilization of this bridging strategy have improved over time. There are several issues the intensivist must consider when managing a patient with advanced lung disease that requires MV, including the evaluation of pulmonary hypertension (PH), nutritional support, and avoidance of deconditioning.

We use transthoracic echocardiography to evaluate for PH before intubation. If there is evidence of pulmonary hypertension or right ventricular failure, we frequently arrange for ECMO backup at the time of intubation or consider ECMO cannulation before intubation. Low compliance due to advanced fibrotic lung disease is expected and we typically use pressure control or pressure support ventilation strategies.

Frailty is associated with death and delisting before transplant and with increased 1-year mortality after lung transplant.[31–34] The need for MV may portend debility and deconditioning and some centers may consider deep sedation and paralysis grounds for delisting. Early tracheostomy and ECMO should be considered to allow for mobilization before lung transplant. Adequate nutrition is paramount and nasojejunal feeding should be considered early, even ahead of need for MV.

Our practice is to intubate when medically indicated in terms of hypoxemia and/or hypercarbia and to proceed with early tracheostomy to allow for the lightning of sedation and mobilization ahead of lung transplant.

EXTRACORPOREAL MEMBRANE OXYGENATION AS A BRIDGE TO LUNG TRANSPLANT

The benefit of ECMO in the management of hypoxemic respiratory failure was first demonstrated in the neonate population and over the last 15 years has been increasingly adapted to the care of adult patients with acute respiratory distress syndrome as a bridge to recovery.[35] The CESAR trial, published during the H1N1 pandemic in 2009, showed benefit among patients with ARDS cared for in ECMO-capable centers; however, mortality

benefit in the ECMO group was not observed in a 2018 randomized, controlled trial.[36,37]

The use of ECMO as a bridge to lung transplant (BTT) has increased significantly over time. Between 2005 and 2011, 1% of all US lung transplant recipients were bridged using ECMO. This increased to 5% between 2012 and 201,719. ECMO is indicated to prolong the pretransplant life expectancy of patients awaiting lung transplant and to improve the likelihood of survival after transplant.[7]

Who Is a Candidate For Extracorporeal Membrane Oxygenation Bridge To Transplant?

The criteria for ECMO BTT vary by center. Current ISHLT guidelines recommend the consideration of ECMO for younger patients without multi-organ dysfunction and with good potential for rehabilitation.[7]

We prefer to use ECMO BTT in patients who have been fully evaluated for lung transplant and are actively listed. The decision to place a patient on ECMO is based on clinical criteria including the inability to sustain oxygenation or ventilation on maximal MV or evidence of progressive RV dysfunction. Some centers advocate for early ECMO cannulation before overt decompensation to prevent deconditioning and ensure continued rehabilitation.[38]

There is a subset of critically ill patients who are referred to transplant who were not evaluated as outpatients. These patients may progress rapidly and necessitate ECMO cannulation and support before completing the evaluation for lung transplant. This clinical scenario is becoming increasingly salient in the era of the COVID pandemic whereby patients with severe COVID-19 ARDS are placed on ECMO initially as bridge to recovery but ultimately develop irreversible progressive fibrotic lung disease. The use of ECMO in the not-yet-listed patient should be considered on a case-by-case basis.

Outcomes After Bridge To Transplant With Extracorporeal Membrane Oxygenation

Similar to MV, the need for ECMO support was historically considered to be a contraindication to lung transplant. Early studies identified ECMO as a risk factor for mortality after lung transplant with 44% survival at 1 year.[39] To date, there have been no randomized, controlled trials evaluating the efficacy of ECMO in the prelung transplant population and data largely come from registries and case series. A single-center, retrospective cohort study showed favorable outcomes using ECMO BTT.[40] Successful ECMO BTT was achieved in 68% of patients overall, 71% among actively listed, and 60% among emergently listed patients. Thirty-day survival for ECMO BTT was 98% overall and 1-year survival conditional on discharge was 97% overall. There was no difference in 30-day or 1-year survival between those already wait-listed and those emergently listed.[40] As reviewed previously, contemporary literature suggests no difference in mortality between patients bridged with MV versus ECMO.[19,21]

Survival from ECMO is improving with time, center experience, and advances in ECMO technology.[19,21,41,42] A study using UNOS registry data from 2000 to 2011 showed that while 1-year survival after lung transplant remains higher among patients who did not require ECMO BTT, 1-year survival for patients necessitating ECMO BTT improved significantly over the 11-year study period.[43] Single-center case series have demonstrated improvement in survival for ECMO BTT with 1-year survival of 85% to 100%.[38,44–46] Significantly, higher center volume correlates with higher survival likelihood using ECMO BTT.[41]

Types of Extracorporeal Membrane Oxygenation

Venous-venous-ECMO (VV-ECMO) is used in the patient with hypoxemic or hypercarbic respiratory failure without evidence of RV dysfunction.[47] We prefer the placement of dual-lumen cannula in the internal jugular vein to allow for awake, ambulatory ECMO; however, this is not always technically or physiologically feasible. Venous-arterial ECMO (VA-ECMO) is used in the patient with evidence of RV dysfunction.[47] This typically requires femoral-internal jugular cannulation. Central ECMO cannulation may also be used.

Awake and ambulatory ECMO facilitates activity and rehab while awaiting lung transplant (**Fig. 1**). Some centers prefer ECMO without MV although this has not been adequately studied.[38,46] At our center, most of the patients bridged to transplant with ECMO are also on MV and ultimately undergo tracheostomy. We recommend and routinely use ECMO as a method of bridge to transplant in the appropriate patient. At our center, we do not typically offer ECMO to patients above age 65.

CARE OF THE IMMEDIATE POSTLUNG TRANSPLANT PATIENT IN THE INTENSIVE CARE UNIT
Ventilation Strategy

The optimal ventilation strategy after lung transplantation is not established as no randomized, controlled trials exist. Practice has largely been extrapolated from ARDS literature, animal studies,

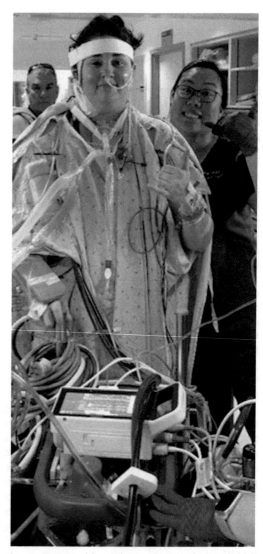

Fig. 1. 33-year-old waitlist patient ambulatory with ECMO + MV bridge to transplant.

and small case series.[48] The overall goal of ventilation postlung transplant is to protect the graft from ventilator-induced lung injury, prevent primary graft dysfunction (PGD), a type of acute lung injury secondary to reperfusion injury that occurs within 72 hours after lung transplant, and allow for the weaning of sedation to optimize mobilization.[48] In practice, this equates with lung-protective ventilation. An international survey of transplant centers found that most centers used lung-protective approaches to mechanical ventilation based on recipient characteristics (as donor characteristics are typically unknown).[49] The survey also found that low Fio_2 strategies are preferred over minimizing PEEP.[49]

Murine models have demonstrated that lung-protective ventilation using low tidal volumes is associated with a lower incidence of PGD.[50,51] Similarly, a single-center study demonstrated that the hyperinflation of the undersized allograft is associated with an increased risk of graft failure.[52] This may be due to ventilation based on recipient characteristics rather than donor characteristics and resultant nonlung protective ventilation, so it is important to consider size mismatch when thinking about ventilation strategies. High peak pressures should also be avoided: a small, single-center, retrospective study found that peak pressures $\geq$ 25 cm H2O in the first 6-hours postoperatively was associated with worse outcomes.[53]

Extubation after lung transplantation may occur as early as postoperative day zero depending on the center. If patients are unable to be extubated within a few days postoperatively, or if they fail extubation, early tracheostomy should be considered to facilitate mobilization. A small, retrospective, single-center study evaluated outcomes with early (<3 days) versus late tracheostomy and found the early tracheostomy group had decreased ICU and hospital length of stay, shorter duration of mechanical ventilation, and earlier mobilization.[54]

It is our practice to use lung-protective ventilation strategies posttransplant. We typically use 6 cc/kg (ideal recipient body weight), volume assists control ventilation mode, PEEP of 5 to 10, lowest Fio_2 to maintain Pao_2 > 60 mm Hg, and early extubation to NIPPV.[48] We also pursue early tracheostomy to optimize rehabilitation in patients who are unable to be extubated.

Single-lung Transplantation

For patients who have undergone single-lung transplantation, the physiologic characteristics of the native lung may significantly impact ventilation strategy.[48] In the patient with fibrotic ILD, the native lung will have markedly reduced compliance compared with the graft and ventilation will preferentially be distributed to the more compliant graft increasing the risk of hyperinflation and injury to the graft.[48] Additionally, exacerbations of ILD can be seen in the native lung after single-lung transplant. Lung-protective ventilation is optimal in this setting.

In contrast, the patient with COPD will have disproportionally higher compliance in the native lung as well as a high degree of airflow obstruction resulting in hyperinflation and the development of auto-PEEP.[48] This is managed with ventilatory strategies used in the management of severe obstructive lung disease including decreased respiratory rate and prolonged expiratory time.[48] The

impact of airflow obstruction and auto-PEEP can be profound and in severe cases may require ECMO or double-lumen ET tube to perform single-lung ventilation.[48,55]

Bronchial Anastomoses

During lung transplant surgery, the bronchial circulation is not reanastomosed; consequently, the bronchi and bronchial anastomoses depend on retrograde flow from the lower pressure pulmonary arterial system for weeks after lung transplantation.[48,56,57] This can result in airway ischemia and mucosal sloughing immediately after lung transplantation and longer-term airway complications including dehiscence, stenosis, and malacia.[48,56,57] It is our practice to perform daily bronchoscopy the first 5 days after lung transplant to manage mucosal sloughing and inspect the anastomoses. New-onset air leak in the early posttransplant patient should prompt evaluation for dehiscence, among other etiologies.

Primary Graft Dysfunction

Primary graft dysfunction (PGD) is a form of acute lung injury that results from ischemia-reperfusion injury during the lung transplant surgery with an incidence of 10% to 30%.[51,58–60] PGD occurs within the first 72 hours after lung transplantation. PGD is diagnosed clinically by the presence of diffuse alveolar infiltrates on chest imaging (in both lungs if a bilateral lung transplant, and in multiple lobes of the transplanted lung if a single transplant) and exclusion of other causes, such as pulmonary edema or pneumonia. PGD is graded by the degree of hypoxemia as defined by Pao_2/Fio_2 ratio, analogous to ARDS (**Table 1**: PGD stages). PGD is graded at four-time points after lung transplantation: 0 hours, 24 hours, 48 hours, and 72 hours.

Table 1
Primary graft dysfunction stages

Grade	Pao_2/Fio_2 Ratio	Radiographic Infiltrates
0	>300	Absent
1	>300	Present
2	200–300	Present
3	<200	Present

Data from Diamond JM, Arcasoy S, Kennedy CC, et al. Report of the International Society for Heart and Lung Transplantation Working Group on Primary Lung Graft Dysfunction, part II: Epidemiology, risk factors, and outcomes—A 2016 Consensus Group statement of the International Society for Heart and Lung Tran. The Journal of Heart and Lung Transplantation. 2017;36(10):1104 to 1113.

PGD is a significant cause of both early and late morbidity and mortality in lung transplant recipients. PGD is associated with the development of chronic lung allograft dysfunction (CLAD).[51,60–63] Risk factors for the development of PGD have been well-described. A ten-center, prospective, cohort study between 2002 and 2010 identified independent risk factors for the development of grade 3 PGD as donor smoking history, diagnosis of ILD, pulmonary hypertension, large-volume blood product transfusion, obesity, use of cardiopulmonary bypass, and elevated Fio_2 during reperfusion.[51] While obesity has been identified as a risk factor for PGD, it is subcutaneous but not visceral adiposity which is associated with PGD.[64] Among patients with pulmonary hypertension, female sex, high right atrial pressure, and creatinine at the time of transplant have all been identified as additional risk factors for the development of PGD.[65] The transplantation of an undersized graft has been associated with a higher risk of severe PGD as well as increased 1-year mortality.[48,66–70]

The treatment of PGD is largely supportive.[71] There have been no randomized, controlled trials evaluating the optimal management of PGD; however, lung-protective ventilation and fluid-conservative strategy are generally used.[48,58,71,72] A small, single-center study demonstrated that the implementation of an evidence-based guideline for the management of postlung transplant ventilation and fluid balance (based on ARDS data and conservative fluid management guided by central venous pressure) was associated with reduced severity of PGD and less fluid administration.[73,74] Inhaled nitric oxide is frequently used as both prophylaxis for and treatment of PGD as it reduces pulmonary artery pressures, although there is no evidence to show definitive benefit in preventing or improving PGD.[71,75–78] It is our practice to use inhaled nitric oxide in all postlung transplant patients as prophylaxis for PGD. Inhaled nitric oxide is then slowly down-titrated based on clinical course, with a slower taper if patients had preexisting pulmonary hypertension.

The initiation of early ECMO (typically VV-ECMO), defined as within 24 hours from the onset of PGD, for severe PGD (PGD 3), has been shown to improve outcomes.[71,79–82] Notably, the initiation of late ECMO is associated with worsened mortality highlighting the importance of the early recognition and management of severe PGD.[71,79–82] Patients considered at high risk for PGD may come out of the OR on ECMO.

Retransplantation for severe PGD can be considered but is generally not recommended due to poor outcomes.[83]

IMMUNOSUPPRESSION AFTER LUNG TRANSPLANT

The goals of immunosuppression after lung transplant are to protect the vulnerable graft from the immune system while simultaneously minimizing adverse effects of immunosuppression.[84,85] The backbone of modern immunosuppression includes a calcineurin inhibitor (CNI), an antiproliferative agent, and a corticosteroid.[84,85] mTOR (mammalian target of rapamycin) inhibitors are commonly used as adjunctive therapy. mTOR inhibitors are typically not added early after transplant because of the significant impact on wound healing.[84,85]

There are 2 CNI used in practice today, cyclosporine and tacrolimus.[85,86] Tacrolimus is currently the most widely used CNI,[86] because of data showing a higher incidence of chronic lung allograft dysfunction (CLAD) observed with cyclosporine at 3 years after transplant compared with tacrolimus, although there was no survival difference.[87] Adverse effects are similar between the 2 agents (**Table 2**: Immunosuppressive Agents).[84,85] Both agents require close monitoring of drug levels (typically troughs) to avoid adverse effects. Target trough is dependent on time from transplant and other factors including comorbidities (chronic kidney disease, malignancy, and CLAD).[84,85]

Our practice is to use tacrolimus, prednisone, and mycophenolate mofetil as the backbone of immunosuppression. We will add mTOR inhibitor if there is renal dysfunction, malignancy, CLAD, or CNI intolerance.

CARE OF THE LATER LUNG TRANSPLANT PATIENT IN THE INTENSIVE CARE UNIT

There are a vast number of complications that can affect the postlung transplant patient and it is useful to consider these in terms of time from transplant. The differential of hypoxemic respiratory failure in a postlung transplant patient is akin to nontransplant patients, although there are some specific posttransplant complications that should be considered. This includes rejection and atypical infections, which are described later in discussion. In the posttransplant patient, bronchoscopy is commonly used early to exclude infection along with transbronchial biopsies to evaluate for rejection if patients can tolerate the procedure. The differential of altered mental status in a postlung transplant patient is also similar to nontransplant patients; however, transplant-specific causes should also be considered.

Table 2
Commonly used immunosuppressive agents and adverse effects

	Calcineurin Inhibitors	Antiproliferative Agents	Corticosteroid	mTOR Inhibitor
Drugs	Tacrolimus Cyclosporine	MMF Azathioprine	Prednisone Methylprednisolone	Everolimus Sirolimus
Adverse Effects	Nephrotoxicity Hypertension Mg wasting Hyperkalemia Tremor Malignancy PRES TMA Headache	Leukopenia Thrombocytopenia Hepatotoxicity Malignancy	Diabetes mellitus Weight gain Hair loss Osteoporosis	Decreased wound healing Proteinuria DVT Pneumonitis Hypertriglyceridemia

Abbreviations: mTOR, mammalian target of rapamycin; Mg, magnesium; PRES, posterior reversible encephalopathy syndrome; TMA, thrombotic microangiopathy; MMF, mycophenolate mofetil; DVT, deep venous thrombosis.

Acute Cellular Rejection

Acute cellular rejection (ACR) is diagnosed by the presence of perivascular and interstitial mononuclear cell infiltrates in the alveoli.[88,89] ACR is relatively common, affecting 27% of lung transplant recipients one or more times within the first year after lung transplant, although it can occur at any point after lung transplant.[2] Clinically, ACR may be asymptomatic or present with acute or subacute dyspnea, cough, fever, and frequently a decrease in lung function measured by spirometery.[89] Radiographically, ACR typically presents with ground-glass opacities and interlobular septal thickening.[89,90]

ACR is typically diagnosed via transbronchial biopsy although in severe presentations, when transbronchial biopsy is not feasible, a clinical diagnosis may be made. Severe ACR may result in hypoxemic respiratory failure due to acute lung injury necessitating mechanical ventilation. ACR is treated with pulse-dose intravenous corticosteroids.[89] Protocols vary based on transplant center. It is our practice to treat moderate and severe ACR

with intravenous methylprednisolone for 3 days followed by oral prednisone taper.

Antibody-mediated rejection (AMR) is a complex pathologic, serologic, and clinical process caused by donor-specific HLA antibodies resulting in allograft dysfunction.[91] AMR can be severe and is an important cause of hypoxemic respiratory failure in the postlung transplant patient. Typically, AMR is treated with high-dose steroids, plasmapheresis, and IVIG, with the consideration of rituximab as additional therapy.

Infections

Immunosuppression puts lung transplant recipients at high risk of infection. For this reason, when there is a concern for severe infection or sepsis, we typically empirically treat with broad-spectrum antibiotics and deescalate based on cultures. Lung transplant recipients are also vulnerable to opportunistic infections including invasive fungal infections and cytomegalovirus (**Table 3**). Invasive fungal infections are common: 8.6% of patients develop

Table 3
Risk factors and sequelae of infection after lung transplant

	Invasive Fungal Infection	CMV Infection

Risk Factors	Single-lung transplant
	Early airway ischemia
	CMV viremia
	Augmented
	  immunosuppression
	Hypogammaglobulinemia
	Aspergillus colonization
		Serostatus
		• Greatest risk = high-risk mismatch
		  (donor positive, recipient negative)
		Recent use of ATG

Sequelae of Infection	2nd most common cause of death CLAD	ACR CLAD

invasive fungal infection during the first year after lung transplant coinciding with when immunosuppression is at its peak.[92] Treatment is targeted at the fungal species. *Aspergillus spp* is the most common cause of invasive fungal infection after lung transplant, although mucormycosis and scedosporium are also common pathogens.[92,93] Infection with cytomegalovirus (CMV) is also associated with morbidity and mortality after lung transplant.[94] CMV infection is typically treated with valganciclovir or ganciclovir; however, it is notable that CMV resistance to valganciclovir is increasingly common.[95]

Community-acquired viral infections (CARVI) can also be devastating for lung transplant recipients. CARVI have been associated with increased risk of CLAD and mortality.[96,97] Respiratory viral panel PCR should be checked early in the course and antiviral therapy, if indicated, should be initiated. Some centers empirically give a prednisone pulse and taper to avoid immune activation from the viral infection.

Chronic lung Allograft Dysfunction

Long-term survival in lung transplantation is limited by the development of CLAD, the most common cause of death after the first year of lung transplantation.[98] The prevalence of CLAD is 50% at 5 years after lung transplant.[98–100]

CLAD is defined as a sustained decline in FEV1 of $\geq$ 20% from baseline, with or without a decline in FVC by $\geq$ 20%.[99] CLAD can be predominantly obstructive, restrictive, or mixed[101] (**Table 4**). Two predominant phenotypes of CLAD have emerged. BOS, bronchiolitis obliterans syndrome, is an obstructive phenotype and RAS, restrictive allograft syndrome, is a restrictive phenotype. In BOS, remodeling causes the obliteration of terminal bronchioles resulting in severe obstruction.[99,102]

Treatment of both obstructive and restrictive CLAD is limited and centers on augmenting immunosuppression, photopheresis, azithromycin prophylaxis, use of antifibrotics for the restrictive phenotype, and in some patients, retransplantation.[100]

Altered Mental Status

Calcineurin inhibitors are a well-known cause of posterior reversible encephalopathy syndrome (PRES) which can present with altered mental status, difficult-to-control hypertension, headache, blindness, confusion, and coma.[103] Treatment for PRES is the discontinuation of the offending CNI, with subsequent alteration of the immunosuppression regimen, either switching to an mTOR inhibitor (which does not cause PRES) or using a different CNI (ie, cyclosporine instead of tacrolimus) with very close observation. Notably, PRES can occur at any level of CNI.

Calcineurin inhibitors are also an important cause of thrombotic microangiopathy (TMA) including thrombotic thrombocytopenic purpura/ hemolytic uremic syndrome (TTP/HUS).[104] TTP/ HUS classically presents as altered mental status, fever, acute kidney injury, microangiopathic hemolytic anemia, and thrombocytopenia. Treatment for CNI-induced TTP/HUS is the discontinuation of the offending CNI agent.

TREND: LUNG TRANSPLANT FOR COVID-19

The COVID-19 pandemic emerged in early 2020 and resulted in a surge of cases of ARDS, overwhelming hospital systems worldwide, and ushering in an era of uncharted territory for both the intensive care unit and the field of lung transplantation. Lung transplant as a therapeutic option for severe COVID-19-associated ARDS has been increasingly discussed and pursued over the last year.

Historically, ARDS has been an uncommon indication for lung transplantation and there is little data regarding candidate selection in patients with ARDS and regarding outcomes in this population.[105] Severe COVID-19 infection can be associated with the need for deep sedation and paralysis making it difficult to have an informed

Table 4
Phenotypes of chronic lung allograft dysfunction[99,101,102]

	Definition	Sequelae
Obstructive CLAD	↓ in FEV1 by $\geq$ 20%	Severe airflow obstruction, obstructive lung disease
Restrictive CLAD	↓ FEV1 ± FVC by $\geq$ 20%, ↓ in TLC to < 90%, AND Opacities on imaging	Severe restrictive lung disease Portends worse outcome

Abbreviations: CLAD, chronic lung allograft dysfunction; FEV1, forced expiratory volume in 1 s; TLC, total lung capacity.

conversation about transplant, as well as limiting rehabilitation potential. Further, lung recovery after ARDS, including severe COVID-ARDS, is difficult to prognosticate and may take time; therefore, the timing of proceeding with lung transplant is tricky. There are also ethical considerations due to the impact on patients with end-stage lung disease who are already waiting for lung transplantation while there is a constant shortage of acceptable donors.

Despite these considerations, lung transplantation has been increasingly pursued as a therapeutic option for severe COVID-19 ARDS[109–112]. A recently published *Lancet* case series examined the short-term outcomes of 12 patients with severe COVID-19 ARDS who underwent lung transplantation at 6 centers worldwide.[106] This was a high-acuity cohort of patients, with a median LAS of 85.7 [106]. Eleven of 12 were on VV-ECMO at the time of listing and the remaining patient was on mechanical ventilation.[106] Survival thus far has been acceptable with 100% 30-day survival and only one death at posttransplant day 61.[106]

To date, we have transplanted 6 patients with severe COVID-19 ARDS at our center. Five of the 6 patients were transplanted from ECMO. Multidrug-resistant infections were common. Hospitalizations are prolonged and discharge to acute rehabilitation facility is common.

We believe transplant for severe COVID-19 ARDS should be considered on a case-by-case basis and generally agree with the criteria proposed by Bharat and colleagues, which include patients ≤ 55 years of age, single organ system failure, BMI ≤ 32, COVID-19 PCR negative, ability to be awake and show rehab potential (can be on ECMO), and demonstrate lack of recoverability of lung function after a minimum of 4 weeks into illness course.[106]

FUTURE DIRECTIONS

Critical care is a pillar of the care of the lung transplant recipient. Future studies should focus on refining criteria for critically ill patients with advanced lung disease requiring transplant, particularly with the recent COVID-19 pandemic. More information is needed regarding the short- and long-term outcomes of COVID-19 ARDS lung transplant recipients. Consensus is also needed regarding timing and appropriate candidate selection.

A major limitation in lung transplantation and cause of wait list mortality is donor shortage. Novel approaches to organ donation are needed to expand the donor pool and allow more patients to successfully get to lung transplantation. A recent study out of Brigham and Women's Hospital, for example, demonstrated the successful

Table 5
Clinics care points: Postlung transplant complications over time

Immediate (<1 mo)	Early (>1 mo)	Late
Primary Graft Dysfunction	Acute cellular rejection Antibody mediated rejection	Chronic Lung Allograft Dysfunction
Postoperative hemorrhage and hematoma Hyperacute rejection Infection: • Pretransplant colonization • Donor derived • Hospital acquired	Infection: • Opportunistic: CMV, EBV, PJP, invasive fungal, toxoplasmosis • Atypical infections: NTM, TB, nocardia, actinomyces • Community and hospital acquired • CARVI TMA	Infection: • Opportunistic: CMV, EBV, PJP, invasive fungal, toxoplasmosis • Atypical infections: NTM, TB, nocardia, actinomyces • Community and hospital acquired • CARVI Malignancy
Anastomotic dehiscence Pleural effusions	PRES Anastomotic stenosis	• PTLD • Skin cancer: SCC, BCC, melanoma
	Pleural effusions	Pleural effusions
		TMA
		PRES

Abbreviations: CMV, cytomegalovirus; EBV, Epstein–Barr virus; PJP, pneumocystis jirovecii; NTM, nontuberculous mycobacterium; TB, tuberculosis; CARVI, community-acquired respiratory viral infection; TMA, thrombotic microangiopathy; PRES, posterior reversible encephalopathy syndrome; PTLD, posttransplant lymphoproliferative disorder; SCC, squamous cell carcinoma; BCC, basal cell carcinoma.

transplantation of patients without hepatitis C with hepatitis C-positive organs.[107] Initiation of treatment with antivirals within a few hours of transplantation, and continued for 4 weeks, prevented the development of hepatitis C infection in recipients.[107] Routinely using hepatitis C-positive organs has the potential to greatly expand the donor pool.

Further understanding of PGD including pathogenesis, risk factors, as well as prevention and treatment is also needed as PGD remains a significant source of morbidity and mortality after lung transplantation. Similarly, there is a need for a better understanding of the pathogenesis of CLAD as well as better and more targeted treatment modalities. CLAD remains a limiting factor of longevity after lung transplantation and the most common cause of death after the first year.[6,102,108,109]

We expect that as knowledge evolves, the number and survival of lung transplant recipients will continue to increase (**Table 5**).

DISCLOSURE

A.A. Perez has no disclosures. R.J. Shah has no disclosures.

REFERENCES

1. Singer JP, Katz PP, Soong A, et al. Effect of lung transplantation on health-related quality of life in the era of the lung allocation score: a U.S. Prospective cohort study. Am J Transplant 2017;17(5):1334–45.
2. Chambers DC, Cherikh WS, Harhay MO, et al. The international Thoracic organ transplant registry of the international Society for Heart and lung transplantation: Thirty-sixth adult lung and heart-lung transplantation report—2019; focus theme: donor and recipient size match. J Heart Lung Transplant 2019;38(10):1042–55.
3. Valapour M, Lehr CJ, Skeans MA, et al. OPTN/SRTR 2018 Annual data report: lung. Am J Transplant official J Am Soc Transplant Am Soc Transpl Surgeons. 2020;20(Suppl s):427–508.
4. Hall DJ, Jeng EI, Gregg JA, et al. The impact of donor and recipient age: older lung transplant recipients do not require younger lungs. Ann Thorac Surg 2019;107(3):868–76.
5. Yusen RD, Christie JD, Edwards LB, et al. The registry of the international Society for heart and lung transplantation: Thirtieth adult lung and heart-lung transplant report – 2013; focus theme: age. The J Heart Lung Transplant 2013;32(10):965–78.
6. Bos S, Vos R, van Raemdonck DE, et al. Survival in adult lung transplantation: where are we in 2020? Curr Opin Organ Transplant 2020;25(3):268–73.
7. Weill D, Benden C, Corris PA, et al. A consensus document for the selection of lung transplant candidates: 2014–an update from the pulmonary transplantation Council of the international Society for heart and lung transplantation. J Heart Lung Transplant official Publ Int Soc Heart Transplant 2015;34(1):1–15.
8. Egan TM. How should lungs Be allocated for transplant? Semin Respir Crit Care Med 2018;39(2):126–37.
9. Egan TM, Edwards LB. Effect of the lung allocation score on lung transplantation in the United States. The J Heart Lung Transplant 2016;35(4):433–9.
10. Egan TM, Murray S, Bustami RT, et al. Development of the new lung allocation system in the United States. Am J Transplant official J Am Soc Transplant Am Soc Transpl Surgeons. 2006;6(5 Pt 2):1212–27.
11. Valapour M, Lehr CJ, Skeans MA, et al. OPTN/SRTR 2019 Annual data report: lung. Am J Transplant 2021;21(S2):441–520.
12. Crawford TC, Grimm JC, Magruder JT, et al. Lung transplant mortality is improving in recipients with a lung allocation score in the upper Quartile. Ann Thorac Surg 2017;103(5):1607–13.
13. Valapour M, Skeans MA, Smith JM, et al. OPTN/SRTR 2015 Annual data report: lung. Am J Transplant official J Am Soc Transplant Am Soc Transpl Surgeons. 2017;17(Suppl 1):357–424.
14. Lyu DM, Goff RR, Chan KM. The lung allocation score and its Relevance. Semin Respir Crit Care Med 2021;42(3):346–56.
15. Kilic A, Merlo CA, Conte J v, et al. Lung transplantation in patients 70 years old or older: have outcomes changed after implementation of the lung allocation score? J Thorac Cardiovasc Surg 2012;144(5):1133–8.
16. Lehr CJ, Blackstone EH, McCurry KR, et al. Extremes of age decrease survival in adults after lung transplant. Chest 2020;157(4):907–15.
17. Barac YD, Mulvihill MS, Cox ML, et al. Implications of blood group on lung transplantation rates: a propensity-matched registry analysis. The J Heart Lung Transplant 2019;38(1):73–82.
18. Tague LK, Witt CA, Byers DE, et al. Association between allosensitization and waiting list outcomes among adult lung transplant candidates in the United States. Ann Am Thorac Soc 2019;16(7):846–52.
19. Hayanga JWA, Hayanga HK, Holmes SD, et al. Mechanical ventilation and extracorporeal membrane oxygenation as a bridge to lung transplantation: Closing the gap. The J Heart Lung Transplant 2019;38(10):1104–11.
20. Smits JMA, Mertens BJA, Van Houwelingen HC, et al. Predictors of lung transplant survival in eurotransplant. Am J Transplant 2003;3(11):1400–6.

21. Hayanga AJ, Du AL, Joubert K, et al. Mechanical ventilation and extracorporeal membrane oxygenation as a bridging strategy to lung transplantation: significant Gains in survival. Am J Transplant 2018;18(1):125–35.

22. Fuehner T, Kuehn C, Welte T, et al. ICU care before and after lung transplantation. Chest 2016;150(2): 442–50.

23. Elizur A, Sweet SC, Huddleston CB, et al. Pre-transplant mechanical ventilation increases short-term morbidity and mortality in pediatric patients with cystic fibrosis. The J Heart Lung Transplant 2007;26(2):127–31.

24. Mason DP, Thuita L, Nowicki ER, et al. Should lung transplantation be performed for patients on mechanical respiratory support? The US experience. J Thorac Cardiovasc Surg 2010;139(3):765–73.e1.

25. Gebistorf F, Karam O, Wetterslev J, et al. Inhaled nitric oxide for acute respiratory distress syndrome (ARDS) in children and adults. Cochrane database Syst Rev 2016;2016(6):CD002787.

26. Porteous MK, Lee JC, Lederer DJ, et al. Clinical risk factors and prognostic model for primary graft dysfunction after lung transplantation in patients with pulmonary hypertension. Ann Am Thorac Soc 2017;14(10):1514–22.

27. Network IPFCR, Zisman DA, Schwarz M, et al. A controlled trial of sildenafil in advanced idiopathic pulmonary fibrosis. New Engl J Med 2010; 363(7):620–8.

28. Prins KW, Duval S, Markowitz J, et al. Chronic use of PAH-specific therapy in World health Organization group III pulmonary hypertension: a systematic review and meta-analysis. Pulm Circ 2017;7(1):145–55.

29. Han MK, Bach DS, Hagan PG, et al. Sildenafil preserves exercise capacity in patients with idiopathic pulmonary fibrosis and right-sided ventricular dysfunction. Chest 2013;143(6):1699–708.

30. Thenappan T, Ormiston ML, Ryan JJ, et al. Pulmonary arterial hypertension: pathogenesis and clinical management. BMJ (Clinical research ed) 2018;360:j5492.

31. Singer JP, Diamond JM, Gries CJ, et al. Frailty phenotypes, disability, and outcomes in adult candidates for lung transplantation. Am J Respir Crit Care Med 2015;192(11):1325–34.

32. Venado A, Kolaitis N, Huang C, et al. Frailty after lung transplantation is associated with impaired health related quality of life and mortality. Thorax 2020;75(8):669–78.

33. Singer JP, Diamond JM, Anderson MR, et al. Frailty phenotypes and mortality after lung transplantation: a prospective cohort study. Am J Transplant 2018;18(8):1995–2004.

34. Venado A, McCulloch C, Greenland JR, et al. Frailty trajectories in adult lung transplantation: a cohort study. The J Heart Lung Transplant 2019; 38(7):699–707.

35. Keller SP. Contemporary approaches in the use of extracorporeal membrane oxygenation to support patients waiting for lung transplantation. Ann Cardiothorac Surg 2020;9(1):29–41.

36. Peek GJ, Mugford M, Tiruvoipati R, et al. Efficacy and economic assessment of conventional ventilatory support versus extracorporeal membrane oxygenation for severe adult respiratory failure (CESAR): a multicentre randomised controlled trial. Lancet 2009;374(9698):1351–63.

37. Combes A, Hajage D, Capellier G, et al. Extracorporeal membrane oxygenation for severe acute respiratory distress syndrome. New Engl J Med 2018;378(21):1965–75.

38. Biscotti M, Gannon WD, Agerstrand C, et al. Awake extracorporeal membrane oxygenation as bridge to lung transplantation: a 9-year experience. Ann Thorac Surg 2017;104(2):412–9.

39. Russo MJ, Davies RR, Hong KN, et al. Who is the high-risk recipient? Predicting mortality after lung transplantation using pretransplant risk factors. J Thorac Cardiovasc Surg 2009;138(5):1234–8.e1.

40. Kukreja J, Tsou S, Chen J, et al. Risk factors and outcomes of extracorporeal membrane oxygenation as a bridge to lung transplantation. Semin Thorac Cardiovasc Surg 2020;32(4):772–85.

41. Hayanga JWA, Lira A, Aboagye JK, et al. Extracorporeal membrane oxygenation as a bridge to lung transplantation: what lessons might we learn from volume and expertise? Interactive Cardiovasc Thorac Surg 2016;22(4):406–10.

42. Hayanga JA, Lira A, Vlahu T, et al. Procedural volume and survival after lung transplantation in the United States: the need to look beyond volume in the establishment of quality metrics. Am J Surg 2016;211(4):671–6.

43. Hayanga AJ, Aboagye J, Esper S, et al. Extracorporeal membrane oxygenation as a bridge to lung transplantation in the United States: an evolving strategy in the management of rapidly advancing pulmonary disease. J Thorac Cardiovasc Surg 2015;149(1):291–6.

44. Rehder KJ, Turner DA, Hartwig MG, et al. Active rehabilitation during extracorporeal membrane oxygenation as a bridge to lung transplantation. Respir Care 2013;58(8):1291 LP–1298.

45. Hoopes CW, Kukreja J, Golden J, et al. Extracorporeal membrane oxygenation as a bridge to pulmonary transplantation. J Thorac Cardiovasc Surg 2013;145(3):862–8.

46. Hakim AH, Ahmad U, McCurry KR, et al. Contemporary outcomes of extracorporeal membrane oxygenation used as bridge to lung transplantation. Ann Thorac Surg 2018;106(1):192–8.

47. Biscotti M, Sonett J, Bacchetta M. ECMO as bridge to lung transplant. Thorac Surg Clin 2015;25(1): 17–25.

48. Barnes L, Reed RM, Parekh KR, et al. Mechanical ventilation for the lung transplant recipient. Curr pulmonology Rep 2015;4(2):88–96.

49. Beer A, Reed RM, Bölükbas S, et al. Mechanical ventilation after lung transplantation. An international survey of practices and preferences. Ann Am Thorac Soc 2014;11(4):546–53.

50. de Perrot M, Imai Y, Volgyesi GA, et al. Effect of ventilator-induced lung injury on the development of reperfusion injury in a rat lung transplant model. J Thorac Cardiovasc Surg 2002;124(6): 1137–44.

51. Diamond JM, Lee JC, Kawut SM, et al. Clinical risk factors for primary graft dysfunction after lung transplantation. Am J Respir Crit Care Med 2013; 187(5):527–34.

52. Kozower BD, Meyers BF, Ciccone AM, et al. Potential for detrimental hyperinflation after lung transplantation with application of negative pleural pressure to undersized lung grafts. J Thorac Cardiovasc Surg 2003;125(2):430–2.

53. Thakuria L, Davey R, Romano R, et al. Mechanical ventilation after lung transplantation. J Crit Care 2016;31(1):110–8.

54. Miyoshi R, Chen-Yoshikawa TF, Hamaji M, et al. Effect of early tracheostomy on clinical outcomes in critically ill lung transplant recipients. Gen Thorac Cardiovasc Surg 2018;66(9):529–36.

55. Lucangelo U, Del Sorbo L, Boffini M, et al. Protective ventilation for lung transplantation. Curr Opin anaesthesiology 2012;25(2):170–4.

56. Crespo MM, McCarthy DP, Hopkins PM, et al. ISHLT Consensus Statement on adult and pediatric airway complications after lung transplantation: Definitions, grading system, and therapeutics. The J Heart Lung Transplant 2018; 37(5):548–63.

57. Machuzak M, Santacruz JF, Gildea T, et al. Airway complications after lung transplantation. Thorac Surg Clin 2015;25(1):55–75.

58. Snell GI, Yusen RD, Weill D, et al. Report of the ISHLT Working group on primary lung graft dysfunction, part I: Definition and grading—a 2016 consensus group statement of the international Society for heart and lung transplantation. The J Heart Lung Transplant 2017;36(10):1097–103.

59. Shah RJ, Diamond JM. Primary graft dysfunction (PGD) following lung transplantation. Semin Respir Crit Care Med 2018;39(2):148–54.

60. Christie JD, Kotloff RM, Ahya VN, et al. The effect of primary graft dysfunction on survival after lung transplantation. Am J Respir Crit Care Med 2005; 171(11):1312–6.

61. Huang HJ, Yusen RD, Meyers BF, et al. Late primary graft dysfunction after lung transplantation and bronchiolitis obliterans syndrome. Am J Transplant 2008;8(11):2454–62.

62. Daud SA, Yusen RD, Meyers BF, et al. Impact of immediate primary lung allograft dysfunction on bronchiolitis obliterans syndrome. Am J Respir Crit Care Med 2007;175(5):507–13.

63. Kreisel D, Krupnick AS, Puri V, et al. Short- and long-term outcomes of 1000 adult lung transplant recipients at a single center. J Thorac Cardiovasc Surg 2011;141(1):215–22.

64. Anderson MR, Udupa JK, Edwin E, et al. Adipose tissue quantification and primary graft dysfunction after lung transplantation: the Lung Transplant Body Composition study. The J Heart Lung Transplant 2019;38(12):1246–56.

65. Porteous MK, Lee JC, Lederer DJ, et al. Clinical risk factors and prognostic model for primary graft dysfunction after lung transplantation in patients with pulmonary hypertension. Ann Am Thorac Soc 2017;14(10):1514–22.

66. Eberlein M, Reed RM, Bolukbas S, et al. Lung size mismatch and primary graft dysfunction after bilateral lung transplantation. The J Heart Lung Transplant 2015;34(2):233–40.

67. Eberlein M, Bolukbas S, Reed RM. Bilateral lobar lung transplantation and size mismatch by pTLC-ratio. Eur J cardio-thoracic Surg official J Eur Assoc Cardio-thoracic Surg 2013;44(2):394–5.

68. Eberlein M, Permutt S, Chahla MF, et al. Lung size mismatch in bilateral lung transplantation is associated with allograft function and bronchiolitis obliterans syndrome. Chest 2012;141(2):451–60.

69. Eberlein M, Reed RM, Permutt S, et al. Parameters of donor-recipient size mismatch and survival after bilateral lung transplantation. The J Heart Lung Transplant 2012;31(11):1207–13.e7.

70. Eberlein M, Reed RM, Maidaa M, et al. Donor-recipient size matching and survival after lung transplantation. A cohort study. Ann Am Thorac Soc 2013;10(5):418–25.

71. Shargall Y, Guenther G, Ahya VN, et al. Report of the ISHLT Working group on primary lung graft dysfunction Part VI: treatment. The J Heart Lung Transplant 2005;24(10):1489–500.

72. Geube MA, Perez-Protto SE, McGrath TL, et al. Increased Intraoperative fluid Administration is associated with severe primary graft dysfunction after lung transplantation. Anesth analgesia 2016; 122(4):1081–8.

73. Currey J, Pilcher DV, Davies A, et al. Implementation of a management guideline aimed at minimizing the severity of primary graft dysfunction after lung transplant. J Thorac Cardiovasc Surg 2010;139(1):154–61.

74. Pilcher DV, Scheinkestel CD, Snell GI, et al. High central venous pressure is associated with prolonged mechanical ventilation and increased mortality after lung transplantation. J Thorac Cardiovasc Surg 2005;129(4):912–8.

75. Cornfield DN, Milla CE, Haddad IY, et al. Safety of inhaled nitric oxide after lung transplantation. J Heart Lung Transplant 2003;22(8):903–7.

76. Ardehali A, Laks H, Levine M, et al. A prospective trial of inhaled nitric oxide in clinical lung transplantation. Transplantation 2001;72(1):112–5.

77. Botha P, Jeyakanthan M, Rao JN, et al. Inhaled nitric oxide for modulation of ischemia-reperfusion injury in lung transplantation. The J Heart Lung Transplant 2007;26(11):1199–205.

78. Meade MO, Granton JT, Matte-Martyn A, et al. A randomized trial of inhaled nitric oxide to prevent ischemia-reperfusion injury after lung transplantation. Am J Respir Crit Care Med 2003;167(11): 1483–9.

79. Wigfield CH, Lindsey JD, Steffens TG, et al. Early institution of extracorporeal membrane oxygenation for primary graft dysfunction after lung transplantation improves outcome. The J Heart Lung Transplant 2007;26(4):331–8.

80. Fischer S, Bohn D, Rycus P, et al. Extracorporeal membrane oxygenation for primary graft dysfunction after lung transplantation: analysis of the extracorporeal life support Organization (ELSO) registry. The J Heart Lung Transplant 2007; 26(5):472–7.

81. Bermudez CA, Adusumilli PS, McCurry KR, et al. Extracorporeal membrane oxygenation for primary graft dysfunction after lung transplantation: long-term survival. Ann Thorac Surg 2009;87(3):854–60.

82. Bellier J, Lhommet P, Bonnette P, et al. Extracorporeal membrane oxygenation for grade 3 primary graft dysfunction after lung transplantation: long-term outcomes. Clin Transplant 2019;33(3):e13480.

83. Diamond JM, Arcasoy S, Kennedy CC, et al. Report of the international Society for heart and lung transplantation Working group on primary lung graft dysfunction, part II: Epidemiology, risk factors, and outcomes—a 2016 consensus group statement of the international Society for heart and lung tran. The J Heart Lung Transplant 2017; 36(10):1104–13.

84. Chung PA, Dilling DF. Immunosuppressive strategies in lung transplantation. Ann translational Med 2020;8(6):409.

85. Scheffert JL, Raza K. Immunosuppression in lung transplantation. J Thorac Dis 2014;6(8):1039–53.

86. Christie JD, Edwards LB, Kucheryavaya AY, et al. The registry of the international Society for heart and lung transplantation: 29th adult lung and heart-lung transplant report—2012. The J Heart Lung Transplant 2012;31(10):1073–86.

87. Treede H, Glanville AR, Klepetko W, et al. Tacrolimus and cyclosporine have differential effects on the risk of development of bronchiolitis obliterans syndrome: results of a prospective, randomized international trial in lung transplantation. The J Heart Lung Transplant 2012;31(8):797–804.

88. Stewart S, Fishbein MC, Snell GI, et al. Revision of the 1996 Working Formulation for the Standardization of Nomenclature in the diagnosis of lung rejection. The J Heart Lung Transplant 2007;26(12): 1229–42.

89. Greer M, Werlein C, Jonigk D. Surveillance for acute cellular rejection after lung transplantation. Ann translational Med 2020;8(6):410.

90. di Piazza A, Mamone G, Caruso S, et al. Acute rejection after lung transplantation: association between histopathological and CT findings. La radiologia Med 2019;124(10):1000–5.

91. Levine DJ, Glanville AR, Aboyoun C, et al. Antibody-mediated rejection of the lung: a consensus report of the international Society for heart and lung transplantation. The J Heart Lung Transplant 2016;35(4):397–406.

92. Pappas PG, Alexander BD, Andes DR, et al. Invasive fungal infections among organ transplant recipients: results of the transplant-associated infection surveillance Network (TRANSNET). Clin Infect Dis 2010;50(8):1101–11.

93. Arthurs SK, Eid AJ, Deziel PJ, et al. The impact of invasive fungal diseases on survival after lung transplantation. Clin Transplant 2010;24(3):341–8.

94. Alsaeed M, Husain S. Infections in heart and lung transplant recipients. Crit Care Clin 2019;35(1): 75–93.

95. Chang A, Musk M, Lavender M, et al. Cytomegalovirus viremia in lung transplantation during and after prophylaxis. Transpl Infect Dis 2019;21(3): e13069.

96. Fisher CE, Preiksaitis CM, Lease ED, et al. Symptomatic respiratory virus infection and chronic lung allograft dysfunction. Clin Infect Dis 2016; 62(3):313–9.

97. Peghin M, Los-Arcos I, Hirsch HH, et al. Community-acquired respiratory Viruses are a risk factor for chronic lung allograft dysfunction. Clin Infect Dis official Publ Infect Dis Soc America 2019; 69(7):1192–7.

98. Yusen RD, Edwards LB, Kucheryavaya AY, et al. The registry of the international Society for heart and lung transplantation: Thirty-second Official adult lung and heart-lung transplantation report—2015; focus theme: early graft failure. The J Heart Lung Transplant 2015;34(10):1264–77.

99. Verleden GM, Raghu G, Meyer KC, et al. A new classification system for chronic lung allograft dysfunction. The J Heart Lung Transplant 2014; 33(2):127–33.

100. Benden C, Haughton M, Leonard S, et al. Therapy options for chronic lung allograft dysfunction–bronchiolitis obliterans syndrome following first-line immunosuppressive strategies: a systematic review. The J Heart Lung Transplant 2017;36(9):921–33.

101. Verleden GM, Glanville AR, Lease ED, et al. Chronic lung allograft dysfunction: Definition, diagnostic criteria, and approaches to treatment—A consensus report from the Pulmonary Council of the ISHLT. The J Heart Lung Transplant 2019;38(5):493–503.

102. Meyer KC, Raghu G, Verleden GM, et al. An international ISHLT/ATS/ERS clinical practice guideline: diagnosis and management of bronchiolitis obliterans syndrome. Eur Respir J 2014;44(6):1479–503.

103. Dhar R. Neurologic complications of transplantation. Neurocrit Care 2018;28(1):4–11.

104. Boyer NL, Niven A, Edelman J. Tacrolimus-associated thrombotic microangiopathy in a lung transplant recipient. BMJ case Rep 2013;2013. bcr2012007351.

105. Chang Y, Lee SO, Shim TS, et al. Lung transplantation as a therapeutic option in acute respiratory distress syndrome. Transplantation 2018;102(5):829–37.

106. Bharat A, Machuca TN, Querrey M, et al. Early outcomes after lung transplantation for severe COVID-19: a series of the first consecutive cases from four countries. Lancet Respir Med 2021;9(5):487–97.

107. Woolley AE, Singh SK, Goldberg HJ, et al. Heart and lung transplants from HCV-infected donors to Uninfected recipients. New Engl J Med 2019;380(17):1606–17.

108. Allyn PR, Duffy EL, Humphries RM, et al. Graft Loss and CLAD-onset is Hastened by viral pneumonia after lung transplantation. Transplantation 2016;100(11):2424–31.

109. Kulkarni HS, Cherikh WS, Chambers DC, et al. Bronchiolitis obliterans syndrome-free survival after lung transplantation: an international Society for heart and lung transplantation Thoracic transplant registry analysis. J Heart Lung Transplant 2019;38(1):5–16.

Obstetric Disorders and Critical Illness

Kelly M. Griffin, MD[a],*, Corrina Oxford-Horrey, MD[b], Ghada Bourjeily, MD[c]

KEYWORDS

- Obstetric critical care • Postpartum hemorrhage • Hypertensive disorders of pregnancy
- HELLP syndrome • Acute fatty liver of pregnancy • Peripartum cardiomyopathy
- Amniotic fluid embolism • Pulmonary embolism

KEY POINTS

- Pregnant women may become critically ill due to obstetric or nonobstetric illness. The intensivists caring for them must have a fundamental understanding of maternal physiology.
- The most common obstetric-related conditions that lead to critical illness include postpartum hemorrhage; the hypertensive disorders of pregnancy; hemolysis, elevated liver enzymes, and low platelets syndrome; acute fatty liver of pregnancy; amniotic fluid embolism; and peripartum cardiomyopathy.
- Two nonobstetric conditions that cause life-threatening illness in pregnant women include pulmonary embolism and Covid-19.
- An understanding of the physiology and best management of these conditions is essential for providing best care to one's patients. We provide presentations, physiology and management of these conditions in this review.

INTRODUCTION

Pregnant and postpartum women rarely need the involvement of intensivists in their care. When they do, it is crucial for their critical care physicians to be prepared to provide the best, most well-informed care by an interdisciplinary team including the patient's obstetrician, maternal–fetal medicine (MFM) specialist, obstetric anesthesiologist, and other relevant specialties.

There are over 3.5 million live births per year in the United States,[1] and UNICEF estimates over 130 million annual births worldwide. Globally, maternal mortality shows a great variation among countries, but it approaches 216 per 100,000 births.[2] Similarly, severe maternal morbidity (SMM) also varies greatly between more- and less-resourced regions. In the United States, maternal mortality has been on the rise, nearing 17.4 per 100,000 live births, with significant ethnic and racial variability[3] and cardiovascular diseases as the most common causes.[4] Maternal mortality is higher in the United States than in all other developed countries and is justifiably considered a crisis, hence the need to act swiftly to identify causes for this rise and educate providers on the care of pregnant women. There are clear racial discrepancies in maternal morbidity and mortality in the United States. Black women in this country have a maternal mortality rate 2.5 times that of white women.[5] Black women are also more likely to be readmitted with severe morbidity in the postpartum period than white women.[6] This warrants particular awareness and recognition of structural and intrinsic biases when assessing patients for ICU admission and care and ongoing work to eliminate these disparities.

a Department of Medicine, Division of Pulmonary and Critical Care, Weill Cornell Medical College, 525 East 68th Street, New York, NY 10065, USA; b Department of Obstetrics and Gynecology, Division of Maternal Fetal Medicine, Weill Cornell Medical College, 525 East 68th, Street, New York, NY 10065, USA; c Department of Medicine, Divisions of Pulmonary, Critical Care and Sleep Medicine and Obstetric Medicine, Warren Alpert Medical School of Brown University, 146 West River Street, Providence, RI 02904, USA
* Corresponding author.
E-mail address: keg2007@med.cornell.edu

Clin Chest Med 43 (2022) 471–488
https://doi.org/10.1016/j.ccm.2022.04.008

Abbreviations	
ICU	intensive care unit
IM/IV	intramuscular/ intravenous
ARDS	acute respiratory distress syndrome
DIC	disseminated intravascular coagulation
SBP	systolic blood pressure
DBP	diastolic blood pressure
BP	blood pressure
LDH	lactate dehydrogenase
AST	aspartate transaminase
ALT	alanine transaminase
PT	prothrombin time
PTT	partial thromboplastin time
APTT	activated partial thromboplastin time
ECMO	extracorporeal membrane oxygenation
INR	international normalized ratio
TTE	transthoracic echocardiogram
TEE	transesophageal echocardiogram
ECMO	extracorporeal membrane oxygenation
RV	right ventricle
VA	venoarterial
IF	insulin-like growth factor
CHEST	the official publication of the American College of Chest Physicians
NIH	National Institutes of Health
UNICEF	United Nations International Children's Emergency Fund
WHO	World Health Organization

Obstetric patients may become critically ill due to either obstetric or non-obstetric illness. The most common causes for pregnant and peripartum women to be admitted to an ICU—with variations depending on the robustness of health care systems and resources available therein—include postpartum hemorrhage (PPH), hypertensive disorders of pregnancy (HDP), sepsis, and pulmonary embolism (PE).[7–10] A fundamental knowledge of obstetric critical illness and specific aspects of maternal care and physiology is essential.

In this article, we will discuss some of the more common obstetric-related conditions that can lead to critical illness and require management in an ICU. We will also discuss PE and Covid-19. Despite not being specific to obstetric patients, PE is a common, life-threatening diagnosis in pregnancy with particular risks and management aspects. Covid-19 does not seem to occur with higher frequency in pregnant women, but it does lead to higher rates of ICU admissions and mechanical ventilation in pregnant women than in

their nonpregnant peers.[11] Its prevalence during our current global pandemic makes it important to discuss in this article.

PHYSIOLOGIC CHANGES IN PREGNANCY MOST RELEVANT TO CRITICAL CARE

This section highlights physiologic changes most relevant to the assessment and care of critically ill obstetric patients—specifically, those affecting hemodynamic and respiratory states—and is not intended as a comprehensive review.

Hemodynamics

Pregnancy is associated with profound hemodynamic changes. **Table 1** illustrates some of these.[12–14] Blood volume increases by approximately 50% above baseline,[13,15] reflecting increases in both plasma volume and erythrocytes. As a result, there is an ability to tolerate 500 to 1000 mL rapid blood loss without significant hemodynamic compromise.[16,17] This may lead to a

Table 1
Hemodynamic changes in normal pregnancies

	Direction of Change in Pregnancy	% Change
Blood volume	⬆	40%–50%
Cardiac output	⬆	30%–50%
Heart rate	⬆	15%–20%
Blood pressure	⬇	—
Systematic vascular resistance	⬇	20%–30%

false assessment of the severity of blood loss in a pregnant patient if judging by the hemodynamic state.

In the supine position, by mid-pregnancy, the enlarging uterus compresses the aorta and vena cava. This leads to decreased venous return and a drop in maternal cardiac output. To counter this, critically ill gravid patients should typically be positioned with a left lateral tilt to 15° to 20°, displacing the uterus laterally and offsetting the aortocaval compromise.[18] This is particularly true in instances of clinically significant hemodynamic compromise.

Airways and Ventilation

Functional residual capacity decreases by about 20% in pregnancy. By approximately 12 weeks gestational age, ligamental relaxation leads to widening of the rib cage, pulling the diaphragm upward.[19] As the fetus grows, the enlarging uterus creates cephalad pressure on the diaphragm with resultant further elevation of the diaphragm,[19] and the chest wall becomes less compliant.[20] At the same time, oxygen demand increases due to increases in both metabolic rate and oxygen consumption.[21] As a result, the tolerance for hypoventilation and apnea in pregnancy is reduced as compared with nonpregnant patients.[22]

Endotracheal intubation in pregnant patients is challenging. Rates of failed intubation are eight times higher than in the general population.[23] The intolerance of hypoventilation or apnea, combined with airways that are difficult in pregnancy due to airway edema and hyperemia, necessitates that intubation be performed by the most experienced provider available. Preoxygenation is essential.

Laboratory differences in pregnancy must be factored into the assessments of patients. Arterial blood gases (ABGs), commonly used in the assessment of critically ill patients, normally indicate mild respiratory alkalosis in pregnancy, with a physiologic $PaCO_2$ of 28 to 32 mm Hg. In compensation for this, the serum bicarbonate level falls to 18 to 21 meq/L.

Some of the conditions requiring ICU admission in pregnant women may be specific to or worsen in pregnancy, whereas others are not. Here, we focus primarily on the obstetric-specific conditions associated with high maternal mortality that lead to ICU admissions.

POSTPARTUM HEMORRHAGE

PPH is the leading cause of maternal death worldwide. It accounts for 27.1% of maternal fatalities and occurs with a much higher frequency in developing countries.[24] Between 1993 and 2014, the United States had a precipitous 4- to 5-fold rise in the rate of PPH.[25] This coincided with the

- Leading cause of maternal death worldwide
- Etiologies: the 4 Ts—tone, trauma, tissue, and thrombin
- Management:
  - Uterotonics
    - Oxytocin 10 IU IM/IV for all births, can repeat up to 40 IU for continued hemorrhage
    - Secondary agents such as methylergonovine
  - Transexamic acid (TXA) 1g in 10 mL IV, can repeat if ongoing bleeding after 30 minutes
  - Removal of retained tissues
  - Repair of trauma
  - Transfusion of blood and blood products, using a massive transfusion protocol where appropriate and available

- Most frequent nonhemorrhagic diagnoses requiring ICU admission in pregnancy/peripartum
- HDP can present de novo postpartum
- Gestational hypertension: blood pressure greater than 140/90 mm Hg at greater than 20 weeks gestational age in a patient without prior hypertension
- Hypertensive emergency: systolic blood pressure greater than 160/110 mm Hg for greater than 15 minutes
- Preeclampsia: hypertension with proteinuria or other measures of organ dysfunction
- Eclampsia: preeclampsia plus seizures or coma
- Management:
  ○ Antihypertensives
    ■ Initial management with nifedipine, labetalol, or hydralazine (suggested dosing in **Table 2**)
    ■ Refractory management with nicardipine, labetalol, esmolol, or sodium nitroprusside (suggested dosing in **Table 3**)
  ○ Magnesium for seizure prophylaxis, 4–6 g IV loading dose, and then 1–2 g/h continuous infusion
  ○ Delivery

increased rates of cesarean deliveries, leading both to increased obstetric interventions and instrumentation, but also to increased risk for intra-abdominal scar tissue and abnormal placentation, leading in turn to the increased risk of PPH in future pregnancies.[26]

PPH is defined differently by various national obstetric societies, but most recently the American College of Obstetrics and Gynecology (ACOG) defines it as cumulative blood loss of 1000 mL or more, or blood loss associated with clinical evidence of hypovolemia, regardless of route of delivery.[27]

Risk factors for PPH include advanced maternal age, grand multiparity, previous cesarean delivery, suspected or proven placental abruption, placenta previa, and preeclampsia or gestational hypertension. Uterine fibroids, multiple pregnancy, fetal macrosomia, instrumental vaginal delivery, cervical laceration, and uterine rupture also increase risk of PPH.[28]

Etiologies can be categorized according to the "4 Ts" mnemonic by order of frequency: tone (uterine atony, accounting for 70% of all cases), trauma, tissue (retained tissue, invasive placenta), and thrombin (coagulopathies).[27] Because of the prevalence of uterine atony as a cause, the World Health Organization (WHO) recommends prophylactic administration of oxytocin 10 IU IM or IV for all births during the third stage of labor to stimulate uterine contraction.[29]

Uterine atony can be managed medically, mechanically, or failing those conservative measures, surgically. This management is mainly led by the obstetric team. The initial management of hemorrhage due to uterine atony includes bimanual uterine massage and the routine administration of oxytocin. Further dosing of oxytocin, not to exceed 40 IU, can be infused at a rate necessary to control uterine atony. Following that, a secondary uterotonic agent can be administered, often methylergonovine. If these measures fail, mechanical attempts to control atony-related hemorrhage may include balloon tamponade of the uterus, placement of an internal uterine suction device,[30] or uterine compression sutures. If these methods are unsuccessful, surgical interventions, including bilateral uterine artery ligation, internal iliac ligation, or ultimately hysterectomy, can be lifesaving procedures for the mother.[27]

The uterus must be inspected for retained placental tissue, with evacuation as needed. The uterus and genital tract are inspected for trauma, with repair of any lacerations.

The mainstays of management by the ICU team are achieving hemostasis and transfusion support, including the utilization of a massive transfusion protocol. The administration of large volumes of clear fluids has been associated with more severe deterioration of coagulation parameters, suggesting that restrictive fluid resuscitation in women with PPH is advisable.[31] Blood and blood products should be administered at ratios based on local and institutional thresholds and massive transfusion protocols. There are no clear obstetric guidelines on a recommended ratio of administration of packed red blood cells, fresh frozen plasma, and platelets. These data have been extrapolated from trauma literature,[32,33] and institutions develop their own massive transfusion protocols. As with all bleeding, the indication for transfusion may be guided by targeting certain laboratory values (ie, hemoglobin > 7, platelets >50, INR >1.5) or by the clinical scenario. Lack of hemodynamic instability may be misleading, as mentioned previously. Thromboelastography or rotational thromboelastometry, where available, may be beneficial in helping guide blood and blood products' administration.[34]

Table 2
Suggested initial management for severe intrapartum or postpartum Hypertension

If SBP ≥ 160 mm Hg or BBP ≥ 110 mm Hg, start fetal surveillance if undelivered and the fetus is viable
If this degree of hypertension is maintained for >15 min, start...

Choice of initial medication	IV labetalol (intermittent)	IV hydralazine	Oral nifedipine
	Labetalol 10–20 mg IV over 2 min	Hydralazine 5–10 mg IV over 2 min	Immediate-release nifedipine capsules, 10 mg orally
Repeat BP in ...	10 min	20 min	20 min
If SBP still ≥160 mm Hg or DBP ≥110 mm Hg....	Labetalol 40 mg IV over 2 min	Hydralazine 10 mg IV over 2 min	Immediate-release nifedipine capsules, 20 mg orally
Repeat BP in ...	10 min	20 min	20 min
If SBP still ≥160 mm Hg or DBP ≥ 110 mm Hg....	Labetalol 80 mg IV over 2 min	Labetalol 20 mg IV over 2 min	Immediate-release nifedipine capsules, 20 mg orally
Repeat BP in ...	10 min	10 min	20 min
If SBP still ≥ 160 mm Hg or DBP ≥ 110 mm Hg....	Hydralazine 10 mg IV over 2 min	Labetalol 40 mg IV over 2 min consult MFM internal medicine, anesthesia, or critical care subspecialists	Labetalol 20 mg IV over 2 min and consult MFM, internal medicine, anesthesia, or critical care subspecialist
Repeat BP in ...	20 min		
If SBP still ≥ 160 mm Hg or DBP ≥ 110 mm Hg....	Consult MFM, internal medicine, anesthesia, or critical care subspecialists		

- Variant of severe preeclampsia
- Women may have any or all of the elements of the triad of HELLP syndrome
- Differential diagnosis: idiopathic thrombocytopenic purpura (ITP), acute fatty liver of pregnancy (AFLP), hemolytic uremic syndrome (HUS), thrombotic thrombocytopenia purpura (TTP), and systemic lupus erythematosus (SLE)
- Management
  - Delivery
  - Corticosteroids for fetal lung maturity if < 34 weeks gestational age, and it is felt safe to defer immediate delivery
- Complications:
  - DIC, hepatic infarction, subcapsular hematomas, hepatic intraparenchymal hemorrhage, intracranial hemorrhage, placental abruption, acute renal failure, pulmonary edema, and seizures

TXA inhibits the breakdown of fibrinogen and fibrin clots. In 2017, the WHO recommended its use within 3 hours of delivery in women diagnosed with PPH in addition to standard care.[35,36] The recommended dose is 1g in 10 mL (100 mg/mL) IV at 1 mL/min, with a second dose of 1g IV given if bleeding continues after 30 minutes (WHO). There is a reduction in benefit of TXA with time from delivery, with no benefit in its administration after 3 hours from birth.

SMM due to PPH remains a significant problem worldwide, with patients developing multisystem organ failure, shock, ARDS, and DIC. Management of each of these is unchanged from their management in non-obstetric patients, and intensivists' expertise managing those patients who progress to severe illness after PPH is invaluable.

HYPERTENSIVE DISORDERS OF PREGNANCY: HYPERTENSIVE EMERGENCIES, PREECLAMPSIA, AND ECLAMPSIA

The HDP are the most frequent nonhemorrhagic diagnoses requiring ICU admission in pregnant

Table 3
Suggested secondary management for severe intrapartum or postpartum hypertension

Choice of Initial Infusion Medication	Labetalol (Continuous Infusion)	Nicardipine	Esmolol	Sodium Nitroprusside
Starting dose	1–2 mg/min	5 mg/h	Bolus: 500 µg/kg Maintenance: 50 µg/kg/min	0.25 µg/kg/min
Titration dose and frequency	Increase by 1-mg/min every 10 min as needed	Increase by 2.5 mg/h every 5–15 min as needed	Increase by 50 µg/kg/min every 4 min as needed	Increase by 0.25–0.5 µg/kg/min every 2–3 min as needed
Maximum dose	300 mg/d IV	15 mg/h	300 µg/kg/min	5 µg/kg/min * potential risk for cyanide/thiocyanate toxicity if used for >4 h

and peripartum women.[7,37] They are the second-leading cause of maternal death worldwide.[24]

Gestational hypertension is defined as a blood pressure greater than 140/90 at greater than 20 weeks gestational age in a woman who was not hypertensive before 20 weeks. Preeclampsia is the same degree of hypertension but with the additional finding of proteinuria and/or any of the

Box 1
Preeclampsia

Preeclampsia: SBP $\geq$ 140 mm Hg and/or DBP $\geq$ 90 mm Hg after 20 weeks gestation in a woman without chronic hypertension, accompanied by proteinuria ($\geq$300 mg protein/24 h urine collection; protein: creatinine $\geq$ 0.3 mg/dL; or urine dipstick reading of 2+ if quantitative measures are unavailable) or any of the features listed below.

Any of the following criteria in the setting of preeclampsia with severe features:

- SBP $\geq$160 mm Hg and/or DPB $\geq$110 more than 4 hours apart (unless antihypertensive therapy has begun)
- Thrombocytopenia (plt < 100,000 × 10^9/L)
- Transaminases >2X upper limit of normal
- Severe right upper quadrant or epigastric pain without an alternative diagnosis
- Serum creatinine greater than 1.1 mg/dL or twice baseline, without other kidney disease
- Pulmonary edema
- New-onset headache unresponsive to acetaminophen and without other diagnosis or visual symptoms

features listed in **Box 1**.[38–40] Those other features, or a severely elevated blood pressure (greater than 160/110 mm Hg on at least two separate assessments) with proteinuria or the listed findings, define preeclampsia with severe features. Eclampsia is the disease state when preeclampsia is accompanied by seizures or coma. The syndrome of hemolysis, elevated liver enzymes, and low platelets (HELLPs) is considered a variant of HDP and will be discussed separately.

The presence of acute, severe hypertension (>160/110 mm Hg) measured accurately more than 15 minutes apart is a hypertensive emergency, with the greatest risk to the mother of a central nervous system injury. Pregnant women with severe systolic or diastolic hypertension, or both, require urgent therapy.[39] ACOG has published guidelines for the emergency management of acute, severe hypertension during pregnancy and the postpartum period.[38]

The definitive treatment of preeclampsia and eclampsia is delivery of the fetus. When hypertension is associated with severe features at or beyond 34 weeks gestational age, delivery is recommended. At earlier gestational ages, expectant management may be considered, with guidance available from ACOG.[38]

These recommendations include the choice of IV labetalol, IV hydralazine, or oral nifedipine when IV access is unavailable. The target blood pressure should be an initial range of 140 to 150/90 to 100 mm Hg. There is no single accepted first line agent, but see **Table 2** for first-choice options and suggested dosing and intervals.[38,39,41–43]

Guidance is less clear on medications to use when the initial antihypertensive therapies fail. See **Table 3** for alternatives, dosing and intervals.[41,42]

Table 4
Mississippi and Tennessee criteria for hemolysis, elevated liver enzymes, and low platelet syndrome

Tennessee Criteria	Missisippi-Triple Class System
• Evidence of hemolysis on a peripheral smear • Decreased haptoglobin • Increased serum bilirubin ($\geq$20.5 μmol/L or) or $\geq$ 1.2 mg/100 mL) • Elevated LDH (>600 units/L_ • Platelets $\leq$ 100 × 10^9/L • AST $\geq$ 70 IU/L (ref)	Class 1 • LDH $\geq$ 600 IU/L • ALT or AST $\geq$70 IU/L • platelets $\leq$50 × 10^9/L
	Class 2 • LDH $\geq$ 600 IU/L • ALT or AST $\geq$ 70 IU/L • platelets $\geq$ 50 × 10^9/L but $\leq$ 150 × 10^9/L
	Class 3 • LDH $\geq$ 600 IU/L • ALT or AST $\geq$ 40 IU/L • platelets $\geq$ 100 × 10^9/L but $\leq$ 150 × 10^9/L

• More true hepatic dysfunction than HELLP, evidenced by hypoglycemia, coagulopathies, and encephalopathy
• Many women have coexisting preeclampsia
• Management:
  ○ Delivery
  ○ Supportive care—close monitoring, transfusions as needed, mechanical ventilation if needed
• Most patients recover within 1 to 2 weeks after delivery
• Evaluation for orthotopic liver transplantation, though rarely needed, is indicated if liver failure is severe or progressive.

Box 2
Diagnostic criteria for acute fatty liver of pregnancy

Swansea criteria

Six or more of the following, without an alternative etiology, are needed for a diagnosis of AFLP:

• Nausea/vomiting
• Abdominal pain
• Polydipsia/polyuria
• Encephalopathy
• Ascites or "bright-appearing" liver on ultrasound
• Hyperbilirubinemia (>14 μmol/L or >0.82 mg/dL)
• Hypoglycemia (<4 mmol/L or <72 mg/dL)
• Hyperuricemia (>340 μmol/L or >5.7 mg/dL)
• Leukocytosis (>11 × 10/L)
• Transaminitis (AST or ALT >42 IU/L)
• Hyperammonemia (>47 μmol/L or 66 μg/dL)
• Renal dysfunction (creatinine >150 μmol/L or >1.7 mg/dL)
• Coagulopathy (PT > 14 sec or APTT> 34 sec)
• If liver biopsy is performed, +microvesicular steatosis

Magnesium is also recommended for seizure prophylaxis, and per ACOG guidelines should be started in a pregnant or postpartum patient with gestational hypertension with severe features, preeclampsia with severe features, or those with eclampsia.[38] For the first two, it is more effective than other agents in reducing the risk of eclampsia.[44] A suggested regimen is a loading dose of 4-6g IV of magnesium sulfate followed by 1-2 g/h maintenance infusion.[38]

If the patient requires induction of general anesthesia and endotracheal intubation, blood pressure monitoring and management are critical, as induction and intubation themselves can raise blood pressures dramatically.

It is also important to recognize that approximately 1/3 of eclampsia develops postpartum. A postpartum patient with hypertension accompanied by headaches and/or vision changes is at high risk of serious complications. Half of intracerebral hemorrhage caused by preeclampsia occurs postpartum.[40] Last, patients with preeclampsia tend to have baseline intravascular depletion and do not tolerate the same degree of blood loss as patients without preeclampsia.

HEMOLYSIS, ELEVATED LIVER ENZYMES, AND LOW PLATELETS (HELLP SYNDROME)

- Presents with a clinical triad of dyspnea and/or hypoxia; cardiovascular collapse; DIC
- Management
  - Supportive, including clearly cardiopulmonary resuscitation (CPR) in event of cardiac arrest
  - Fetal delivery (if not already delivered) within 5 minutes of starting CPR if there has been no return of spontaneous circulation
  - Vasopressors are preferred over crystalloid fluid infusions for BP support
  - Pulmonary vasodilator such as inhaled nitric oxide
- Patients with refractory heart or lung failure should be considered for ECMO
- Differential diagnosis includes PE, high spinal anesthesia, and magnesium toxicity

---

The HELLP syndrome is characterized by the triad of HELLPs. There is no consensus for specific laboratory values, and women may have one, two, or all three components of the syndrome.

HELLP syndrome is considered a variant of severe preeclampsia, though it can occur in women with normal blood pressure. It is rare, occurring in 0.2% to 0.9% of all pregnancies[45–47] and 10% to 20% of women with severe preeclampsia.[47] The diagnosis carries an increased risk of complications for both mother and fetus,[45,46] and its recognition and appropriate management are therefore paramount.

There are two classification systems for HELLP, the Tennessee criteria and the Mississippi Triple

Class System, as shown in **Table 4**, which define and classify HELLP based on degrees of hemolysis, thrombocytopenia, and degree of liver dysfunction.

The differential diagnosis of HELLP is broad as mentioned above. ITP is not more common in or exacerbated by pregnancy, and even with quite low platelet counts, the incidence of maternal or fetal morbidity or mortality is low.[48] HUS and TTP are thrombotic microangiopathies with some similar features to HELLP syndrome. HUS, when present in peripartum patients, tends to develop postpartum and presents with symptoms of renal failure.[47] TTP is exceedingly rare in pregnancy but presents with neurologic dysfunction, fever, abdominal pain, and bleeding.[47] SLE can affect multiple organ systems, but patients with lupus nephritis may present with clinical and laboratory findings similar to patients with severe preeclampsia.[47]

If HELLP manifests at ≥34 weeks gestational age, or if there are concerning and potentially dangerous additional findings in the mother including multiorgan dysfunction, DIC, liver hemorrhage or infarction, renal failure, suspected placental abruption, or nonreassuring fetal status, there is general consensus to deliver the fetus.[46,49,50]

In pregnancies less than 34 weeks gestational age, glucocorticoids are used for fetal lung maturity if it is felt to be safe to delay delivery. Glucocorticoids have no benefit in regard to maternal morbidity/mortality or perinatal or infant death.[51]

Decisions regarding timing of delivery will necessarily be made in close collaboration with the patient's obstetrician and MFM specialists.

Potential complications include DIC, hepatic infarction, subcapsular hematomas, hepatic intraparenchymal hemorrhage, intracranial hemorrhage, placental abruption, acute renal failure, pulmonary edema, and seizures.[47,52–54]

Particular mention is warranted of the complication of hepatic rupture, as it can be catastrophic. Abdominal pain, particularly in the epigastric or right upper quadrant and/or radiating to the right shoulder, with either hypertension or shock, should trigger consideration of prompt abdominal imaging with ultrasound or CT if the patient is stable enough to allow it.[52–54] Treatment may include conservative management with aggressive support of coagulation, transfusion of blood products, and prophylactic antibiotics if the hematoma is contained.[52] Embolization may also be considered at that point. Hemodynamic instability should trigger either hepatic artery embolization, surgical packing of the liver, or a combination of these therapies.[52–54]

ACUTE FATTY LIVER OF PREGNANCY

This is a relatively rare but potentially fatal complication of pregnancy characterized histologically by microvesicular fatty infiltration of hepatocytes. It demonstrates more true hepatic dysfunction than preeclampsia or HELLP, which manifests clinically as hypoglycemia as well as coagulopathies, encephalopathy, and DIC.[55]

The diagnosis is often clinical, based on symptoms and laboratory values. Liver biopsy is the gold standard for diagnosis but is rarely performed. The clinical and laboratory findings included in the diagnosis are combined in the Swansea criteria, as shown in **Box 2**.

Treatment is primarily supportive, including transfusions, ICU monitoring, and mechanical ventilation if indicated. Delivery of the fetus is critical. Most patients' liver function returns to normal after delivery, typically within 1 to 2 weeks.

In rare cases, orthotopic liver transplantation is pursued.[56,57] A small review of patients referred to a UK liver transplant center between 1997 and 2008 with severe pregnancy associated liver dysfunction from AFLP or HELLP revealed that elevated lactate and the presence of hepatic encephalopathy were the only admission parameters predictive of death or need for liver transplant. King's college criteria did *not* predict outcome.[56]

AMNIOTIC FLUID EMBOLISM

- Presents in late pregnancy or postpartum with symptoms of HF or more rarely with catastrophic complications
- Management
  - Standard therapy for HF, with modifications for fetal and breastfeeding safety
  - Anticoagulation
  - Ventricular assist devices or ECMO for severe decompensated HF
  - Consideration of wearable defibrillators while awaiting possible cardiac recovery
  - Consideration of implantable cardioverter/defibrillators (ICDs) for prolonged, severe LV dysfunction

---

Amniotic fluid embolism (AFE) is a rare entity, with a wide range of reported incidence based on different reporting methodologies. It carries a high morbidity and mortality ranging between less than 20% to more than 60%. The pathophysiology seems to be a combination of fetal components entering the maternal circulation and an abnormal, anaphylactoid, immune response to those fetal components. Fetal components can be found in the maternal circulation of pregnant and postpartum women without AFE; the immune response is a key component of the clinical syndrome.[58,59]

AFE classically encompasses a triad of dyspnea and/or hypoxia followed by cardiovascular collapse and severe coagulopathy, with significant oozing and frank bleeding at suture lines, vaginal tears, and venipuncture sites. Patients may also demonstrate neurologic changes that include altered mentation and seizures. These physical signs and symptoms typically occur during labor and delivery, cesarean delivery, dilation and evacuation, or immediately postpartum without an alternative explanation. There also seems to be a version of AFE that presents as isolated DIC and hemorrhage, without or with only minimal maternal hypoxia or hemodynamic instability or collapse.[60]

Physiologically, there is a transient initial period of pulmonary and systemic hypertension, with intense pulmonary vasoconstriction leading to hypoxia and right heart failure (HF).[61] This is followed by profound depression of left ventricular (LV) function with normal PA pressures. The myocardial dysfunction may be due to myocardial ischemia from hypoxia due to lung injury or cardiac arrest imposed by AFE or there may be myocardial ischemia due to coronary artery spasm.[58]

In women who suffer cardiac arrest from AFE, all three of the lethal dysrhythmias have been described—ventricular fibrillation, pulseless electrical activity, and asystole. These likely reflect different physiologic mechanisms of arrest: hypoxia, direct myocardial depression, and exsanguination.[62] Survivors of cardiac arrest often develop multisystem organ failure, including hypoxic brain injury.[58]

The differential diagnosis includes PE, anaphylaxis, aortic dissection, septic shock, air or fat embolism, eclampsia, adverse reaction to medications, and hemorrhagic shock, among others.[63] In classic AFE, ABGs will reflect hypoxemia but are not specific enough to really aid in diagnosis. Chest x-rays are also nonspecific, often appearing consistent with pulmonary edema. PT/INR/PTT and fibrinogen should be evaluated. For patients with suspected AFE who experience hemodynamic collapse, bedside echocardiogram (TTE or TEE if an experienced provider is immediately available) can be useful in demonstrating RV failure, though this may not help differentiate between AFE and some of the alternative diagnoses, particularly PE. The presence of the acute, often profound, coagulopathy seen in AFE can help differentiate between these two diagnoses. Various serum markers have been examined as clues to the diagnosis, including C1 esterase inhibitor and IGF, but do not seem particularly useful in acute diagnosis and management. The diagnosis is a clinical one.

Other diagnoses in the differential include high spinal anesthesia, which can complicate spinal or epidural anesthesia and can present with dyspnea or apnea, profound hypotension, and bradycardia. It is managed with aggressive fluid resuscitation, hemodynamic and respiratory support, and intralipid. Magnesium toxicity is also in the differential as it can present with hemodynamic collapse. It is treated with IV calcium.

The management of AFE is supportive. CPR is indicated in the event of cardiac arrest, and delivery is indicated within 5 minutes if there is no response to CPR or if non-reassuring fetal status remains despite correction of maternal hypoxia.

Blood pressure support with vasopressors is recommended over volume expansion (excepting blood and blood products to manage hemorrhage)

- One of the leading causes of maternal deaths in the United States
- Pregnant women have a significantly higher incidence of thromboembolic disease than their nonpregnant peers, with highest risk postpartum
- Management:
  - Anticoagulation
  - Systemic or catheter-directed thrombolysis
  - Surgical thrombectomy
  - Salvage therapy with ECMO should be considered for patients with circulatory collapse or refractory hypoxemia

---

due to the presence of acute right HF. Inotropic support and pulmonary vasodilators may also be indicated.[64] Patients with refractory HF should be evaluated for VA ECMO.[65]

Transfusion of blood and blood products is indicated for the coagulopathy and secondary hemorrhage that develop.[66] Recombinant factor VIIa has been associated with worse outcomes compared with blood and blood products alone; thus, it is not a recommended therapy.[67] Experimental therapies include administration of C1 esterase inhibitor concentrate,[68,69] TXA, aminocaproic acid, and aprotinin. They remain investigational and

are not currently recommended therapies, and aprotinin is no longer on the market.

PERIPARTUM CARDIOMYOPATHY

Peripartum cardiomyopathy (PPCM) is defined as "an idiopathic condition with LV systolic dysfunction (ejection fraction [EF] <45%) toward the end of pregnancy or following delivery, when no other cause of HF is found."[70]

The incidence varies greatly in different studies, with variability between different populations. Of note, women of African descent have a much higher incidence of PPCM than white women.[71–73] There is also a strong association between the HDP and PPCM.[74–76] Risk factors for PPCM include African ancestry, preeclampsia and hypertension, multiparity, and advanced maternal age[70,77–79].

The pathophysiology of PPCM is unclear and likely multifactorial. It does not seem to be a response to the physiologic hemodynamic demands of pregnancy. For most patients, presenting symptoms of PPCM include the symptoms of HF, which can unfortunately overlap with some of the symptoms—particularly dyspnea—typically seen in pregnancy. A minority of patients may present in cardiogenic shock or with arrhythmias or complications of thromboembolism.[80] There are no specific laboratory markers for this condition, but the B-type natriuretic peptide is markedly elevated in PPCM and is not elevated in typical pregnancy, which makes this a useful test in this diagnosis.[81–83] Echocardiography reveals a reduced EF and may demonstrate left and right ventricular dilatation and/or dysfunction, valvular dysfunction, left or bi-atrial enlargement, or pulmonary hypertension.[80]

Mortality in this diagnosis can be due to arrhythmias and thromboembolic disease as well as decompensated HF.

Management includes the management of decompensated HF; diuresis, beta blockade, and sometimes inotropes, all with the caveats of taking medication safety in pregnancy and breastfeeding into account. There is a high reported incidence of LV thrombosis and thromboembolism,[84,85] so anticoagulation has been recommended from diagnosis through 6 to 8 weeks after delivery.[86] Both the American Heart Association and the European Society of Cardiology suggest anticoagulation in PPCM with EF < 30 or 35%, respectively,[87–89] but there are no published guidelines to determine therapeutic versus prophylactic anticoagulation. Prolactin inhibition has been studied, specifically with the use of

- Pregnant women with Covid-19 have higher rates of ICU admission, need for mechanical ventilation, and death than their nonpregnant peers.
- Management of critically ill pregnant women with Covid-19 pneumonia and ARDS should include:
  - Latest medical therapies in accordance with infectious disease guidelines
  - Neuromuscular blockade, prone positioning, and inhaled nitric oxide should all be considered for refractory hypoxemia
  - Prone positioning can be safely performed even in later stages of pregnancy
  - For truly refractory hypoxemia, hypercarbia, or cardiopulmonary failure, patients should be evaluated for ECMO

bromocriptine, but it remains experimental, especially given a concern for increased risk of thrombosis with bromocriptine and the importance of retaining the ability to breastfeed.[80,90]

The increased risk of thrombosis and thromboembolism are thought to be due to a combination of factors, including hemostasis in a poorly contracting ventricle, the hypercoagulable state of pregnancy, and relative immobility for many patients (particularly those recovering from cesarean sections or complicated vaginal deliveries).

Patients with severe HF due to PPCM may require mechanical support with ventricular assist devices or cardiopulmonary support with ECMO.[91–93]

For patients who present with PPCM while still pregnant, the planning for labor and delivery should be multidisciplinary, involving obstetricians, cardiologists, MFM specialists, obstetric internists, anesthesiologists, nursing, pharmacologists, and social workers.

Many patients demonstrate recovery in their LV function, often within the first 6 months, with a significantly higher likelihood of recovery in those patients whose EF is greater than 30% at their time of diagnosis.[94] Because of frequent recovery of cardiac function, ICDs are generally not recommended initially, though there may be a consideration of wearable defibrillators.[74,95] There are no clear guidelines on when, or in which patients, ICDs should be considered. These decisions should be guided by the patient's cardiologist as they are followed after initial diagnosis.

PULMONARY EMBOLISM

PE is one of the leading causes of death in the United States, accounting for 9.5% of

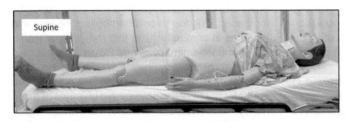
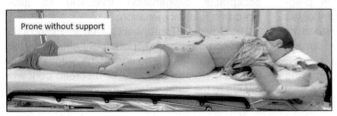
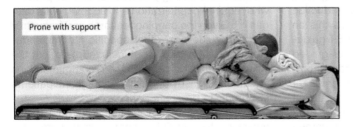

Fig. 1. Prone positioning of the pregnant patient with key areas of support. *(From* Oxford-Horrey C, Savage M, Prabhu M, Abramovitz S, Griffin K, LaFond E, Riley L, Easter SR. Putting It All Together: Clinical Considerations in the Care of Critically Ill Obstetric Patients with COVID-19. Am J Perinatol. 2020 Aug;37(10):1044-1051.)

pregnancy-related deaths there.[5,96,97] During pregnancy, there are increases in procoagulant factors, resistance to activated protein C, and decreases in circulating protein S,[98] with simultaneous decreases in fibrinolysis, leading to a state of hypercoagulability. Pregnancy yields a triad of this hypercoagulability, venous stasis, and vascular injury[99] that together significantly increase the incidence of PE in pregnant women compared with their nonpregnant peers.[100–102]

We focus here on the acute management of high-risk submassive and massive PEs. The mortality rate for untreated submassive and massive PEs is high in the general population.[103–105] Treatment with anticoagulation reduces the mortality risk, and at minimum, this should be started in all patients without a contraindication[106–108] as soon as the PE is diagnosed. With high-risk submassive and massive PEs, however, consideration should be given to the more aggressive therapies, including systemic or catheter-guided thrombolysis, surgical or catheter-based thrombectomy or fragmentation, and support with ECMO.[106,107,109–111] Evidence-based data supporting one management strategy over another are exceedingly limited, with most of the literature encompassing limited case series. There is also a concern for publication bias suggesting a higher than actual success rate. Despite those caveats, we present what is known of the therapeutic options for these potentially catastrophic PEs.

The 2016 CHEST guidelines on antithrombotic and thrombolytic therapy in the general population recommend thrombolysis for treatment of a PE with hypotension (SBP<90 mm Hg), but pregnancy is included as a relative contraindication.[107] However, a 2020 systematic review of thrombolysis in pregnancy and the immediate puerperium concluded that there was in fact *not* a prohibitive risk to thrombolytic therapy for PE in pregnancy.[112] The risks of hemorrhage in thrombolysis are higher in pregnant and particularly postpartum patients than in the general population, but the risks of morbidity and mortality from massive PE outweigh the risks from thrombolysis, making this a justifiable intervention.[109,110,112]

Although data are limited, the theoretic decreased risk of bleeding with catheter-guided lysis,[113,114] due to its two-third dose reduction compared with systemic lysis,[115] makes this an attractive option to explore further. CHEST guidelines still recommend reserving catheter-guided lysis for patients at increased risk of bleeding complications, with no specific comment on pregnant patients. The very limited case reports on patients for whom catheter directed therapy was used in massive and submassive PEs in pregnant women

seem to show good outcomes with few complications.[116,117].

In cases of refractory hypoxemia or circulatory collapse, pregnant women with massive or submassive PE may be evaluated for VV or VA ECMO. This is a promising strategy under scrutiny in the general population, with data supporting its consideration.[118–120] Data on its use in pregnant women are quite limited, but they have been reported with favorable outcomes.[121–124]

COVID-19 AND ARDS MANAGEMENT

Covid-19 is clearly not an obstetric disease. Nevertheless, given its current prevalence around the world and the increased risk for severe illness that pregnant women face from the SARS-CoV2 virus, a brief section on severe Covid-19 in pregnant women is included in this article.

Pregnant women with Covid-19 have higher rates of ICU admission, need for mechanical ventilation, need for ECMO, and death than their age-matches, nonpregnant peers.[11,125] In pregnant and recently pregnant women with Covid-19 compared with pregnant and recently pregnant women without Covid-19, all-cause mortality and ICU admission rates were significantly higher in the patients with the disease. Some of the speculated reasons for this include physiologic changes of pregnancy such as increased heart rate and oxygen consumption, decreased lung capacity, increased risk for thromboembolic disease, and changes in immunity[11] but this remains unclear.

The management of severe Covid-19 and Covid ARDS in pregnancy has few differences from nonpregnant patients, but providers need to account for some of the physiologic changes of pregnancy and remain mindful of that higher acceptable oxygenation threshold to allow adequate fetal oxygenation.

The Covid-19 Treatment Guidelines Panel of the NIH recommends that "potentially effective treatment for Covid-19 should not be withheld from pregnant women because of theoretic concerns related to the safety of therapeutic agents in pregnancy."[126] Included in these guidelines, dexamethasone is strongly recommended for patients who require hospitalization and supplemental oxygen.[126] Given the ongoing research and frequently updated guidelines, other specific recommendations for treatment are not included here, but the NIH states that "In general, the recommendations for managing Covid-19 in nonpregnant patients also apply to pregnant patients."

In the event that a patient's Covid-19 progresses to ARDS, some reminders for management of ARDS in pregnancy are included. Maternal oxygenation should be maintained at a PaO2 greater than 70, corresponding to an oxygen saturation of $\geq$95%, to maintain adequate fetal oxygenation. A recent study suggested that an SpO$_2$ of 93% is normal in pregnancy and may be a reasonable acceptable threshold,[127] but this has not yet been widely adopted.

The acceptable range for pCO$_2$ in permissive hypercapnia is also altered, with allowance of pCO$_2$ rising only to 60 mm Hg out of concern for decreased placental perfusion at higher ranges.[128] This contrasts with much higher accepted ranges of pCO$_2$ in nonpregnant patients with ARDS.

For refractory hypoxemia, neuromuscular blocking agents should be added to sedatives to facilitate lung-protective ventilation, and inhaled pulmonary vasodilators such as inhaled nitric oxide and epoprostenol should be considered for hypoxemia that is refractory to standard management.[129] Prone positioning in ARDS has a demonstrated mortality benefit[130] and has been widely used to improve gas exchange in patients with Covid-19 ARDS. Accordingly, this strategy should also be used in pregnant patients with Covid-19 ARDS when indicated. Prone positioning can be challenging in later stages of pregnancy given the gravid uterus, but with proper support (**Fig. 1**), it can be achieved and provide benefit.[131,132]

For truly refractory hypoxemia and/or hypercarbia, pregnant women with Covid ARDS should be evaluated for ECMO by an experienced ECMO team.[121,122,133,134] There may be cannulation challenges in later stages of pregnancy related to the degree of uterine enlargement, which will require close communication and coordination with the ECMO team.

SUMMARY

Pregnant and peripartum women rarely require the care of intensivists. However, they may need ICU level care for a variety of conditions—some unrelated to pregnancy, and some that are directly related to pregnancy. We have discussed the diagnosis and management of these obstetric critical illnesses here, as they may be somewhat less familiar to medical intensivists than the nonobstetric indications for ICU admission (septic shock, for example) and also a few non-obstetric conditions that create significant morbidity and mortality in pregnant patients. Although the care of critically ill pregnant and peripartum women should remain a collaborative effort between the intensivists, obstetricians, MFM, and other relevant specialists involved with a given patient, our hope is that this article has provided a framework to guide more informed, medically sophisticated conversations among all participants in the care team.

CLINICS CARE POINTS

- Maternal physiology in a normal, healthy pregnancy includes changes in blood volume, heart rate, cardiac output, blood pressure, and systemic vascular resistance.

- Airways and ventilation change as well, with a decrease in functional residual capacity and an increase in oxygen demand. The tolerance for hypoventilation and apnea is decreased in pregnant women as compared to nonpregnant patients.

- Postpartum hemorrhage is the leading cause of maternal death in the world. Management recommendations include prophylactic oxytocin for all births, with further medical, mechanical, and surgical management options if it develops despite the oxytocin.

- The hypertensive disorders of pregnancy are the most common nonhemorrhagic ICU-requiring diagnoses in pregnancy and the peripartum period. Management includes antihypertensive medications, magnesium, and for refractory conditions, delivery.

- HELLP syndrome is a variant of preeclampsia. If it manifests at 34 weeks gestational age or the mother develops dangerous adverse effects from this syndrome, delivery is recommended.

- Acute fatty liver of pregnancy is managed with delivery and with supportive care, with rare referrals for orthotopc liver transplantation.

- Amniotic fluid embolism is a rare entity, though with high morbidity and mortality, that is managed supportively but must be recognized immediately for appropriate management.

- Peripartum cardiomyopathy is managed similarly to decompensated heart failure and is best managed in close collaboration with cardiologists.-Pulmonary embolism is one of the leading causes of maternal deaths in the United States. It is most often managed with anticoagulation, but other treatment options, depending on the clinical picture, include thrombolysis, thrombectomy, or salvage therapy with ECMO.

- Covid-19 does not infect pregnant women more than others, but does convey a higher risk of ICU admission, need for mechanical ventilation, and death than in nonpregnant patients. Management of Covid-19 ARDS in pregnant women is similar to management in nonpregnant patients, with some alterations based on the physiologic changes of pregnancy, including a higher threshold of acceptable PaO2 to allow adequate fetal oxygenation.

- The care of critically ill pregnant women is best managed by a multidisciplinary team that includes intensivists, obstetricians, maternal-fetal-medicine specialists, and other relevant specialists depending on the specific situation.

ACKNOWLEDGMENTS

Dr. Ghada Bourjeily has this grant funding number: NHLBI R01-HL130702Dr. Corrina Oxford-HorreyDr. Kelly Griffin has no funding to declare.

DISCLOSURE

The authors have nothing to disclose.

REFERENCES

1. Hamilton BE, Martin JA, OstermanMJK. Births: Provisional data for 2020.Vital Statistics Rapid Release; no 12.Hyattsville, MD: National Center forHealth Statistics. May 2021. https://doi.org/10.15620/cdc:104993.
2. Alkema L, Chou D, Hogan D, et al. Global, regional, and national levels and trends in maternal mortality between 1990 and 2015, with scenario-based projections to 2030: a systematic analysis by the UN Maternal Mortality Estimation Inter-Agency Group. Lancet 2016;387(10017):462–74.
3. Hoyert DL. Maternal mortality rates in the United States, 2020. NCHS Health E-Stats. 2022. https://dx.doi.org/10.15620/cdc:113967external icon.
4. Howell EA. Reducing disparities in severe maternal morbidity and mortality. Clin Obstet Gynecol 2018; 61(2):387–99.
5. Hoyert DLM, Arialdi M. Maternal mortality in the United States: changes in coding, publication, and data release, 2018. Natl Vital Stat Rep 2020; 69(2):1–18.
6. Aziz A, Gyamfi-Bannerman C, Siddiq Z, et al. Maternal outcomes by race during postpartum re-admissions. Am J Obstet Gynecol 2019;220(5): 484. e481-e410.
7. Pollock W, Rose L, Dennis CL. Pregnant and post-partum admissions to the intensive care unit: a systematic review. Intensive Care Med 2010;36(9): 1465–74.
8. Wanderer JP, Leffert LR, Mhyre JM, et al. Epidemiology of obstetric-related ICU admissions in Maryland: 1999-2008*. Crit Care Med 2013;41(8): 1844–52.
9. Yi HY, Jeong SY, Kim SH, et al. Indications and characteristics of obstetric patients admitted to the intensive care unit: a 22-year review in a tertiary care center. Obstet Gynecol Sci 2018;61(2): 209–19.
10. Zieleskiewicz L, Chantry A, Duclos G, et al. Intensive care and pregnancy: epidemiology and general principles of management of obstetrics ICU patients during pregnancy. Anaesth Crit Care Pain Med 2016;35(Suppl 1):S51–7.
11. Allotey J, Stallings E, Bonet M, et al. Clinical manifestations, risk factors, and maternal and perinatal outcomes of coronavirus disease 2019 in pregnancy: living systematic review and meta-analysis. BMJ 2020;370:m3320.
12. Clark SL, Cotton DB, Lee W, et al. Central hemodynamic assessment of normal term pregnancy. Am J Obstet Gynecol 1989;161(6):1439–42.
13. Sanghavi M, Rutherford JD. Cardiovascular physiology of pregnancy. Circulation 2014;130(12): 1003–8.
14. Hegewald MJ, Crapo RO. Respiratory physiology in pregnancy. Clin Chest Med 2011;32(1):1–13.
15. Pritchard Jack A. Changes in the blood volume during pregnancy and delivery. Anesthesiology 1965;26(4):393–9.
16. Chesnutt AN. Physiology of normal pregnancy. Crit Care Clin 2004;20(4):609–15.
17. Yeomans ER, Gilstrap LC 3rd. Physiologic changes in pregnancy and their impact on critical care. Crit Care Med 2005;33(10 Suppl):S256–8.
18. Lee SW, Khaw KS, Ngan Kee WD, et al. Haemodynamic effects from aortocaval compression at different angles of lateral tilt in non-labouring term pregnant women. Br J Anaesth 2012; 109(6):950–6.
19. Cohen ME, Thomson KJ. Studies on the circulation in pregnancy. I. The velocity of blood flow and related aspects of the circulation in normal pregnant women. J Clin Invest 1936;15(6):607–25.
20. Marx GF, Pushpa MK, Orkin LR. Static compliance before and after vaginal delivery. Br J Anaesth 1970;42(12):1100–4.
21. Soma-Pillay P, Nelson-Piercy C, Tolppanen H, et al. Physiological changes in pregnancy. Cardiovasc J Afr 2016;27(2):89–94.
22. Archer GW Jr, Marx GF. Arterial oxygen tension during apnoea in parturient women. Br J Anaesth 1974;46(5):358–60.
23. Quinn AC, Milne D, Columb M, et al. Failed tracheal intubation in obstetric anaesthesia: 2 yr national case-control study in the UK. Br J Anaesth 2013; 110(1):74–80.

24. Say L, Chou D, Gemmill A, et al. Global causes of maternal death: a WHO systematic analysis. Lancet Glob Health 2014;2(6):e323–33.

25. Data on Pregnancy Complications | Pregnancy | Maternal and Infant Health | CDC.pdf.

26. Silver RM, Landon MB, Rouse DJ, et al. Maternal morbidity associated with multiple repeat cesarean deliveries. Obstet Gynecol 2006;107(6):1226–32.

27. Practice bulletin No. 183: postpartum hemorrhage. Obstet Gynecol 2017;130(4):e168–86.

28. Kramer MS, Berg C, Abenhaim H, et al. Incidence, risk factors, and temporal trends in severe postpartum hemorrhage. Am J Obstet Gynecol 2013; 209(5):449 e441–447.

29. WHO. WHO recommendations: uterotonics for the prevention of postpartum haemorrhage. In: WHO recommendations: uterotonics for the prevention of postpartum haemorrhage. Geneva (Switzerland): World Health Organization; 2018. Licence: CC BY-NC-SA 3.0 IGO.2018.

30. D'Alton ME, Rood KM, Smid MC, et al. Intrauterine vacuum-induced hemorrhage-control device for rapid treatment of postpartum hemorrhage. Obstet Gynecol 2020;136(5):882–91.

31. Gillissen A, van den Akker T, Caram-Deelder C, et al. Association between fluid management and dilutional coagulopathy in severe postpartum haemorrhage: a nationwide retrospective cohort study. BMC Pregnancy Childbirth 2018;18(1):398.

32. Holcomb JB, Tilley BC, Baraniuk S, et al. Transfusion of plasma, platelets, and red blood cells in a 1:1:1 vs a 1:1:2 ratio and mortality in patients with severe trauma: the PROPPR randomized clinical trial. JAMA 2015;313(5):471–82.

33. Young PP, Cotton BA, Goodnough LT. Massive transfusion protocols for patients with substantial hemorrhage. Transfus Med Rev 2011;25(4):293–303.

34. Toffaletti JG, Buckner KA. Use of earlier-reported rotational thromboelastometry parameters to evaluate clotting status, fibrinogen, and platelet activities in postpartum hemorrhage compared to surgery and intensive care patients. Anesth Analg 2019;128(3):414–23.

35. World Health Organization (WHO). Updated WHO Recommendation on Tranexamic Acid for the Treatment of Postpartum Haemorrhage. Geneva, Switzerland: WHO; 2017.

36. Shakur H, Roberts I, Fawole B, et al. Effect of early tranexamic acid administration on mortality, hysterectomy, and other morbidities in women with postpartum haemorrhage (WOMAN): an international, randomised, double-blind, placebo-controlled trial. Lancet 2017;389(10084):2105–16.

37. Guntupalli KK, Hall N, Karnad DR, et al. Critical illness in pregnancy: part I: an approach to a pregnant patient in the ICU and common obstetric disorders. Chest 2015;148(4):1093–104.

38. Gestational hypertension and preeclampsia. Obstet Gynecol 2020;135(6):e237–60.

39. Khedagi AM, Bello NA. Hypertensive disorders of pregnancy. Cardiol Clin 2021;39(1):77–90.

40. Bateman BT, Schumacher HC, Bushnell CD, et al. Intracerebral hemorrhage in pregnancy. Neurology 2006;67(3):424–9.

41. Too GT, Hill JB. Hypertensive crisis during pregnancy and postpartum period. Semin Perinatol 2013;37(4):280–7.

42. Vadhera RB, Simon M. Hypertensive emergencies in pregnancy. Clin Obstet Gynecol 2014;57(4): 797–805.

43. Olson-Chen C, Seligman NS. Hypertensive emergencies in pregnancy. Crit Care Clin 2016;32(1): 29–41.

44. Euser AG, Cipolla MJ. Magnesium sulfate for the treatment of eclampsia: a brief review. Stroke 2009;40(4):1169–75.

45. Weinstein L. Syndrome of hemolysis, elevated liver enzymes, and low platelet count: a severe consequence of hypertension in pregnancy. 1982. Am J Obstet Gynecol 2005;193(3 Pt 1):859 [discussion: 860].

46. Sibai BM. Diagnosis, controversies, and management of the syndrome of hemolysis, elevated liver enzymes, and low platelet count. Obstet Gynecol 2004;103(5 Pt 1):981–91.

47. Haram K, Svendsen E, Abildgaard U. The HELLP syndrome: clinical issues and management. A Review. BMC Pregnancy Childbirth 2009;9:8.

48. Parnas M, Sheiner E, Shoham-Vardi I, et al. Moderate to severe thrombocytopenia during pregnancy. Eur J Obstet Gynecol Reprod Biol 2006;128(1–2): 163–8.

49. Sibai BM, Ramadan MK, Usta I, et al. Maternal morbidity and mortality in 442 pregnancies with hemolysis, elevated liver enzymes, and low platelets (HELLP syndrome). Am J Obstet Gynecol 1993; 169(4):1000–6.

50. Haddad B, Barton JR, Livingston JC, et al. Risk factors for adverse maternal outcomes among women with HELLP (hemolysis, elevated liver enzymes, and low platelet count) syndrome. Am J Obstet Gynecol 2000;183(2):444–8.

51. Woudstra DM, Chandra S, Hofmeyr GJ, et al. Corticosteroids for HELLP (hemolysis, elevated liver enzymes, low platelets) syndrome in pregnancy. Cochrane Database Syst Rev 2010;9:CD008148.

52. Westbrook RH, Dusheiko G, Williamson C. Pregnancy and liver disease. J Hepatol 2016;64(4): 933–45.

53. Tran TT, Ahn J, Reau NS. ACG clinical guideline: liver disease and pregnancy. Am J Gastroenterol 2016;111(2):176–94 [quiz: 196].

54. Grand'Maison S, Sauve N, Weber F, et al. Hepatic rupture in hemolysis, elevated liver enzymes, low

platelets syndrome. Obstet Gynecol 2012;119(3): 617–25.

55. Liu J, Ghaziani TT, Wolf JL. Acute fatty liver disease of pregnancy: updates in pathogenesis, diagnosis, and management. Am J Gastroenterol 2017; 112(6):838–46.

56. Westbrook RH, Yeoman AD, Joshi D, et al. Outcomes of severe pregnancy-related liver disease: refining the role of transplantation. Am J Transplant 2010;10(11):2520–6.

57. Ma K, Berger D, Reau N. Liver diseases during pregnancy. Clin Liver Dis 2019;23(2):345–61.

58. Clark SL. Amniotic fluid embolism. Obstet Gynecol 2014;123(2 Pt 1):337–48.

59. Tamura N, Farhana M, Oda T, et al. Amniotic fluid embolism: pathophysiology from the perspective of pathology. J Obstet Gynaecol Res 2017;43(4): 627–32.

60. Hasegawa A, Murakoshi T, Otsuki Y, et al. Clinical course of disseminated intravascular coagulopathy-type amniotic fluid embolism: a report of three cases. J Obstet Gynaecol Res 2016;42(12):1881–5.

61. Aurangzeb I, George L, Raoof S. Amniotic fluid embolism. Crit Care Clin 2004;20(4):643–50.

62. Clark SLHG, Dudley DA, Dildy GA, et al. Amniotic fluid embolism: analysis of the national registry. Am J Obstet Gynecol 1995;172(4):1158–67.

63. Kaur K, Bhardwaj M, Kumar P, et al. Amniotic fluid embolism. J Anaesthesiol Clin Pharmacol 2016; 32(2):153–9.

64. Dildy GA, Belfort MA, Clark SL. Amniotic fluid embolism. In: Dildy, Gary A, Belfort, et al, editors. "Amniotic fluid embolism." critical care obstetrics. Chichester (UK): John Wiley & Sons; 2018. p. 653–69. Web.

65. Pacheco LD, Clark SL, Klassen M, et al. Amniotic fluid embolism: principles of early clinical management. Am J Obstet Gynecol 2020;222(1):48–52.

66. Tanaka H, Katsuragi S, Osato K, et al. Efficacy of transfusion with fresh-frozen plasma:red blood cell concentrate ratio of 1 or more for amniotic fluid embolism with coagulopathy: a case-control study. Transfusion 2016;56(12):3042–6.

67. Leighton BL, Wall MH, Lockhart EM, et al. Use of recombinant factor VIIa in patients with amniotic FLuid embolism A systematic review of case reports. Anesthesiology 2011;115(6):1201–8.

68. Todo Y, Tamura N, Itoh H, et al. Therapeutic application of C1 esterase inhibitor concentrate for clinical amniotic fluid embolism: a case report. Clin Case Rep 2015;3(7):673–5.

69. Akasaka M, Osato K, Sakamoto M, et al. Practical use of C1 esterase inhibitor concentrate for clinical amniotic fluid embolism. J Obstet Gynaecol Res 2018;44(10):1995–8.

70. Sliwa K, Hilfiker-Kleiner D, Petrie MC, et al. Current state of knowledge on aetiology, diagnosis,

management, and therapy of peripartum cardiomyopathy: a position statement from the Heart Failure Association of the European Society of Cardiology Working Group on peripartum cardiomyopathy. Eur J Heart Fail 2010;12(8):767–78.

71. Harper MA, Meyer RE, Berg CJ. Peripartum cardiomyopathy: population-based birth prevalence and 7-year mortality. Obstet Gynecol 2012;120(5):1013–9.

72. Brar SS, Khan SS, Sandhu GK, et al. Incidence, mortality, and racial differences in peripartum cardiomyopathy. Am J Cardiol 2007;100(2):302–4.

73. Sinkey RG, Rajapreya IN, Szychowski JM, et al. (2020): Racial disparities in peripartum cardiomyopathy: eighteen years of observations, The Journal of Maternal-Fetal & Neonatal Medicine 2022; 35(10). DOI: 10.1080/14767058.2020.1773784

74. Elkayam U. Clinical characteristics of peripartum cardiomyopathy in the United States: diagnosis, prognosis, and management. J Am Coll Cardiol 2011;58(7):659–70.

75. Mielniczuk LM, Williams K, Davis DR, et al. Frequency of peripartum cardiomyopathy. Am J Cardiol 2006;97(12):1765–8.

76. Bello N, Rendon ISH, Arany Z. The relationship between pre-eclampsia and peripartum cardiomyopathy: a systematic review and meta-analysis. J Am Coll Cardiol 2013;62(18):1715–23.

77. Pearson GD, Veille JC, Rahimtoola S, et al. Peripartum cardiomyopathy: National Heart, Lung, and Blood Institute and Office of Rare Diseases (National Institutes of Health) Workshop Recommendations and Review. JAMA 2000;283(9):1183–8.

78. Kao DP, Hsich E, Lindenfeld J. Characteristics, adverse events, and racial differences among delivering mothers with peripartum cardiomyopathy. JACC Heart Fail 2013;1(5):409–16.

79. Pillarisetti J, Kondur A, Alani A, et al. Peripartum cardiomyopathy: predictors of recovery and current state of implantable cardioverter-defibrillator use. J Am Coll Cardiol 2014;63(25 Pt A):2831–9.

80. Davis MB, Arany Z, McNamara DM, et al. Peripartum cardiomyopathy: JACC state-of-the-art review. J Am Coll Cardiol 2020;75(2):207–21.

81. Dockree S, Brook J, Shine B, et al. Pregnancy-specific reference intervals for BNP and NT-pro BNP-changes in natriuretic peptides related to pregnancy. J Endocr Soc 2021;5(7):bvab091.

82. Resnik JL, Hong C, Resnik R, et al. Evaluation of B-type natriuretic peptide (BNP) levels in normal and preeclamptic women. Am J Obstet Gynecol 2005;193(2):450–4.

83. Li W, Li H, Long Y. Clinical characteristics and long-term predictors of persistent left ventricular systolic dysfunction in peripartum cardiomyopathy. Can J Cardiol 2016;32(3):362–8.

84. Sliwa K, Mebazaa A, Hilfiker-Kleiner D, et al. Clinical characteristics of patients from the worldwide

registry on peripartum cardiomyopathy (PPCM): EURObservational Research Programme in conjunction with the Heart Failure Association of the European Society of Cardiology Study Group on PPCM. Eur J Heart Fail 2017;19(9):1131–41.

85. Kolte D, Khera S, Aronow WS, et al. Temporal trends in incidence and outcomes of peripartum cardiomyopathy in the United States: a nationwide population-based study. J Am Heart Assoc 2014; 3(3):e001056.

86. Arany Z, Elkayam U. Peripartum cardiomyopathy. Circulation 2016;133(14):1397–409.

87. Bauersachs J, Arrigo M, Hilfiker-Kleiner D, et al. Current management of patients with severe acute peripartum cardiomyopathy: practical guidance from the Heart Failure Association of the European Society of Cardiology Study Group on peripartum cardiomyopathy. Eur J Heart Fail 2016;18(9): 1096–105.

88. Bozkurt B, Colvin M, Cook J, et al. Current diagnostic and treatment strategies for specific dilated cardiomyopathies: a scientific statement from the American Heart Association. Circulation 2016; 134(23):e579–646.

89. Regitz-Zagrosek V, Roos-Hesselink JW, Bauersachs J, et al. 2018 ESC Guidelines for the management of cardiovascular diseases during pregnancy. Eur Heart J 2018;39(34):3165–241.

90. Honigberg MC, Givertz MM. Peripartum cardiomyopathy. BMJ 2019;364:k5287.

91. Bouabdallaoui N, Demondion P, Leprince P, et al. Short-term mechanical circulatory support for cardiogenic shock in severe peripartum cardiomyopathy: La Pitie-Salpetriere experience. Interact Cardiovasc Thorac Surg 2017;25(1): 52–6.

92. Loyaga-Rendon RY, Pamboukian SV, Tallaj JA, et al. Outcomes of patients with peripartum cardiomyopathy who received mechanical circulatory support. Data from the Interagency Registry for Mechanically Assisted Circulatory Support. Circ Heart Fail 2014;7(2):300–9.

93. Zimmerman H, Bose R, Smith R, et al. Treatment of peripartum cardiomyopathy with mechanical assist devices and cardiac transplantation. Ann Thorac Surg 2010;89(4):1211–7.

94. McNamara DM, Elkayam U, Alharethi R, et al. Clinical outcomes for peripartum cardiomyopathy in North America: results of the IPAC study (Investigations of Pregnancy-Associated Cardiomyopathy). J Am Coll Cardiol 2015;66(8):905–14.

95. Goland S, Elkayam U. Peripartum cardiomyopathy: approach to management. Curr Opin Cardiol 2018; 33(3):347–53.

96. Davis NLS, Ashley N, Goodman DA. Pregnancy-related deaths: data from 14 U.S. Maternal Mortality Review Committees, 2008-2017. Centers for Disease Control and Infection, U.S. Department of Health and Human Services; 2019.

97. Marik PE, Plante LA. Venous thromboembolic disease and pregnancy. N Engl J Med 2008;359: 2025–33.

98. Clark P, Brennand J, Conkie JA, et al. Activated protein C sensitivity, protein C, protein S and coagulation in normal pregnancy. Thromb Haemost 1998;79:1166–70.

99. Bourjeily G, Paidas M, Khalil H, et al. Pulmonary embolism in pregnancy. Lancet 2010;375(9713): 500–12.

100. Heit JA, Kobbervig CE, James AH, et al. Trends in the incidence of venous thromboembolism during pregnancy or postpartum: a 30-year population-based study. Ann Intern Med 2005;143(10): 697–706.

101. Pomp ER, Lenselink AM, Rosendaal FR, et al. Pregnancy, the postpartum period and prothrombotic defects: risk of venous thrombosis in the MEGA study. J Thromb Haemost 2008;6(4):632–7.

102. Abe K, Kuklina EV, Hooper WC, et al. Venous thromboembolism as a cause of severe maternal morbidity and mortality in the United States. Semin Perinatol 2019;43(4):200–4.

103. Jaff MR, McMurtry MS, Archer SL, et al. Management of massive and submassive pulmonary embolism, iliofemoral deep vein thrombosis, and chronic thromboembolic pulmonary hypertension: a scientific statement from the American Heart Association. Circulation 2011;123(16):1788–830.

104. Dentali F, Riva N, Turato S, et al. Pulmonary embolism severity index accurately predicts long-term mortality rate in patients hospitalized for acute pulmonary embolism. J Thromb Haemost 2013; 11(12):2103–10.

105. Kasper W, Konstantinides S, Geibel A, et al. Management strategies and determinants of outcome in acute major pulmonary embolism: results of a multicenter registry. J Am Coll Cardiol 1997;30(5): 1165–71.

106. Becattini CAG. Risk stratification and management of acute pulmonary embolism. Hematol Am Soc Hematol Educ Program 2016;1:404–12.

107. Kearon C, Akl EA, Ornelas J, et al. Antithrombotic therapy for VTE disease: CHEST guideline and expert Panel report. Chest 2016;149(2):315–52.

108. Konstantinides SV, Torbicki A, Agnelli G, et al. 2014 ESC guidelines on the diagnosis and management of acute pulmonary embolism. Eur Heart J 2014; 35(43):3033–69, 3069a-3069k.

109. te Raa GD, Ribbert LS, Snijder RJ, et al. Treatment options in massive pulmonary embolism during pregnancy; a case-report and review of literature. Thromb Res 2009;124(1):1–5.

110. Martillotti G, Boehlen F, Robert-Ebadi H, et al. Treatment options for severe pulmonary embolism

during pregnancy and the postpartum period: a systematic review. J Thromb Haemost 2017; 15(10):1942–50.

111. Pasrija C, Shah A, George P, et al. Triage and optimization: a new paradigm in the treatment of massive pulmonary embolism. J Thorac Cardiovasc Surg 2018;156(2):672–81.

112. Rodriguez D, Jerjes-Sanchez C, Fonseca S, et al. Thrombolysis in massive and submassive pulmonary embolism during pregnancy and the puerperium: a systematic review. J Thromb Thrombolysis 2020;50(4):929–41.

113. Sharifi M, Bay C, Skrocki L, et al. Moderate pulmonary embolism treated with thrombolysis (from the "MOPETT" Trial). Am J Cardiol 2013; 111(2):273–7.

114. Piazza G, Hohlfelder B, Jaff MR, et al. A prospective, single-arm, multicenter trial of ultrasound-facilitated, catheter-directed, low-dose fibrinolysis for acute massive and submassive pulmonary embolism: the SEATTLE II Study. JACC Cardiovasc Interv 2015;8(10):1382–92.

115. Heavner MS, Zhang M, Bast CE, et al. Thrombolysis for massive pulmonary embolism in pregnancy. Pharmacotherapy 2017;37(11):1449–57.

116. Compadre AJ, Kohi M, Lokken RP, et al. Catheter-directed thrombolysis for submassive pulmonary embolism in the third trimester of pregnancy. JACC: Case Rep 2020;2(12):1899–904.

117. Gowda N, Nwabuobi CK, Louis JM. Catheter-directed thrombolytic therapy in the management of massive pulmonary embolism in pregnancy. Obstet Gynecol 2019;134(5):1002–4.

118. Pasrija C, Kronfli A, George P, et al. Utilization of veno-arterial extracorporeal membrane oxygenation for massive pulmonary embolism. Ann Thorac Surg 2018;105(2):498–504.

119. Ghoreishi M, DiChiacchio L, Pasrija C, et al. Predictors of recovery in patients supported with venoarterial extracorporeal membrane oxygenation for acute massive pulmonary embolism. Ann Thorac Surg 2020;110(1):70–5.

120. Malekan R, Saunders PC, Yu CJ, et al. Peripheral extracorporeal membrane oxygenation: comprehensive therapy for high-risk massive pulmonary embolism. Ann Thorac Surg 2012;94(1):104–8.

121. Sebastian NA, Spence AR, Bouhadoun S, et al.(2020) Extracorporeal membrane oxygenation in pregnant and postpartum patients: a systematic review, The Journal of Maternal-Fetal & Neonatal Medicine 2020. DOI: 10.1080/14767058.2020.1860932

122. Webster CM, Smith KA, Manuck TA. Extracorporeal membrane oxygenation in pregnant and postpartum women: a ten-year case series. Am J Obstet Gynecol MFM 2020;2(2):100108.

123. Agerstrand C, Abrams D, Biscotti M, et al. Extracorporeal membrane oxygenation for cardiopulmonary failure during pregnancy and postpartum. Ann Thorac Surg 2016;102(3):774–9.

124. Ünver SS, Kalkan A, Demirel A, et al. Extracorporeal membrane oxygenation for pulmonary embolism during pregnancy and postpartum. Eur Arch Med Res 2020;36(1):1–7.

125. Zambrano LD, Ellington S, Strid P. Update: characteristics of symptomatic women of reproductive age with laboratory-confirmed SARS-CoV-2 infection by pregnancy status — United States, January 22–October 3, 2020. MMWR Morb Mortal Wkly Rep 2020;69:1641–7.

126. COVID-19 Treatment Guidelines Panel. Coronavirus disease 2019 (COVID-19) treatment guidelines. National Institutes of Health. 2020. Available at. https://www.covid19treatmentguidelines.nih.gov/. Accessed July 14, 2021.

127. Green LJ, Mackillop LH, Salvi D, et al. Gestation-specific vital sign reference ranges in pregnancy. Obstet Gynecol 2020;135(3):653–64.

128. Guntupalli KK, Karnad DR, Bandi V, et al. Critical illness in pregnancy: Part II: common medical conditions complicating pregnancy and puerperium. Chest 2015;148(5):1333–45.

129. COVID-19 Treatment Guidelines Panel Coronavirus disease 2019 (COVID-19) treatment guidelines. National Institutes of Health. Available at: https://www.covid19treatmentguidelines.nih.gov/. Accessed July 14, 2021.

130. Guérin C, Reignier J, Richard JC, et al. Prone positioning in severe acute respiratory distress syndrome. N Engl J Med 2013;368(23):2159–68.

131. Oxford-Horrey C, Savage M, Prabhu M, et al. Putting it all together: clinical considerations in the care of critically ill obstetric patients with COVID-19. Am J Perinatol 2020;37(10):1044–51.

132. Vogel JP, Tendal B, Giles M, et al. Clinical care of pregnant and postpartum women with COVID-19: living recommendations from the National COVID-19 Clinical Evidence Taskforce. Aust N Z J Obstet Gynaecol 2020;60(6):840–51.

133. Saad AF, Rahman M, Maybauer DM, et al. Extracorporeal membrane oxygenation in pregnant and postpartum women with H1N1-related acute respiratory distress syndrome: a systematic review and meta-analysis. Obstet Gynecol 2016; 127(2):241–7.

134. Barrantes JH, Ortoleva J, O'Neil ER, et al. Successful treatment of pregnant and postpartum women with severe COVID-19 associated acute respiratory distress syndrome with extracorporeal membrane oxygenation. ASAIO J 2021;67(2):132–6.

Advances in Sepsis Care

Karen E. Jackson, MD[a], Matthew W. Semler, MD, MSc[b],*

KEYWORDS

• Sepsis • Septic shock • Critical care

KEY POINTS

- For most patients presenting with sepsis or septic shock, empiric broad-spectrum antibiotics should be administered as soon as feasible and narrowed after 48 to 72 hours as information on the causative organism becomes available.
- Recent large, randomized trials found that the use of balanced crystalloids may result in better outcomes than saline for patients with sepsis and septic shock; the role in albumin infusion remains uncertain.
- For patients with septic shock, treatment with corticosteroids decreases the dose of catecholamines required to maintain blood pressure, increases the number of vasopressor-free days, and may decrease the risk of death.
- Early renal replacement therapy and high-dose vitamin C have been demonstrated to not improve clinical outcomes for patients with sepsis or septic shock.

INTRODUCTION

Sepsis–life-threatening organ dysfunction in response to severe infection[1] – affects more than 48 million people globally each year.[2] Early recognition and appropriate management improve sepsis outcomes. Although more than 30 years have passed since the first formal definition of sepsis and more than 15 years since the Surviving Sepsis Campaign (SSC) first published broadly adopted management guidelines, the understanding of sepsis and its treatment continues to evolve rapidly. This article reviews the key history of and recent advances in sepsis treatment, including new research in the domains of antibiotics, fluids, vasopressors, and adjunctive therapies, such as corticosteroids and renal replacement therapy. We also highlight the remaining areas of clinical uncertainty and areas for future research.

DEFINITION

Sepsis, first formally defined in 1991,[3] has since 2016 been defined according to the Third

International Consensus Definition for Sepsis and Septic Shock (Sepsis-3) as life-threatening organ dysfunction caused by a dysregulated host response to infection.[1] The organ dysfunction component of the definition may be operationalized as an increase of 2 or more points in the Sequential Organ Failure Assessment (SOFA) score. The SOFA score assesses the function of 6 major organ systems (neurologic, cardiovascular, respiratory, hepatic, renal, and hematologic) on a scale of 0 (no dysfunction) to 4 (most severe dysfunction).[1] In the current definition, septic shock is defined as the presence of sepsis and circulatory, cellular, and metabolic abnormalities that are associated with a greater risk of mortality than sepsis alone (receipt of vasopressors and serum lactate >2 mmoL/L in the absence of hypovolemia).[1]

THERAPIES

Because sepsis is a common, complex, and life-threatening illness, recommendations regarding treatments have often preceded research to understand their effectiveness and safety. Moreover,

Sources of Funding: M.W. Semler was supported in part by the NHLBI (K23HL143053).
a Division of Pulmonary, Critical Care and Sleep Medicine, Rush University Medical Center, 1725 West Harrison Street, Suite 010, Chicago, IL 60612, USA; b Division of Allergy, Pulmonary and Critical Care Medicine, Vanderbilt University Medical Center, T-1218 MCN, 1161 21st Avenue South, Nashville, TN 37232, USA
* Corresponding author.
E-mail address: matthew.w.semler@vumc.org

Clin Chest Med 43 (2022) 489–498
https://doi.org/10.1016/j.ccm.2022.05.003
0272-5231/22/© 2022 Elsevier Inc. All rights reserved.

sepsis research of different designs conducted in different contexts has frequently produced conflicting results. Although supportive therapies like the administration of intravenous antibiotics, fluid, and vasopressors have been central to sepsis therapy for 2 decades, only in recent years has evidence from detailed studies of sepsis phenotyping and large, randomized clinical trials started to make clear the complex picture of how these simple-seeming therapies may affect sepsis outcomes.

Antibiotics

Since 2004, sepsis management guidelines have recommended the initiation of antimicrobial therapy within an hour of presentation to patients with severe sepsis and septic shock. In 2006, Kumar and colleagues[4] observed that among 2731 patients with septic shock at hospitals in Canada and the United States, each hour of delay in the initiation of effective antimicrobial therapy was associated with a mean decrease in survival of 7.6% (95% CI, 3.6%–9.9%).[4] Similarly, a retrospective analysis of 28,150 patients with severe sepsis and septic shock[5] found that the risk of mortality increases linearly for each 1 hour delay in antibiotic administration.[5] After the New York State Department of Health required hospitals to follow protocols for early treatment of severe sepsis and septic shock in 2013, a study of 49,331 patients found that longer time to the administration of antibiotics was associated with higher risk-adjusted in-hospital mortality (odds ratio, 1.04 per hour).[6] Results were similar among children presenting with sepsis.[7]

Although observational studies have consistently demonstrated an association between early antibiotic administration and improved outcomes for patients with sepsis and hypotension, results have been less consistent in studies of patients with sepsis without hypotension and in prospective randomized trials attempting to assess the causal effect of decreased time-to-antimicrobial therapy on sepsis outcomes. The PHANTASi (Prehospital Antibiotics against Sepsis) multicenter randomized trial examined whether prehospital administration of antibiotics increased survival for patients with sepsis, severe sepsis, or septic shock.[8] The trial found that antibiotic administration in the ambulance did not improve survival regardless of illness severity. Interpretation of the trial, however, was limited by the small number of patients with shock, lower than expected mortality rate, and a significant number of randomization violations.[8]

Recent research has shifted focus to minimizing risks associated with antibiotic administration, particularly antibiotic stewardship and the optimal

choice of antibiotics. The Surviving Sepsis Campaign Guidelines recommend initiating therapy with one or more antibiotics for patients presenting with sepsis or septic shock covering all likely pathogens and narrowing antibiotic coverage once a pathogen is identified.[9] Questions about when to narrow empiric therapy remain unanswered. A recent study found that, among critically ill adults whose cultures ultimately grew methicillin-resistant Staphylococcus aureus (MRSA), 98% of blood cultures demonstrated gram-positive cocci by 48 hours, whereas only 85% of respiratory cultures were positive by 48 hours.[10] A similar study among critically ill adults whose cultures ultimately grew Gram-negative rods (GNRs)[11] found that (1) 54.2% of respiratory cultures and 18.6% of blood cultures demonstrated resistance to ceftriaxone and (2) 87% of respiratory cultures and 85% of blood cultures that ultimately grew GNRs resistant to ceftriaxone had demonstrated growth by 48 hours.[11] The rapid evolution of methods for early molecular identification of pathogens for patients with sepsis offers the potential to significantly expedite identification of the causal organism and facilitate early narrowing of antibiotic therapy in the near future.[12]

In current practice, most patients with septic shock receive empiric antibiotic therapy with activity against Pseudomonas aeruginosa and resistant GNRs.[9,13] Anti-pseudomonal penicillins and cephalosporins are 2 of the most commonly administered classes of antibiotic for empiric coverage of resistant GNRs in patients with sepsis.[9,13] Recent observational data have suggested that concurrent receipt of piperacillin-tazobactam and vancomycin may be associated with elevations in serum creatinine concentration and that receipt of cefepime or ceftazidime may cause neurotoxicity.[14–20] Prospective randomized trials are urgently needed to compare effectiveness and safety of antipseudomonal penicillins versus antipseudomonal cephalosporins for initial empiric antibiotic therapy in patients with sepsis.

Intravenous Fluid Administration

In addition to antibiotics, the administration of intravenous (IV) fluid is a fundamental component of early sepsis management.[21] The physiologic rationale for administering IV fluids to patients with sepsis and hypotension is to increase venous return, increase stroke volume and cardiac output, and increase organ perfusion and oxygen delivery to reverse tissue hypoxia. Despite tens of millions of patients receiving IV fluid therapy for sepsis over the last 20 years, our understanding of the optimal approach to fluid therapy in sepsis, overall and for specific subsets of patients, remains limited. Fundamental questions are only recently beginning to be answered regarding the optimal timing, dose, duration, and composition of IV fluid for patients with sepsis.[22,23]

The concept that early IV fluid administration might improve outcomes for patients with sepsis was first popularized by a 2001 study of early goal-directed therapy (EGDT) by Rivers and colleagues[24] In this landmark trial, 263 patients presented to a single ED with severe sepsis or septic shock were randomized to usual care or EGDT. In the usual care group, patients were to receive a central venous catheter and an arterial catheter, administration of 500 mL boluses of IV fluid every 30 minutes to achieve a central venous pressure of 8 to 12 mm Hg, and vasopressor administration as required to achieve a mean arterial pressure goal of 65 mm Hg. Patients in the EGDT group were to receive the same therapies plus central venous oxygen saturation monitoring (ScvO2) and, for patients with a ScvO2 less than 70%, transfusion of red blood cells to achieve a hematocrit of at least 30% and infusion of dobutamine. During the 6 hours of intervention, patients in the EGDT group received significantly more fluid than patients in the usual care group (4981 ± 2984 L vs 3499 ± 2438 L, $P < .001$), and more frequently received blood transfusion (64.1% vs 18.5%, $P < .001$) and inotropic support (13.7% vs 0.8%, $P < .001$). In-hospital mortality rates were significantly lower in the EGDT group compared with the usual care group (38% vs 46.5%, $P = .009$).[24]

Based on the results of the Rivers EGDT study, and dozens of before-after studies of EGDT implementation, the Surviving Sepsis Campaign recommended fluid bolus administration as a foundational component of early sepsis management. Three subsequent large, multicenter trials, ProCESS,[25] ARISE,[26] and ProMISe,[27] randomized a combined 4201 patients to EGDT or usual care across 138 centers in 7 countries. Each of the 3 trials found no difference in clinical outcomes between EGDT and usual care (Fig. 1A). A meta-analysis of the individual patient data did not identify benefits in any of the prespecified subgroups.[28] Several possible explanations exist for the difference in findings between the trial by Rivers and colleagues and ProCESS, ARISE, and ProMISe trials. First, in the decade between the trial by Rivers and colleagues and the subsequent 3 trials, the administration of IV fluid boluses for early sepsis became more common in usual care and the separation between groups in the volume of IV fluid received may not have been sufficient to contribute to differences in outcome in the subsequent 3 trials. Second, the trial by Rivers and colleagues occurred in a single ED in a specific setting, and the average SvO2 values at presentation were much lower in this trial than in the subsequent 3 trials (eg, 46.6 ± 11.2 in Rivers and colleagues vs 71 ± 13 in ProCESS). This suggests that differences in patient population, severity, or phase of illness may have accounted for differences in the effect of early fluid therapy on outcomes. Third, the differences in outcomes between groups in the 263-patient single-center trial may have occurred due to chance imbalances.

Significant uncertainty remains regarding the optimal volume of IV fluid for patients with early sepsis and septic shock. In addition to the studies of EGDT in high-income countries, recent studies evaluating EGDT and fluid administration for infection in low- and middle-income countries have reported worse clinical outcomes with early IV fluid administration for patients with acute infection.[29–31] How the results of these trials apply to the patient populations and care settings in high-income countries remain uncertain. The ongoing NHLBI PETAL Network's CLOVERS trial (NCT03434028) is a large, multicenter, randomized trial comparing liberal versus restrictive IV fluid administration in early sepsis, the results of which may provide the first rigorous data comparing these common approaches to early sepsis fluid management.

In the absence of definitive evidence, guidelines differ in their recommendations. The most recent Surviving Sepsis Campaign Guidelines suggest early administration of 30 mL/kg IV fluid for septic shock or sepsis-induced hypoperfusion,[9] whereas the guidelines from the American College of Emergency Physicians Take Force agree with delivering an intravenous fluid bolus during the initial management of patients with hypotension or findings of hypoperfusion but does "not support a prespecified volume of body mass-adjusted volume of fluid for all patients."[32] While the optimal use of IV fluid boluses or vasopressors in early sepsis management remains unclear, the results of the ProCESS, ARISE, and ProMISe trials do make clear that many patients with early sepsis may be safely managed without invasive monitoring. In recent clinical practice, patients with sepsis and even septic shock on low doses of vasopressors are cared for without a central venous catheter or arterial catheter in many settings.[33] Future research must address whether the use of dynamic measures of fluid responsiveness, such as the assessment of stroke volume change in response to a passive leg raise or stroke volume variation during invasive mechanical ventilation, can improve outcomes by balancing the risks and benefits of fluid therapy in early sepsis.

The choice of IV fluid composition for sepsis resuscitation has generated significant recent

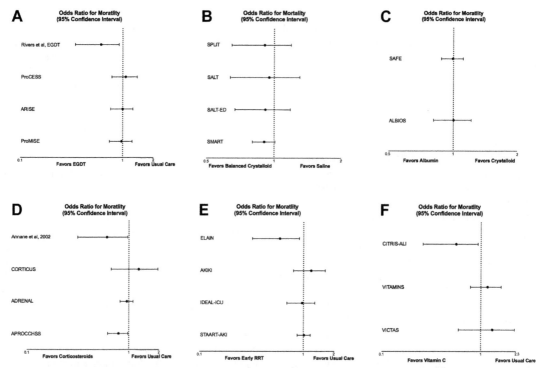

Fig. 1. Effect of sepsis therapies on mortality in large, randomized trials. *Odds ratios are unadjusted and calculated from raw data reported in trials unless specified otherwise.* (*A*) – mortality from the Rivers and ProCESS trials are 60-day mortality, ARISE and ProMISE are 90-day mortality. ProMISE is an adjusted OR. (*B*) – SPLIT, SALT, SALT-ED, and SMART show ORs for in-hospital mortality. (*C*) – SAFE and ALBIOS show ORs for 28-day mortality. (*D*) – Annane and CORTICUS report 28-day mortality in nonresponders, ADRENAL and APROCCHSS report 90-day mortality. Annane and ADRENAL are adjusted ORs. (*E*) – ELAIN, STAART-AKI, and IDEAL-ICU report 90-day mortality, AKIKI reported 60-day mortality. (*F*) – CITRIS ALI and VITAMINS report 28-day mortality, VICTAS reported 180-day mortality.

interest. Historically, the majority of the isotonic crystalloid solution administered to patients with sepsis has been saline (0.9% sodium chloride).[34,35] Saline contains 154 mmol/L of sodium and chloride, whereas isotonic crystalloid solutions referred to as "balanced crystalloids" (eg, lactated Ringer's, Plasma-Lyte, Normosol) contain buffers and a chloride concentration more similar to that of plasma (98–112 mmol/L). The administration of solutions with high chloride concentrations has been associated with hyperchloremic metabolic acidosis, decreased renal perfusion, hypotension, and acute kidney injury.

Four recent randomized trials compared balanced crystalloids to saline among adults (**Fig. 1**B). Two pilot trials, SPLIT (0.9% Saline vs Plasma-lyte 148 [PL-148] for ICU fluid therapy)[36] and SALT (isotonic Solution Administration Logistical Testing),[37] demonstrated the feasibility of comparing balanced crystalloids to saline among acutely ill adults. Two larger trials, the SMART (Isotonic Solutions and Major Adverse Renal Events Trial)[38] and SALT-ED (Saline against Lactated Ringer's or Plasma-Lyte in the Emergency

Department)[39] trials, compared saline to balanced crystalloids among ICU patients and patients with ED, respectively. Among the 15,802 patients in the SMART trial, the use of balanced crystalloid resulted in a lower rate of the composite outcome of death, new renal-replacement therapy, or persistent renal dysfunction, compared with the use of saline. In the SALT-ED trial, among noncritically ill adults treated in the emergency department, there was no difference between groups in the primary outcome of hospital-free days, but fewer patients experienced death, new renal-replacement therapy, or persistent renal dysfunction in the balanced crystalloid group. A secondary analysis of the SMART trial dataset found that, among 1641 patients with a diagnosis of sepsis, the use of balanced crystalloids was associated with an absolute risk reduction in 30-day in-hospital mortality of 4.9% points, compared with saline.[40] The effect of balanced crystalloids versus saline on mortality was greater among patients for whom fluid choice was controlled starting in the ED compared with patients for whom fluid choice was controlled starting in the ICU.[41] These findings raise the hypothesis that the effect of fluid composition on clinical outcomes may be greatest during the initial phase of sepsis resuscitation, when the volume of fluid being administered is greatest, abnormalities in acid–base are most profound, and risk for the development of acute kidney injury is highest.

Although isotonic crystalloid solutions are the most common intravenous fluid administered to patients with sepsis, the potential benefits of colloid solutions have also been investigated. Two basic types of colloid solutions have been evaluated for patients with sepsis: human albumin solution, a purified blood product with oncotic and antiinflammatory effects, and semisynthetic colloid solutions, solutions with fluid, electrolytes, and synthesized high molecular weight molecules. The physiologic rationale for using colloids is the concept that high molecular weight molecules are more likely to retain fluid in plasma rather than moving into the interstitium and contributing to edema and end-organ dysfunction. Recent advances in understanding the manner for which the endothelial glycocalyx regulates the movement of proteins out of the plasma during health and its disruption during disease have raised questions about the applicability of the traditional Starling model of fluid dynamics, specifically whether resuscitation with colloids really requires significantly less fluid volume than resuscitation with crystalloids.

The first major trial to compare colloids to crystalloids among critically ill adults was the Saline versus Albumin Fluid Evaluation (SAFE) trial, which randomized 3497 adult ICU patients to receive 4% albumin and 3500 to receive 0.9% sodium chloride for fluid resuscitation.[42] Mortality did not significantly differ between the albumin group (20.9%) and saline group (21.1%) overall (**Fig. 1**C). In a subgroup analysis of patients with severe sepsis; however, the relative risk of 28-day mortality in the albumin group was 0.87, as compared with 1.05 among patients without severe sepsis (*P* value for interaction = 0.06). The subsequent Albumin Italian Outcome Sepsis (ALBIOS) trial randomized 1818 patients with severe sepsis or septic shock to crystalloid administration alone or crystalloid and 20% albumin (rather than 4% as in SAFE) to maintain a serum albumin level of 30 g/L.[43] Patients in the albumin group experienced a lower heart rate, a higher mean arterial pressure, and lower net fluid balances. Death by day 28 or day 90 did not differ between groups– although a *post hoc* subgroup analysis suggested albumin might benefit patients with septic shock. Meta-analyses have suggested a potential improvement in mortality with albumin administration in patients with sepsis.[44,45] The Surviving Sepsis Campaign Guidelines recommend crystalloids as the initial resuscitation fluid, but encourage consideration of albumin for patients who have received significant volumes of crystalloid. In the absence of definitive data suggesting that the use of albumin improves outcomes, the high relative cost of albumin means crystalloid solutions are likely to remain the first-line therapy for fluid therapy in sepsis.

In an attempt to synthesize colloid solutions less expensive than albumin, starches, dextrans, and gelatins were developed and evaluated in a series of large, randomized trials. Together, these trials suggest that semi-synthetic colloids may cause acute kidney injury and should not be routinely administered to patients with sepsis.[46–49]

Vasoactive Therapy

Patients with sepsis who remain hypotensive after initial fluid resuscitation frequently receive vasopressors to maintain mean arterial pressure (MAP). Historically, dopamine was used as the first-line vasopressor for patients with septic shock. However, a large randomized trial demonstrated that dopamine is associated with more frequent adverse events (particularly tachyarrhythmias) than norepinephrine[50] and a meta-analysis suggested that dopamine may be associated with an increased risk of death.[51]

If blood pressure cannot be maintained at goal with moderate doses of norepinephrine alone, a second vasopressor is often added. The most widely used second vasopressors are vasopressin, epinephrine, and angiotensin II. The Vasopressin and Septic Shock Trial (VASST) examined the addition of vasopressin to norepinephrine among 778 adults with septic shock.[52] VASST found no decrease in mortality with the use of vasopressin overall, but suggested lower mortality in a subgroup of patients who presented with less severe shock.[52] Post hoc analysis of the VASST trial suggested early administration of vasopressin might reduce the need for renal replacement therapy.[52,53] The Vasopressin versus Norepinephrine as Initial Therapy in Septic Shock (VANISH) trial investigated this possibility. VANISH found that early vasopressin administration did not increase the number of renal failure-free days but might have decreased the receipt of renal replacement therapy.[54] Several trials have examined the use of vasopressin analogs such as terlipressin and selepressin. These trials found no difference in key clinical outcomes with selepressin and more serious adverse events associated with the use of terlipressin.[55,56] While the results of trials examining the effect of vasopressin on outcomes of septic shock are inconclusive, vasopressin decreases the required dose of norepinephrine and remains a commonly used second-line vasopressor.[9,52]

The newest vasopressor approved for the treatment of distributive shock is angiotensin II, a potent endogenous vasoconstricting agent. After promising results in a pilot study,[57] the Angiotensin II for the Treatment of High-Output Shock (ATHOS-3) trial randomly assigned patients with vasodilatory shock who were receiving more than 0.2 μg/kg/min norepinephrine or another vasopressor equivalent to receive an infusion of either angiotensin II or placebo.[58] In this trial, patients assigned to angiotensin II were more likely to reach the primary end point, defined as an increase in mean arterial pressure from baseline of at least 10 mm Hg or an increase to at least 75 mm Hg without an increase in the dose of background vasopressors at 3 hours.[58] Whether the use of angiotensin II improves clinical outcomes remains uncertain. How angiotensin II compares to the other available second-line vasopressors, such as vasopressin and epinephrine, remains a key clinical knowledge gap to be addressed in future research.

Other Supportive Therapies: Corticosteroids

Corticosteroid administration for patients with septic shock has been the subject of research and debate for decades. Overt adrenal insufficiency and relative adrenal insufficiency can occur in sepsis and septic shock but are difficult to recognize and diagnose.[59] Administration of corticosteroids to patients with sepsis can increase blood pressure and improve vascular tone.[60] Several large randomized trials have provided evidence regarding the effects of corticosteroid treatment on physiology and outcomes in septic shock (**Fig. 1**D).

In 2002, Annane and colleagues performed a 300-patient randomized, double-blind, parallel-group trial comparing 7 days of hydrocortisone and fludrocortisone to placebo.[61] All patients underwent a 250-μg ACTH stimulation test. The primary analysis found that, among patients who did not experience an increase in cortisol of 9 micrograms/dL after ACTH administration, the 28-day mortality rate in the steroid group was lower than the placebo group (hazard ratio, 0.71; 95% CI, 0.52–0.97).[61]

In 2008, the Corticosteroid Therapy of Septic Shock (CORTICUS) multicenter, randomized, double-blind, placebo-controlled trial assigned patients with septic shock to receive either 50 mg hydrocortisone or placebo every 6 hours for 5 days.[62] They found that hydrocortisone administration was associated with a faster reversal of shock compared with placebo, but no change in mortality at 28 days. Steroid administration was also associated with more episodes of infection, hyperglycemia, and hypernatremia.[62]

In 2018, the Adjunctive Corticosteroid Treatment in Critically Ill Patients with Septic Shock (ADRENAL) trial randomized 3800 patients to receive 200 mg/d of hydrocortisone via continuous infusion for 7 days or placebo. At 90 days, 511 patients (27.9%) in the hydrocortisone group and 526 (28.8%) in the placebo group had died (odds ratio, 0.95; 95% CI 0.82–1.10; $P = .50$).[63] The hydrocortisone group had faster resolution of shock and seemed to experience more days alive and not admitted to an intensive care unit.[63]

Also in 2018, the multicenter, double-blind, randomized Activated Protein C and Corticosteroids for Human Septic Shock (APROCCHSS) trial[64] compared 50 mg of hydrocortisone every 6 hours and 50 μg fludrocortisone by mouth once daily to placebo (in addition to comparing activated drotrecogin alfa vs placebo in a factorial design).[64] Among 1241 patients included in the trial, 90-day mortality was significantly lower in the hydrocortisone and fludrocortisone group (43%) than in the placebo group (49.1%) (relative risk, 0.88; 95% CI, 0.78–0.99).[64] The treatment group also experienced more vasopressor-free days and organ failure-free days. Hyperglycemia was more common in the treatment group but other adverse events did not differ.[64]

Although the optimal approach to steroid administration in sepsis remains uncertain and varies widely in current practice, the currently available data suggest that for patients with sepsis who are requiring moderate or high doses of vasopressors, administration of corticosteroids is a reasonable approach to decreasing catecholamine receipt, shortening the duration of shock, and potentially improving survival for some patients.

Other Supportive Therapies: Renal Replacement Therapy

Acute kidney injury is one of the most common complications of sepsis. When to initiate renal replacement therapy (RRT) for patients without urgent indications have been the subject of significant research (**Fig. 1**E).[65]

The ELAIN randomized, single-center, parallel-group trial compared early initiation (within 8 hours of stage 2 AKI) versus delayed initiation (within 12 hours of stage 3 AKI or no initiation) of RRT for critically ill patients with KDIGO stage 2 AKI and plasma neutrophil gelatinase-associated lipocalin level greater than 150 ng/mL.[65] Early initiation of RRT seemed to reduce 90-day mortality (39.3%) compared with delayed initiation (54.7%) (hazard ratio, 0.66; 95% CI 0.45–0.97).[65]

The Artificial Kidney Initiation in Kidney Injury (AKIKI) multicenter, prospective, two-group randomized trial randomized 620 critically ill adults with AKI at least KDIGO stage 3 who were receiving mechanical ventilation, catecholamine infusion, or both either early (within 6 hours) or delayed (up to 72 hours) initiation of RRT. A total of 250 of 311 patients in the early group and 244 of the 308 patients in the delayed group had a diagnosis of sepsis. Mortality was similar in the early and delayed initiation groups. Catheter-related bloodstream infections occurred more frequently in the early initiation group (10% vs 5%).[66]

The STARRT-AKI trial (Standard vs Accelerated Initiation of Renal-Replacement Therapy in Acute Kidney Injury) compared accelerated versus standard initiation of RRT among patients with stage 2 or 3 AKI by KDIGO classification.[67] Among 3019 patients, 1689 (57.7%) of whom had a diagnosis of sepsis, death by 90 days occurred in 643 (43.9%) in the accelerated initiation group and in 639 (43.7%) in the standard initiation group (relative risk, 1.00; P = .92).[67] Significantly more adverse events occurred in the accelerated initiation group.[67]

The Initiation of Dialysis Early versus Delayed in the Intensive Care Unit (IDEAL-ICU) randomized, open-label, multicenter trial compared early initiation (within 12 hours) versus delayed initiation (within 48 hours) of RRT for severe AKI in patients with early septic shock.[68] The trial was stopped early for futility when 58% of the patients in the early initiation group and 54% of patients in the delayed initiation group had died.[68]

In concert, the results of these 4 large, multicenter, randomized trials demonstrate that nearly half of patients with AKI for whom RRT initiation is delayed ultimately do not require RRT and that early initiation of RRT may increase the risk of adverse events. Therefore, for most patients with sepsis and AKI, delaying the initiation of RRT and carefully watching for the development of urgent indications seems to be the safest approach.

Other Supportive Therapies: High-Dose Vitamin C

Preclinical research has suggested that the administration of vitamin C may attenuate systemic inflammation, improve coagulopathy, and attenuate vascular injury in sepsis.[69–71] Recent randomized clinical trials, however, have not demonstrated benefit from high-dose vitamin C administration in terms of clinical outcomes in sepsis (**Fig. 1**F).[72–74]

SUMMARY

Care for patients with sepsis has improved significantly over the last 2 decades. Early broad-spectrum antibiotics for patients with sepsis-induced hypotension remain the cornerstone of management. Unanswered questions include the optimal choice of initial broad-spectrum antibiotics and the approach to antibiotic deescalation. With regard to fluid therapy, data from recent randomized trials suggest balanced crystalloids may produce better outcomes in sepsis than saline, and the role in albumin remains uncertain. The optimal volume of IV fluid in each phase of sepsis remains unknown. Whether dynamic measures of fluid responsiveness improve outcomes remains an urgent knowledge gap. Norepinephrine is the first-line vasopressor for patients with septic shock. When to initiate vasopressors and which vasopressor should be the second line require additional research. Corticosteroids represent a reasonable adjunctive therapy in septic shock. Early renal replacement therapy and administration of vitamin C have not been shown to improve outcomes in sepsis. Research comparing the effectiveness of available therapies for sepsis and systems to reliably deliver evidence-based sepsis care has the potential to continue to improve sepsis outcomes in the future.

CLINICS CARE POINTS

- Early, broad-spectrum antibiotic therapy remains a cornerstone for the treatment of patients with sepsis and hypotension.
- For initial fluid therapy in sepsis, clinicians should use isotonic crystalloid solutions rather than colloid solutions.
- For patients with sepsis who require vasopressor therapy, norepinephrine is the first-line vasopressor.
- For patient with septic shock, treatment with corticosteroids speeds resolution of shock.

CONFLICTS OF INTEREST

The authors declared no potential conflicts of interest with the current work.

REFERENCES

1. Singer M, Deutschman CS, Seymour CW, et al. The third international consensus definitions for sepsis and septic shock (Sepsis-3). JAMA 2016;315(8):801.
2. Rudd KE, Johnson SC, Agesa KM, et al. Global, regional, and national sepsis incidence and mortality, 1990–2017: analysis for the Global Burden of Disease Study. The Lancet 2020;395(10219):200–11.
3. Levy MM, Fink MP, Marshall JC, et al. 2001 SCCM/ESICM/ACCP/ATS/SIS international sepsis definitions conference. Crit Care Med 2003;31(4):1250–6.
4. Kumar A, Roberts D, Wood KE, et al. Duration of hypotension before initiation of effective antimicrobial therapy is the critical determinant of survival in human septic shock*. Crit Care Med 2006;34(6):1589–96.
5. Ferrer R, Martin-Loeches I, Phillips G, et al. Empiric antibiotic treatment reduces mortality in severe sepsis and septic shock from the first hour: results from a guideline-based performance improvement program. Crit Care Med 2014;42(8):7.
6. Seymour CW, Gesten F, Prescott HC, et al. Time to treatment and mortality during mandated emergency care for sepsis. N Engl J Med 2017;376(23):2235–44.
7. Evans IVR, Phillips GS, Alpern ER, et al. Association between the New York sepsis care mandate and in-hospital mortality for pediatric sepsis. JAMA 2018;320(4):358.
8. Alam N, Oskam E, Stassen PM, et al. Prehospital antibiotics in the ambulance for sepsis: a multicentre, open label, randomised trial. Lancet Respir Med 2018;6(1):40–50.
9. Rhodes A, Evans LE, Alhazzani W, et al. Surviving sepsis campaign: international guidelines for management of sepsis and septic shock. Crit Care Med 2017;45(3):486–552.
10. Melling PA, Noto MJ, Rice TW, et al. Time to first culture positivity among critically ill adults with methicillin-resistant *staphylococcus aureus* growth in respiratory or blood cultures. Ann Pharmacother 2020;54(2):131–7.
11. Buell KG, Casey JD, Noto MJ, et al. Time to first culture positivity for gram-negative rods resistant to ceftriaxone in critically ill adults. J Intensive Care Med 2021;36(1):51–7.
12. Kim J-S, Kang G-E, Kim H-S, et al. Evaluation of verigene blood culture test systems for rapid identification of positive blood cultures. Biomed Res Int 2016;2016:1–6.
13. Magill SS, Edwards JR, Beldavs ZG, et al. Prevalence of antimicrobial use in us acute care hospitals, May-September 2011. JAMA 2014;312(14):1438.
14. Rutter WC, Burgess DR, Talbert JC, et al. Acute kidney injury in patients treated with vancomycin and piperacillin-tazobactam: a retrospective cohort analysis. J Hosp Med 2017;12(2):77–82.
15. Long B, April MD. Are patients receiving the combination of vancomycin and piperacillin-tazobactam at higher risk for acute renal injury? Ann Emerg Med 2018;72(4):467–9.
16. Carreno J, Smiraglia T, Hunter C, et al. Comparative incidence and excess risk of acute kidney injury in hospitalised patients receiving vancomycin and piperacillin/tazobactam in combination or as monotherapy. Int J Antimicrob Agents 2018;52(5):643–50.
17. Bellos I, Karageorgiou V, Pergialiotis V, et al. Acute kidney injury following the concurrent administration of antipseudomonal β-lactams and vancomycin: a network meta-analysis. Clin Microbiol Infect 2020;26(6):696–705.
18. O'Callaghan K, Hay K, Lavana J, et al. Acute kidney injury with combination vancomycin and piperacillin-tazobactam therapy in the ICU: a retrospective cohort study. Int J Antimicrob Agents 2020;56(1):106010.
19. Appa AA, Jain R, Rakita RM, et al. Characterizing cefepime neurotoxicity: a systematic review. Open Forum Infect Dis 2017;4(4):ofx170.
20. Boschung-Pasquier L, Atkinson A, Kastner LK, et al. Cefepime neurotoxicity: thresholds and risk factors. A retrospective cohort study. Clin Microbiol Infect 2020;26(3):333–9.
21. Angus DC, van der Poll T. Severe sepsis and septic shock. N Engl J Med 2013;369(9):840–51.
22. Self WH, Semler MW, Bellomo R, et al. Liberal versus restrictive intravenous fluid therapy for early septic shock: rationale for a randomized trial. Ann Emerg Med 2018;72(4):457–66.
23. Malbrain MLNG, Van Regenmortel N, Saugel B, et al. Principles of fluid management and stewardship in septic shock: it is time to consider the four D's and the four phases of fluid therapy. Ann Intensive Care 2018;8(1):66.
24. Rivers E, Nguyen B, Havstad S, et al. Early goal-directed therapy in the treatment of severe sepsis and septic shock. N Engl J Med 2001;345(19):1368–77.
25. The ProCESS Investigators. A randomized trial of protocol-based care for early septic shock. N Engl J Med 2014;370(18):1683–93.
26. The ARISE Investigators and the ANZICS Clinical Trials Group. Goal-directed resuscitation for patients with early septic shock. N Engl J Med 2014;371(16):1496–506.
27. Mouncey PR, Osborn TM, Power GS, et al. Trial of early, goal-directed resuscitation for septic shock. N Engl J Med 2015;372(14):1301–11.
28. The PRISM Investigators. Early, goal-directed therapy for septic shock — a patient-level meta-analysis. N Engl J Med 2017;376(23):2223–34.
29. Andrews B, Semler MW, Muchemwa L, et al. Effect of an early resuscitation protocol on in-hospital

mortality among adults with sepsis and hypotension: a randomized clinical trial. JAMA 2017;318(13):1233.

30. Andrews B, Muchemwa L, Kelly P, et al. Simplified severe sepsis protocol: a randomized controlled trial of modified early goal–directed therapy in Zambia*. Crit Care Med 2014;42(11):2315–24.

31. Maitland K, Kiguli S, Opoka RO, et al. Mortality after fluid bolus in african children with severe infection. N Engl J Med 2011;364(26):2483–95.

32. Yealy DM, Mohr NM, Shapiro NI, et al. Early care of adults with suspected sepsis in the emergency department and out-of-hospital environment: a consensus-based task force report. Ann Emerg Med 2021. https://doi.org/10.1016/j.annemergmed.2021.02.006.

33. Cardenas-Garcia J, Schaub KF, Belchikov YG, et al. Safety of peripheral intravenous administration of vasoactive medication: peripheral Administration of VM. J Hosp Med 2015;10(9):581–5.

34. Hammond NE, Taylor C, Finfer S, et al. Patterns of intravenous fluid resuscitation use in adult intensive care patients between 2007 and 2014: an international cross-sectional study. In: Moine P, editor. PLoS One 2017;12(5):e0176292.

35. McIntyre L, Rowe BH, Walsh TS, et al. Multicountry survey of emergency and critical care medicine physicians' fluid resuscitation practices for adult patients with early septic shock. BMJ Open 2016;6(7):e010041.

36. Young P, Bailey M, Beasley R, et al. Effect of a buffered crystalloid solution vs saline on acute kidney injury among patients in the intensive care unit: the SPLIT randomized clinical trial. JAMA 2015;314(16):1701.

37. Semler MW, Wanderer JP, Ehrenfeld JM, et al. Balanced crystalloids versus saline in the intensive care unit. the SALT randomized trial. Am J Respir Crit Care Med 2017;195(10):1362–72.

38. Semler MW, Self WH, Wanderer JP, et al. Balanced crystalloids versus saline in critically ill adults. N Engl J Med 2018;378(9):829–39.

39. Self WH, Semler MW, Wanderer JP, et al. Balanced crystalloids versus saline in Noncritically ill adults. N Engl J Med 2018;378(9):819–28.

40. Brown RM, Wang L, Coston TD, et al. Balanced crystalloids versus saline in sepsis: a secondary analysis of the SMART trial. Am J Respir Crit Care Med 2019. https://doi.org/10.1164/rccm.201903-0557OC.

41. Jackson KE, Wang L, Casey JD, et al. Effect of early balanced crystalloids before ICU admission on sepsis outcomes. Chest 2020. https://doi.org/10.1016/j.chest.2020.08.2068.

42. Finfer S, Bellomo R, Boyce N, et al. A comparison of albumin and saline for fluid resuscitation in the intensive care unit. N Engl J Med 2004;350(22):2247–56.

43. Caironi P, Tognoni G, Masson S, et al. Albumin replacement in patients with severe sepsis or septic shock. N Engl J Med 2014;370(15):1412–21.

44. Rochwerg B, Alhazzani W, Sindi A, et al. Fluid resuscitation in sepsis: a systematic review and network meta-analysis. Ann Intern Med 2014;161(5):347.

45. Bansal M, Farrugia A, Balboni S, et al. Relative survival benefit and morbidity with fluids in severe sepsis - a network meta-analysis of alternative therapies. Curr Drug Saf 2013;8(4):236–45.

46. Brunkhorst FM, Engel C, Bloos F, et al. Intensive insulin therapy and pentastarch resuscitation in severe sepsis. N Engl J Med 2008;358(2):125–39.

47. Guidet B, Martinet O, Boulain T, et al. Assessment of hemodynamic efficacy and safety of 6% hydroxyethylstarch 130/0.4 vs. 0.9% NaCl fluid replacement in patients with severe sepsis: the CRYSTMAS study. Crit Care 2012;16(3):R94.

48. Myburgh JA, Finfer S, Bellomo R, et al. Hydroxyethyl starch or saline for fluid resuscitation in intensive care. N Engl J Med 2012;367(20):1901–11.

49. Perner A, Haase N, Guttormsen AB, et al. Hydroxyethyl starch 130/0.42 versus ringer's acetate in severe sepsis. N Engl J Med 2012;367(2):124–34.

50. De Backer D, Biston P, Devriendt J, et al. Comparison of dopamine and norepinephrine in the treatment of shock. N Engl J Med 2010;362(9):779–89.

51. Melzer D. Dopamine versus norepinephrine in the treatment of septic shock: a meta-analysis. J Emerg Med 2012;42(6):751.

52. Russell JA, Walley KR, Singer J, et al. Vasopressin versus norepinephrine infusion in patients with septic shock. N Engl J Med 2008;358(9):877–87.

53. Gordon AC, Russell JA, Walley KR, et al. The effects of vasopressin on acute kidney injury in septic shock. Intensive Care Med 2010;36(1):83–91.

54. Gordon AC, Mason AJ, Thirunavukkarasu N, et al. Effect of early vasopressin vs norepinephrine on kidney failure in patients with septic shock: the VANISH randomized clinical trial. JAMA 2016;316(5):509.

55. Study Group of Investigators, Liu Z-M, Chen J, et al. Terlipressin versus norepinephrine as infusion in patients with septic shock: a multicentre, randomised, double-blinded trial. Intensive Care Med 2018;44(11):1816–25.

56. Laterre P-F, Berry SM, Blemings A, et al. Effect of selepressin vs Placebo on ventilator- and vasopressor-free days in patients with septic shock: the SEPSIS-ACT randomized clinical trial. JAMA 2019;322(15):1476.

57. Chawla LS, Busse L, Brasha-Mitchell E, et al. Intravenous angiotensin II for the treatment of high-output shock (ATHOS trial): a pilot study. Crit Care 2014;18(5):534.

58. Khanna A, English SW, Wang XS, et al. Angiotensin II for the treatment of vasodilatory shock. N Engl J Med 2017;377(5):419–30.

59. Patel GP, Balk RA. Systemic steroids in severe sepsis and septic shock. Am J Respir Crit Care Med 2012;185(2):133–9.

60. Schumer W. Steroids in the treatment of clinical septic shock. Ann Surg 1976;184(3):333–41.

61. Annane D, Sébille V, Charpentier C, et al. Effect of treatment with low doses of hydrocortisone and fludrocortisone on mortality in patients with septic shock. JAMA 2002;288(7):862–71.

62. Sprung CL, Annane D, Kah D, et al. Hydrocortisone therapy for patients with septic shock. N Engl J Med 2008;358(2):111–24.

63. Venkatesh B, Finfer S, Cohen J, et al. Adjunctive glucocorticoid therapy in patients with septic shock. N Engl J Med 2018;378(9):797–808.

64. Annane D, Renault A, Brun-Buisson C, et al. Hydrocortisone plus fludrocortisone for adults with septic shock. N Engl J Med 2018;378(9):809–18.

65. Zarbock A, Kellum JA, Schmidt C, et al. Effect of early vs delayed initiation of renal replacement therapy on mortality in critically ill patients with acute kidney injury: the ELAIN randomized clinical trial. JAMA 2016;315(20):2190.

66. Gaudry S, Hajage D, Schortgen F, et al. Initiation strategies for renal-replacement therapy in the intensive care unit. N Engl J Med 2016;375(2):122–33.

67. The STARRT-AKI Investigators. Timing of initiation of renal-replacement therapy in acute kidney injury. N Engl J Med 2020;383(3):240–51.

68. Barbar SD, Clere-Jehl R, Bourredjem A, et al. Timing of renal-replacement therapy in patients with acute kidney injury and sepsis. N Engl J Med 2018; 379(15):1431–42.

69. Fisher BJ, Seropian IM, Kraskauskas D, et al. Ascorbic acid attenuates lipopolysaccharide-induced acute lung injury*. Crit Care Med 2011;39(6): 1454–60.

70. Fisher BJ, Kraskauskas D, Martin EJ, et al. Mechanisms of attenuation of abdominal sepsis induced acute lung injury by ascorbic acid. Am J Physiol Lung Cell Mol Physiol 2012;303(1):L20–32.

71. Medical Respiratory Intensive Care Unit Nursing, Fowler AA, Syed AA, et al. Phase I safety trial of intravenous ascorbic acid in patients with severe sepsis. J Transl Med 2014;12(1):32.

72. Fowler AA, Truwit JD, Hite RD, et al. Effect of vitamin C infusion on organ failure and biomarkers of inflammation and vascular injury in patients with sepsis and severe acute respiratory failure: the CITRIS-ALI randomized clinical trial. JAMA 2019;322(13): 1261.

73. Fujii T, Luethi N, Young PJ, et al. Effect of vitamin C, hydrocortisone, and thiamine vs hydrocortisone alone on time alive and free of vasopressor support among patients with septic shock: the VITAMINS randomized clinical trial. JAMA 2020;323(5):423.

74. Sevransky JE, Rothman RE, Hager DN, et al. Effect of vitamin C, thiamine, and hydrocortisone on ventilator- and vasopressor-free days in patients with sepsis: the VICTAS randomized clinical trial. JAMA 2021;325(8):742.

Advances in Ventilator Management for Patients with Acute Respiratory Distress Syndrome

Michael C. Sklar, MD[a,b,c], Laveena Munshi, MD, MSc[a,d],*

KEYWORDS

• ARDS • PEEP • Prone positioning • Neuromuscular blockers

KEY POINTS

- Despite decades of research, acute respiratory distress syndrome (ARDS) is not always recognized in ICU practice.
- Low-tidal-volume ventilation, plateau pressure limitations, driving pressure targets, and mechanical ventilation in the prone position for moderate–severe ARDS are strategies shown to minimize harm associated with mechanical ventilation.
- The risk–benefits of spontaneous breathing, optimal and individualized positive end-expiratory pressure titration, and oxygen therapy thresholds are areas of ARDS research that continue to evolve and likely have individualized targets for different phenotypes of patients with ARDS.

INTRODUCTION

The supportive care management of the acute respiratory distress syndrome (ARDS) has remained a cornerstone of therapy in critical care medicine for well over 50 years. Over time, we have seen an evolution in our understanding of the injured lung, its interaction with invasive mechanical ventilation and the optimal approach to supporting the lung while minimizing harm. Recent years have unveiled the heterogeneous nature of ARDS emphasizing the need to more accurately define sub-phenotypes. Given this, research is ongoing to better refine and individualized mechanical ventilatory support (eg, optimal selection of positive end-expiratory pressure [PEEP] and thresholds when spontaneous breathing efforts could be harmful). In this review, we highlight the current evidence-based ventilatory management practices for patients with ARDS and explore some experimental novel ventilation targets (**Fig. 1**).

What Is Acute Respiratory Distress Syndrome?

ARDS is the clinical syndrome consisting of acute hypoxemia, reduced lung compliance, and pulmonary infiltrates which was first described in 1967.[1] The Berlin definition[2] classifies ARDS as respiratory failure that occurs acutely (within 7 days) and is characterized by the onset of bilateral chest radiograph opacities not fully explained by cardiac failure. The severity of the syndrome is classified as mild, moderate, or severe according to the degree of hypoxemia defined by Pao_2/Fio_2. Importantly, this must be fulfilled with patients receiving at least 5 cm H_2O of positive pressure.

[a] Interdepartmental Division of Critical Care Medicine, University of Toronto, Toronto, Canada; [b] Department of Anesthesiology and Pain Medicine, St. Michael's Hospital, Unity Health Toronto, 6th Floor, 30 Bond Street, Toronto M5B 1W8, Ontario, Canada; [c] Department of Anesthesiology and Pain Medicine, University of Toronto, Toronto, Canada; [d] Department of Medicine, Sinai Health System, University of Toronto, Mount Sinai Hospital, 18-206, 600 University Avenue, Toronto M5G1X5, Ontario, Canada.
* Corresponding author. Department of Medicine, Sinai Health System, University of Toronto, Mount Sinai Hospital, 18-206, 600 University Avenue, Toronto M5G1X5, Ontario, Canada.
E-mail address: laveena.munshi@sinaihealth.ca

Clin Chest Med 43 (2022) 499–509
https://doi.org/10.1016/j.ccm.2022.05.002

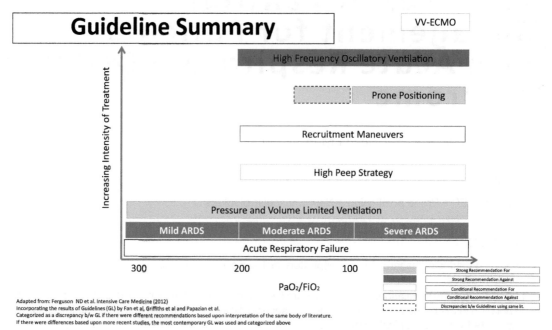

Fig. 1. Guideline summary. Incorporating the results of guidelines (GLs) by Fan and colleagues, Griffiths and colleagues, and Papazian and colleagues categorized as discrepancy between GLs if there were different recommendations based on interpretation of the same body of literature. If there were differences based on more recent studies, the most contemporary GL was used and categorized above. (*Adapted from* Ferguson ND, Fan E, Camporota L, Antonelli M, Anzueto A, Beale R, Brochard L, Brower R, Esteban A, Gattinoni L, Rhodes A, Slutsky AS, Vincent JL, Rubenfeld GD, Thompson BT, Ranieri VM. The Berlin definition of ARDS: an expanded rationale, justification, and supplementary material. Intensive Care Med. 2012 Oct;38(10):1573-82.)

The severity of ARDS correlates strongly with mortality. Contemporary estimates of ARDS mortality were recently described in the LUNGSAFE observational study,[3] where investigators found approximately 25% mortality in mild ARDS and up to 45% in the severe subgroup. More recently and partially driven by the COVID-19 pandemic, there has been an interest in expanding the definition of ARDS, acknowledging the limitations of arterial blood gas measurements in resource-limited settings, and the consideration of high-flow nasal oxygen and noninvasive ventilation as equivalents of mechanical ventilation to satisfy diagnostic criteria.[4]

Ventilator-Induced Lung Injury

The focus of mechanical ventilatory practices in ARDS centers around minimizing ventilator-induced lung injury (VILI). VILI is the consequence of trauma to the lungs secondary to high-tidal-volume ventilation (volutrauma), excessive ventilating pressure (barotrauma) and the cyclic opening and closing of alveoli during tidal ventilation (atelectrauma).[5,6] These deforming and pathologic stresses to the lung architecture cause the release of inflammatory mediators into the systemic circulation (biotrauma).[7] The translocation

of these systemic inflammatory mediators has been implicated in the causal pathway leading to multisystemic organ failure and death that is associated with VILI and ARDS.[8]

Ventilatory Management of Acute Respiratory Distress Syndrome

Lung-protective ventilation

The mainstay of lung-protective mechanical ventilation derives from the seminal ARDSnet trial in 2000.[9] This randomized trial compared ventilating patients at 6 mL/kg of predicted body weight (PBW) 12 mL/kg. Compared with the higher tidal volume (V_T) group, patients ventilated at 6 mL/kg PBW had improved survival, demonstrated important secondary objectives including shortened duration of mechanical ventilation, attenuated systemic inflammation, and reduced the incidence and amount of extrapulmonary organ failure.[9] Current recommendations, based on this trial, suggest limiting both V_T to 4-6 mL/kg of PBW along with limiting plateau pressure (Pplat) to < 30 cmH$_2$O.

Tidal Volume: More than just 6 mL/kg

Although 6 mL/kg of V_T compared with 12 mL/kg has been demonstrated to be effective in preventing VILI,[9] the ideal V_T strategy in ARDS is unknown. In fact, even when V_T is normalized to a patient's PBW, there is experimental evidence to suggest that this too does not guarantee lung protection.[10,11] Conceivably, therefore, ventilating patients below 6 mL/kg may confer even greater lung protection. Two human studies in patients on extracorporeal life support for severe ARDS, in which V_T was below 6 mL/kg demonstrated a reduction in systemic inflammatory mediators.[12,13] However, whether this translates to clinical benefit remains unclear. A recent trial employing the use of extracorporeal CO2 removal to facilitate lower tidal volume ventilation ($\leq$3 mL/kg) did not confer a survival advantage compared with conventional ventilation and there were increased adverse events associated with the device. The trial was stopped early due to futility and feasibility following recommendations from the data safety monitoring committee. More research is needed to evaluate the population, approach, and potential utility to lowering tidal volumes less than 6 mL/kg.

A physiologically derived ventilation target: Driving pressure

A pressure- and volume-limited ventilation strategy neglects the individual respiratory pathophysiology and heterogeneity of ARDS patients. To account for this variability in respiratory mechanics across ARDS patients, investigators evaluated driving pressure (ΔP) as a predictor variable for mortality in ARDS. Compared with set tidal volume, ΔP is a tidal volume normalized to an individual patient's lung compliance. ΔP is measured as the difference between Pplat and total PEEP. There are a few caveats that should be mentioned to ensure the measurement of this value is accurate: the patient should be completely passive on the ventilator (either receiving neuromuscular blockade or deep sedation) and an end-expiratory occlusion maneuver should be performed to ensure there is no additional auto-PEEP.

$$\Delta P = Pplat - PEEPtotal$$

Amato and colleagues performed an individual patient meta-analysis of more than 3000 patients with ARDS from several randomized controlled trials (RCTs) to evaluate the association between ΔP and survival in ARDS.[14] Importantly, these investigators found that increases in ΔP, even in those patients receiving conventionally protective Pplat, were associated with increased mortality. Furthermore, ΔP was found to be the strongest predictor associated with outcome in ARDS patients, potentially explained by the physiologic and individualized nature of this variable.[14] In this analysis,

there was an association toward increased mortality as ΔP became greater than approximately 14 cmH_2O. A pilot, RCT was recently published which established that a ΔP-targeted ventilation approach was safe, feasible, and laid the foundation for a future large-scale RCT.[15,16]

Positive End-Expiratory Pressure Titration and Lung Recruitment

Physiologic impact of positive end-expiratory pressure

PEEP has been a cornerstone of ventilator management for ARDS since its first description.[1,17] However, defining the optimal level of PEEP has been challenging.[18] This is likely due to the fact that no one PEEP strategy is generalizable to all patients with ARDS. PEEP is used primarily to improve oxygenation and prevent atelectrauma (the cyclic opening and closing of alveoli that can occur during tidal ventilation) that contributes to VILI.[5,19] Further mechanistic benefits of PEEP include recruiting collapsed alveoli, thereby improving overall gas exchange,[20] reducing intrapulmonary shunt, and reducing stress and strain on the lung.[21] By recruiting additional alveolar units to participate in gas exchange, this improves the homogeneity of ventilation and reduces VILI by mitigating the effects of stress multipliers on the lung.[22]

PEEP can have a major effect on circulatory function and plays a key role in complex heart–lung interactions in mechanically ventilated patients. PEEP can affect both left and right heart function and depending on volume status and ventricular function can have either beneficial or detrimental effects on cardiovascular and respiratory function. With respect to the compromised left ventricle, PEEP can improve cardiac function by reducing afterload, although PEEP typically increases right ventricular afterload.[23] Conversely, higher levels of applied PEEP via reduction in venous return and therefore preload can significantly reduce cardiac output.[24]

Recruitment maneuvers

Predicated on the physiologic basis that atelectasis is a major contributor to VILI, an "open lung" approach has been advocated for the management of patients with ARDS.[25] One such way to maximally open the lung units is to perform a "recruitment" maneuver. Using a sustained increase in airway pressure, alveolar units are opened, and then a certain amount of applied PEEP is maintained to keep the lungs "open."[26] Two commonly described approaches to delivering a recruitment maneuver involve a sustained inflation and "staircase" increase in positive pressure. Typically, a sustained inflation recruitment maneuver may be executed as a set applied PEEP for a fixed time (30 cmH$_2$O for 30 seconds).[26] The staircase maneuver involves progressive increased airway pressure while maintaining a constant driving pressure up to peak airway pressure of approximately 40 to 60 cmH$_2$O.[27] Although recruitment maneuvers may serve to open atelectatic lung units to improve oxygenation, they may also lead to overdistension or compromise in cardiac output. The overall benefit achieved (improving oxygenation vs overdistension and decrease in cardiac output) depends on the overall recruitability of the lung. Being able to predict which patients will have a favorable response is sometimes difficult to determine at the bedside.

Clinical evidence guiding recruitment maneuvers and positive end-expiratory pressure

Although it has been at least a decade since the publication of RCTs evaluating high versus low PEEP strategies, there is still no clear evidence for the guidance of PEEP in the contemporary management of ARDS. The ALVEOLI trial[28] enrolled 549 patients to receive either high PEEP (mean PEEP 13.2 ± 3.5 cm H$_2$O) or low PEEP (mean PEEP 8.3 ± 3.2 cm H$_2$O) in patients with ARDS. The lung open ventilation study (LOVS)[29] trial enrolled 983 patients randomized to high (mean day 1 PEEP 15.6 ± 3.9 cm H$_2$O) or low (mean day 1 PEEP 10.1 ± 3.0 cm H$_2$O) PEEP strategy. Finally, the EXPRESS trial[30] randomized 767 patients to a moderate PEEP strategy (5–9 cmH$_2$O) or titrated PEEP to reach a Pplat of 28 to 30 cmH$_2$O (mean PEEP 15.8 ± 2.9 cm H$_2$O). All studies individually found no difference in mortality between higher and lower PEEP strategies. However, in a 2299 meta-analysis, high PEEP was associated with a mortality benefit across the subgroup of patients with moderate–severe ARDS.[31]

An RCT of high-intensity recruitment maneuvers, the ART trial,[32] was published in 2017. This trial randomized 1010 patients with moderate or severe ARDS to either a control arm of low PEEP or an experimental arm of lung recruitment maneuvers followed by a decremental PEEP trial incorporating compliance measurements to determine optimal PEEP. The primary outcome of 28-day mortality was higher in the experimental (55%) compared with the control group (49%) contrary to the original hypothesis.

It has been theorized that the excess mortality rate in the experimental arm may be explained by at least two physiologic processes. First, the recruitment maneuvers in the protocol may have

been both excessive and prolonged. Peak pressures upwards of 60 cmH$_2$O and total recruitment maneuver time for as long as 25 minutes may have contributed to barotrauma and VILI, leading to the increased mortality rates.[33] The second concern in this trial was the high proportion of patient–ventilator dyssynchrony in the experimental group. These dyssynchronies have the potential to lead to breath stacking and double triggering, which, effectively, can double tidal volume and/or peak pressures and precipitate further lung injury.

Finally, a reevaluation of high versus low PEEP strategies categorized patients with moderate-to-severe ARDS into hyperinflammatory versus non-hyperinflammatory subphenotypes. The impact of PEEP strategy differed by phenotype for mortality, ventilator-free days, and organ-failure-free days.[34]

Although several questions remain on the contemporary application of PEEP in ARDS, there are several emerging, physiologically based methods proposed to enable clinicians to apply individualized PEEP to their patients.

The future: Personalized positive end-expiratory pressure selection

Esophageal pressure Contemporary ventilator management and guidelines for mechanical ventilation target airway Pplat as surrogates for alveolar distending pressure. Airway pressure, however, reflects the sum of the distending pressures of the lungs and the chest wall. The use of esophageal pressure (Pes) manometer allows for the estimation of pleural pressure and therefore allows for the partitioning of lung and chest wall distending pressures.

Measurement of Pes during mechanical ventilation has been a technique commonly used in the research setting but has had sparse clinical uptake.[35] Pes estimates the changes in pleural pressure[36] and therefore allows estimation of transpulmonary pressure, calculated as the difference between Pplat and Pes.[37] Pes tracings can be used to individually understand and titrate mechanical ventilatory support in patients with ARDS.

$$Ptp = Paw - Pes$$

The most commonly known method to estimate pleural pressure and calculate transpulmonary pressure is by directly estimating pleural pressure from absolute values of Pes.[38]

The absolute value of the Pes method relies on the assumption that Pes is a direct estimate of pleural pressure. A pig and human cadaver study found that absolute measured Pes accurately reflects local pleural pressure in the mid to dependent lung regions,[39] where atelectasis and lung collapse typically occur in ARDS.[40] Thus, titrating PEEP to absolute Pes is physiologically sound, and two RCTs of this approach demonstrated physiologic benefits, but did not demonstrate survival advantage in ARDS patients.[38,41]

An alternative approach is using airway Pplat and the elastance ratio of chest wall to the respiratory system.[42,43] The ratio of chest wall to respiratory system elastance determines the fraction of airway driving pressure consumed to inflate the chest wall, thought to be non-harmful to the lungs. An experimental study found that transpulmonary pressure calculated from the elastance ratio reasonably reflects transpulmonary pressure in the nondependent "baby" lung where it is most vulnerable to VILI.[39]

Perhaps applying both approaches in prospective trials may translate into improved outcomes in patients with ARDS. Pes measurements also have a role in the ARDS recovery phase to monitor spontaneous breathing and the assessment of patient–ventilatory asynchronies.

Recruitment-to-inflation ratio A novel, single-breath maneuver, termed the recruitment-to-inflation (R/I) ratio to assess lung recruitment, was recently described in non-COVID ARDS.[44] Using a drop in PEEP over a single-breath maneuver, investigators measured recruited lung volume over the given range of PEEP change. Mathematically, the R/I ratio represents the proportion of volume distributed to the recruited lung compared with that volume distributed to the baby lung with changes in PEEP. In other terms, the R/I ratio can help clinicians separate patients who may benefit from higher PEEP (recruitment of collapsed alveoli) versus over-distending lung units that are already open (potentially injuring the baby lung).[44] A small prospective study in 24 patients with COVID-related ARDS supported this finding.[45] A multicenter, prospective RCT comparing traditional PEEP titration with PEEP–FiO_2 tables versus PEEP based on the R/I ratio in both COVID and non-COVID ARDS is currently recruiting patients (NCT03963622).

High-frequency oscillation High-frequency oscillatory ventilation was a strategy previously evaluated across patients with moderate–severe ARDS. It was hypothesized that an approach that focuses on optimal lung recruitment with minimal tidal volumes may be the most "lung-protective" approach to ventilation. In two large randomized trials across patients with moderate–severe ARDS, high-frequency oscillation, compared to the standard of care (conventional ventilation targets or an open lung ventilatory strategy), did not improve mortality.[46,47] In an individual patient meta-analysis, however, at a Pao_2/Fio_2 threshold below 64mm Hg, there was a signal toward benefit with the use of high-frequency oscillation.[48]

To Open the Lung or Not

Strategies aimed at fully recruiting or "opening" the lung through recruitment maneuvers, oscillatory ventilation, or higher PEEP strategies have consistently lacked translation to clinically meaningful improvements in patient outcomes. However, many of these studies adopted an approach to opening the lung independent of patient's individual ARDS physiology. Maximal inflation across all patients with ARDS may not be the right approach for all patients. Emerging evidence suggests that the collapsed lung may not be always harmful and may in certain settings be associated less inflammatory compared with aerated lung units.[49–51] Future research evaluating optimal mechanisms of opening/recruiting the lung needs to focus on the identification of which patients would benefit from an open lung strategy and pragmatic methods to execute this at the bedside.

Oxygen Titration

Optimal oxygen thresholds in the setting of ARDS have emerged as a topic receiving much attention in recent years. Liberal oxygen targets (hyperoxia/hyperoxemia), conservative oxygen targets, and permissive hypoxia have all been evaluated yielding conflicting results. The inconsistent findings are likely related to heterogeneous populations being evaluated with different intensities of illness and organ injuries present.

Hyperoxia and hyperoxemia have been associated with local and systemic toxicities. Excess oxygen can result in the development of reactive oxygen species which can precipitate apoptosis, vasoconstriction, inflammation, and multisystem failure. The specific oxygen thresholds and durations at which this may induce harm have yet to be determined. In the OXYGEN-ICU trial of 480 critically ill patients (66%–68% mechanically ventilated), lower oxygen targets (94%–98%, Pao_2 70–100) were associated with lower mortality compared with a liberal oxygen strategy (97%–100%; Pao_2 up to 150 mm Hg).[52] However, this study was not restricted to patients with ARDS and it was stopped early raising concerns about the potential overestimation of treatment effect. In the ICU-ROX trial, 965 mechanically ventilated patients were randomized to a conservative oxygen strategy (91%–96%) compared with a liberal approach (91%–100%).[53] With the exception of patients admitted with anoxic brain injury following cardiac arrest (who did worse overall), there was no difference in mortality or ventilator-free days across the conversative versus liberal strategies. The hypothesis behind the greater harm in the anoxic brain injury group may be related to conservative oxygen-reducing secondary brain injury compared with a more liberal approach. Limitations of the study include concern for heterogeneity of treatment effect across the mechanically ventilated population (ie, potential harm of liberal oxygen in the anoxic encephalopathy cohort vs potential benefit in the septic cohort). It is also important to note that the "liberal arm" of the ICU-ROX trial was not one of "hyperoxia." Furthermore, these trials did not focus on patients with ARDS.[10]

The HOT-ICU trial randomized 2928 critically ill patients with hypoxic respiratory failure (57%–59% invasive ventilation, 13% ARDS) to a lower oxygen target (P_aO_2 60 mm Hg) versus a higher oxygen target (P_aO_2 90 mm Hg).[54] Neither difference was found in 90-day mortality nor any of the secondary outcomes evaluated. This was in contrast to the LOCO2 trial where 201 patients with ARDS were randomized to a conservative oxygen target (P_aO_2 between 55 and 70 mm Hg) compared with a liberal target (90–105 mm Hg).[55] There was no difference in 28-day mortality; however, the trial was stopped early (201/850 original sample size) because of an increased incidence of mesenteric ischemia in the conservative group (5 vs 0). They theorized that pulse oximetry may not be precise enough to avoid unrecognized hypoxic events in those most at risk. There was also a lower incidence of prone positioning in the treatment group which has been shown to improve mortality in ARDS. The trial was also terminated early which might have led to inaccurate estimations of treatment effect.

The ongoing MEGA-ROX trial (NCT01642498) is a platform trial that attempts to further evaluate the question of safe oxygen thresholds and address treatment effects across different populations of critically ill patients. As the evidence continues to evolve, given the totality of the evidence thus far, hyperoxia and hyperoxemia should be avoided, a lower limit saturation of 90% to 91% is likely acceptable and targeting a P_aO_2 between 70 and 100 mmHg has been demonstrated to be safe across patients with ARDS.

Adjunct Therapies to Optimize Mechanical Ventilation

Prone positioning

Prone positioning is one of the few interventions with mortality benefit in patients with moderate–severe ARDS (**Fig. 2**).[56] Prone positioning can improve both oxygenation and ventilation (CO_2) clearance through a variety of mechanisms. Oxygenation is improved principally through improvement in the homogeneity of ventilation and perfusion matching, alveolar recruitment, and alterations in the physical mechanics of the chest wall.[57] Alveolar ventilation may improve with prone positioning because of the above mechanisms as well, which would manifest in a reduction in P_aCO_2.

Although several small trials and physiologic observations supported the concept of prone positioning, the seminal trial informing practice today was PROSEVA. The PROSEVA trial randomized 474 patients with moderate–severe ARDS (P/F < 150 mm Hg) to prone positioning for at least 16 hours per session or to be continuously ventilated in the supine position. Both 28 day and 90 day mortality rates were significantly reduced in the prone positioning group (the 28-day mortality was 16.0% in the prone group and 32.8% in the supine group [P < 0.001], 90-day mortality was 23.6% in the prone group versus 41.0% in the supine group [P < 0.001]).[56] Despite these results, clinical implementation of prone positioning remains poor, as demonstrated in the LUNGSAFE study, where only 16% of patients received prone positioning.[3] Despite concerns of complications[58] (pressure sores, loss of central lines, or endotracheal tubes), there was no such observed difference in the PROSEVA trial.[56]

Prone positioning in spontaneous breathing, non-intubated patients has gained popularity in the context of the COVID-19 pandemic. One clinical trial of 1126 patients requiring HFNC assessed whether prone positioning improved treatment failure as defined as intubation or mortality by 28 days.[59] The primary outcome of interest in this trial was death or intubation at 28 days. Treatment failure (mainly driven by intubation) occurred in 223 (40%) of 564 patients assigned to awake prone positioning and HFNC and 257 (46%) of 557 patients assigned to standard care with HFNC (relative risk 0.86 [95% CI 0.75−0.98]). Physiologic variables (respiratory rate, ROX index, and oxygenation) all improved when moving from the supine to prone position. Importantly, the rates of adverse events were not different between the two groups. More trials are underway evaluating the criteria for consideration of prone positioning and thresholds for intubation.

Neuromuscular blocking agents to facilitate lung-protective ventilation

The contemporary role of neuromuscular blocking agents (NMBAs) in ARDS is evolving. Now more than a decade since its publication, the

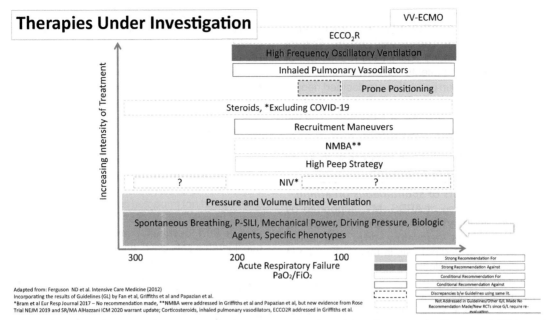

Fig. 2. Therapies under investigation. Incorporating the results of guidelines by Fan and colleagues, Griffiths and colleagues, and Papazian and colleagues. [a]Bram and colleagues Eur Resp Journal 2017—No recommendation made; [b]NMBA were addressed in Griffiths and colleagues and Papazian and colleagues, but new evidence from Rose Trial NEJM 2019 and SR/MA AlHazzani ICM 2020 warrant update; Corticosteroids, inhaled pulmonary vasodilators, and ECCO2R addressed in Griffiths and colleagues. (*Adapted from* Ferguson ND, Fan E, Camporota L, Antonelli M, Anzueto A, Beale R, Brochard L, Brower R, Esteban A, Gattinoni L, Rhodes A, Slutsky AS, Vincent JL, Rubenfeld GD, Thompson BT, Ranieri VM. The Berlin definition of ARDS: an expanded rationale, justification, and supplementary material. Intensive Care Med. 2012 Oct;38(10):1573-82)

ACURASYS trial was the first major RCT which demonstrated a mortality benefit with the use of NMBAs in early ARDS.[60] In this trial, 340 patients with moderate–severe ARDS (P/F < 150 mm Hg) were randomized to 48 hours of NMBA infusion with cisatracurium versus placebo. Importantly, both groups received deep sedation. Investigators demonstrated improved 90 day survival in the NMBA group (23.6% in the prone group vs 41.0% in the supine group [$P < 0.001$]).

The postulated physiologic and survival benefit of NMBA administration are centered around the reduction of patient–ventilator dyssynchrony.[61] It is hypothesized that patient–ventilator dyssynchrony can precipitate VILI due to variable V_T and alveolar distending pressure, with increased risk of breath-stacking. This can lead to further barotrauma, atelectrauma, and biotrauma, resulting in a release of inflammatory mediators and end-organ dysfunction.[8,61] Other physiologic benefits may include reduced respiratory and skeletal muscle oxygen consumption, leading to an increase in mixed venous oxygen[62] and, possibly, anti-inflammatory effects.[63] Despite this sound physiologic rationale and RCT evidence, the clinical use of continuous NMBA in ARDS is not widespread. The LUNGSAFE study demonstrated that

NMBA was used in approximately 7%, 18%, and 38% of patients with mild, moderate, and severe ARDS, respectively.[3] Reservation surrounding adoption may be attributable to concerns of deep sedation in the control arm, which one may argue does not reflect more contemporary sedation targets.

More recently, and based on evolving clinical practices since the publication of ACURASYS, the reevaluation of systemic early neuromuscular blockade (ROSE) trial was performed with a similar intervention arm as ACURASYS. It differed significantly from ACURAYS, however, in the in the timing of enrollment and the design of the control arm.[64] Patients with moderate–severe ARDS (P/F < 150 mm Hg) were randomized either to a deep-sedation arm with 48 hours of NMBA or a light sedation strategy arm. Contrary to ACURASYS, ROSE did not demonstrate a benefit in 90 day survival with routine and early application of NMBA. One possible explanation for the differences in the study findings is that deep sedation without paralysis may precipitate patient–ventilator dyssynchrony, which would not be present under conditions of paralysis, and may be significantly less in cases of light-sedation.[61] Furthermore, the timing of enrollment in ROSE was shorter compared with ACURASYS suggesting that patients in ACURASYS may represent a subset with more "persistent" ARDS. Current guidelines recommend against the routine use of NMBA across all patients; however, NMBA can be considered when paralytics are deemed necessary to facilitate lung-protective ventilation, address refractory hypoxia or hypercapnia, in the setting of ventilator asynchrony.[65]

Spontaneous Breathing in Patients with Acute Respiratory Distress Syndrome

Risks and benefits of spontaneous breathing
Early in the course of ARDS, MV, supported by sedation, and sometimes NMBA will completely suppress patient respiratory drive and effort. Passively ventilated patients in this context are at increased risk of atelectasis and complications of deep sedation including diaphragm and respiratory muscle disuse and atrophy.[66–68] Promoting spontaneous ventilation may mitigate these risks.

However, there may be a threshold of spontaneous ventilation that becomes injurious. Spontaneous ventilation that is excessive can propagate patient self-inflicted lung injury (P-SILI).[69] The mechanisms underlying this have some similarities to VILI.[70] Vigorous spontaneous breathing with large V_T can elevate global and regional lung stress, which precipitates the risk of volutrauma.[71] Importantly, even if V_T is limited by using volume-controlled ventilation, spontaneous effort can still induce injury by increasing local lung stress and overdistension.[72,73] These vigorous efforts can simultaneously induce diaphragm and respiratory muscle injury,[68] which can delay liberation from mechanical ventilation and lead to adverse clinical outcomes.[66,67] Finally, exaggerated spontaneous breathing effort can lead to, or worsen patient–ventilator dyssynchrony, as a consequence of double triggering or flow starvation.[71] It is therefore increasingly recognized that monitoring of patient effort during mechanical ventilation is important to identify the risk of P-SILI.[74]

Monitoring patient effort during mechanical ventilation
Basic interpretation of ventilator waveforms is insufficient in detecting potentially injurious patient efforts for a variety of reasons.[74] For example, airway pressure and flow provide limited direct information about inspiratory effort, but close inspection of flow deformations may be suggestive of patient effort.[71] Furthermore, airway pressure, particularly in the presence of respiratory effort, may underestimate the increased transpulmonary pressure generated by negative pleural pressure swings from the contraction of the inspiratory muscles.[75]

Pes measurements can be used to assess respiratory intensity of spontaneously breathing patients.[40] Unfortunately, Pes measurement is not routinely used at the bedside due to technical challenges, interpretation, and time-constraints.[71] Two simpler techniques have been described to estimate patient drive and effort. First, the airway occlusion pressure (P0.1) is the drop in airway pressure in the first 100 milliseconds after the onset of inspiration during an end-expiratory occlusion of the airway.[76] This measurement has gained recent interest as it is not affected by patient's response to the occlusion, it is independent of respiratory mechanics and not impacted by some degree of respiratory muscle weakness.[77] Although thresholds vary, a P0.1 between 1 and 4 cm H_2O may be considered a safe drive, and below or above these values may be reflective of excessively low or high drive to breathe, respectively.[78] Second, an end-expiratory occlusion maneuver (Pocc) in spontaneously breathing patients can be used to estimate the pressure generated by the respiratory muscles.[71] Pocc can also be used to estimate dynamic transpulmonary driving pressure, which is a measure of the dynamic mechanical stress applied to the lung during inspiration.[79] Although these measurements require prospective analysis, at the bedside, applying a simple end-expiratory hold maneuver, it may be reasonable to consider an estimated muscular pressure > 15 cm H_2O and estimated dynamic transpulmonary driving pressure> 20 cm H_2O as potentially markers of excessive and potentially injurious efforts.[79] There is active ongoing research into prospectively evaluating these measurements (P0.1 and Pocc) to titrate ventilation and sedation to achieve safe spontaneous breathing in mechanically ventilated adults.

SUMMARY

ARDS supportive care has evolved over the past few decades as our understanding of injurious interactions between the ventilator and the lung has improved. Increasingly, the heterogeneous nature of ARDS and individualized lung physiology has proven that a single ventilatory strategy (eg, PEEP, recruitment) is not generalizable to all patients. The future of ARDS ventilatory practice will center around more individualized treatment strategies and targets taking into consideration the subtype of ARDS and evolution of physiology over the course of the disease.

DISCLOSURE

The authors have no financial disclosures.

REFERENCES

1. Ashbaugh DG, Bigelow DB, Petty TL, et al. Acute respiratory distress in adults. Lancet Lond Engl 1967;2(7511):319–23.
2. Ranieri VM, Rubenfeld GD, Thompson BT, et al, ARDS Definition Task Force. Acute respiratory distress syndrome: the Berlin Definition. JAMA 2012;307(23):2526–33.
3. Bellani G, Laffey JG, Pham T, et al. Epidemiology, patterns of care, and mortality for patients with acute respiratory distress syndrome in intensive care units in 50 countries. JAMA 2016;315(8):788–800.
4. Brown SM, Peltan ID, Barkauskas C, et al. What does "ARDS" mean during the COVID-19 pandemic? Ann Am Thorac Soc 2021. https://doi.org/10.1513/AnnalsATS.202105-534PS.
5. Slutsky AS, Ranieri VM. Ventilator-induced lung injury. N Engl J Med 2013;369(22):2126–36.
6. Webb HH, Tierney DF. Experimental pulmonary edema due to intermittent positive pressure ventilation with high inflation pressures. Protection by positive end-expiratory pressure. Am Rev Respir Dis 1974;110(5):556–65.
7. Tremblay LN, Slutsky AS. Ventilator-induced injury: from barotrauma to biotrauma. Proc Assoc Am Physicians 1998;110(6):482–8.
8. Slutsky AS, Tremblay LN. Multiple system organ failure. Is mechanical ventilation a contributing factor? Am J Respir Crit Care Med 1998;157(6 Pt 1):1721–5.
9. Brower RG, Matthay MA, Morris A, et al, Acute Respiratory Distress Syndrome Network. Ventilation with lower tidal volumes as compared with traditional tidal volumes for acute lung injury and the acute respiratory distress syndrome. N Engl J Med 2000; 342(18):1301–8.
10. MacIntyre NR. Lung protective ventilator strategies: beyond scaling tidal volumes to ideal lung size. Crit Care Med 2016;44(1):244–5.
11. Deans KJ, Minneci PC, Cui X, et al. Mechanical ventilation in ARDS: one size does not fit all. Crit Care Med 2005;33(5):1141–3.
12. Bein T, Weber-Carstens S, Goldmann A, et al. Lower tidal volume strategy (3 ml/kg) combined with extracorporeal CO2 removal versus "conventional" protective ventilation (6 ml/kg) in severe ARDS: the prospective randomized Xtravent-study. Intensive Care Med 2013;39(5):847–56.
13. Terragni P, Del Sorbo L, Mascia L, et al. Tidal volume lower than 6 ml/kg enhances lung protection: role of extracorporeal carbon dioxide removal. Anesthesiology 2009;111(4):826–35. https://doi.org/10.1097/ALN.0b013e3181b764d2.
14. Amato MBP, Meade MO, Slutsky AS, et al. Driving pressure and survival in the acute respiratory distress syndrome. N Engl J Med 2015;372(8): 747–55.
15. Pereira Romano ML, Maia IS, Laranjeira LN, et al. Driving pressure-limited strategy for patients with acute respiratory distress syndrome. a pilot randomized clinical trial. Ann Am Thorac Soc 2020;17(5): 596–604.
16. Urner M, Jüni P, Hansen B, et al. Time-varying intensity of mechanical ventilation and mortality in patients with acute respiratory failure: a registry-based, prospective cohort study. Lancet Respir Med 2020;8(9):905–13.
17. Sahetya SK, Goligher EC, Brower RG. Fifty Years of Research in ARDS. Setting positive end-expiratory pressure in acute respiratory distress syndrome. Am J Respir Crit Care Med 2017;195(11):1429–38.
18. Cavalcanti AB, Amato MBP, Serpa-Neto A. The elusive search for "Best PEEP" and whether esophageal pressure monitoring helps. JAMA 2019; 321(9):839–41.
19. Slutsky AS, Drazen JM. Ventilation with small tidal volumes. N Engl J Med 2002;347(9):630–1.
20. Contribution of multiple inert gas elimination technique to pulmonary medicine. 5. Ventilation-perfusion relationships in acute respiratory failure. Thorax 1994;49(12):1251–8.
21. Di Marco F, Devaquet J, Lyazidi A, et al. Positive end-expiratory pressure-induced functional recruitment in patients with acute respiratory distress syndrome. Crit Care Med 2010;38(1):127–32.
22. Lung inhomogeneity in patients with acute respiratory distress syndrome. Am J Respir Crit Care Med 2014;189(02):149–58.
23. Suter PM, Fairley B, Isenberg MD. Optimum end-expiratory airway pressure in patients with acute pulmonary failure. N Engl J Med 1975;292(6):284–9.
24. Dhainaut JF, Devaux JY, Monsallier JF, et al. Mechanisms of decreased left ventricular preload during continuous positive pressure ventilation in ARDS. Chest 1986;90(1):74–80.
25. Lachmann B. Open up the lung and keep the lung open. Intensive Care Med 1992;18(6):319–21.
26. Lung recruitment: the role of recruitment maneuvers. Respir Care 2002;47(03):308–17.
27. Borges JB, Okamoto VN, Matos GFJ, et al. Reversibility of lung collapse and hypoxemia in early acute respiratory distress syndrome. Am J Respir Crit Care Med 2006;174(3):268–78.
28. Brower RG, Lanken PN, MacIntyre N, et al. Higher versus lower positive end-expiratory pressures in patients with the acute respiratory distress syndrome. N Engl J Med 2004;351(4):327–36.
29. Meade MO, Cook DJ, Guyatt GH, et al. Ventilation strategy using low tidal volumes, recruitment maneuvers, and high positive end-expiratory pressure for acute lung injury and acute respiratory distress syndrome: a randomized controlled trial. JAMA 2008;299(6):637–45.

30. Mercat A, Richard J-CM, Vielle B, et al. Positive end-expiratory pressure setting in adults with acute lung injury and acute respiratory distress syndrome: a randomized controlled trial. JAMA 2008;299(6): 646–55.

31. Briel M, Meade M, Mercat A, et al. Higher vs lower positive end-expiratory pressure in patients with acute lung injury and acute respiratory distress syndrome: systematic review and meta-analysis. JAMA 2010;303(9):865–73.

32. Cavalcanti AB, Suzumura ÉA, Laranjeira LN, et al, Writing Group for the Alveolar Recruitment for Acute Respiratory Distress Syndrome Trial (ART) Investigators. Effect of lung recruitment and titrated positive end-expiratory pressure (PEEP) vs low PEEP on mortality in patients with acute respiratory distress syndrome: a randomized clinical trial. JAMA 2017; 318(14):1335.

33. Should the ART trial change our practice? J Thorac Dis 2017;9(12):4871–7.

34. Calfee CS, Delucchi K, Parsons PE, et al. Subphenotypes in acute respiratory distress syndrome: latent class analysis of data from two randomised controlled trials. Lancet Respir Med 2014;2(8): 611–20.

35. Mauri T, Yoshida T, Bellani G, et al. Esophageal and transpulmonary pressure in the clinical setting: meaning, usefulness and perspectives. Intensive Care Med 2016;42(9):1360–73.

36. Agostoni E, Hyatt RE. Static behavior of the respiratory system. Compr Physiol 2011;(Suppl. 12): 113–30.

37. Akoumianaki E, Maggiore SM, Valenza F, et al. The application of esophageal pressure measurement in patients with respiratory failure. Am J Respir Crit Care Med 2014;189(5):520–31.

38. Talmor D, Sarge T, Malhotra A, et al. Mechanical ventilation guided by esophageal pressure in acute lung injury. N Engl J Med 2008;359(20):2095–104.

39. Yoshida T, Amato MBP, Grieco DL, et al. Esophageal manometry and regional transpulmonary pressure in lung injury. Am J Respir Crit Care Med 2018;197(8): 1018–26.

40. Yoshida T, Brochard L. Esophageal pressure monitoring: why, when and how? Curr Opin Crit Care 2018;24(3):216–22.

41. Beitler JR, Sarge T, Banner-Goodspeed VM, et al. Effect of titrating positive end-expiratory pressure (PEEP) with an esophageal pressure-guided strategy vs an empirical high PEEP-Fio2 strategy on death and days free from mechanical ventilation among patients with acute respiratory distress syndrome: a randomized clinical trial. JAMA 2019; 321(9):846–57.

42. Staffieri F, Stripoli T, De Monte V, et al. Physiological effects of an open lung ventilatory strategy titrated on elastance-derived end-inspiratory transpulmonary pressure: study in a pig model*. Crit Care Med 2012;40(7):2124–31.

43. Chiumello D, Cressoni M, Colombo A, et al. The assessment of transpulmonary pressure in mechanically ventilated ARDS patients. Intensive Care Med 2014;40(11):1670–8.

44. Chen L, Del Sorbo L, Grieco DL, et al. Potential for lung recruitment estimated by the recruitment-to-inflation ratio in acute respiratory distress syndrome. a clinical trial. Am J Respir Crit Care Med 2020; 201(2):178–87.

45. Stevic N, Chatelain E, Dargent A, et al. Lung recruitability evaluated by recruitment-to-inflation ratio and lung ultrasound in Covid-19 acute respiratory distress syndrome. Am J Respir Crit Care Med 2021;203(8):1025–7.

46. Young D, Lamb SE, Shah S, et al. High-frequency oscillation for acute respiratory distress syndrome. N Engl J Med 2013;368(9):806–13.

47. Ferguson ND, Cook DJ, Guyatt GH, et al. High-frequency oscillation in early acute respiratory distress syndrome. N Engl J Med 2013;368(9):795–805.

48. Meade MO, Young D, Hanna S, et al. Severity of hypoxemia and effect of high-frequency oscillatory ventilation in acute respiratory distress syndrome. Am J Respir Crit Care Med 2017;196(6): 727–33.

49. Bellani G, Messa C, Guerra L, et al. Lungs of patients with acute respiratory distress syndrome show diffuse inflammation in normally aerated regions: a [18F]-fluoro-2-deoxy-D-glucose PET/CT study. Crit Care Med 2009;37(7):2216–22.

50. Chu EK, Whitehead T, Slutsky AS. Effects of cyclic opening and closing at low- and high-volume ventilation on bronchoalveolar lavage cytokines. Crit Care Med 2004;32(1):168–74.

51. Fanelli V, Mascia L, Puntorieri V, et al. Pulmonary atelectasis during low stretch ventilation: "open lung" versus "lung rest" strategy. Crit Care Med 2009;37(3):1046–53.

52. Girardis M, Busani S, Damiani E, et al. Effect of conservative vs conventional oxygen therapy on mortality among patients in an intensive care unit: the oxygen-ICU randomized clinical trial. JAMA 2016; 316(15):1583–9.

53. Mackle D, Bellomo R, Bailey M, et al, ICU-ROX Investigators and the Australian and New Zealand Intensive Care Society Clinical Trials Group. Conservative oxygen therapy during mechanical ventilation in the ICU. N Engl J Med 2020;382(11):989–98.

54. Schjørring OL, Klitgaard TL, Perner A, et al. Lower or higher oxygenation targets for acute hypoxemic respiratory failure. N Engl J Med 2021;384(14): 1301–11.

55. Barrot L, Asfar P, Mauny F, et al. Liberal or conservative oxygen therapy for acute respiratory distress syndrome. N Engl J Med 2020;382(11):999–1008.

56. Guérin C, Reignier J, Richard J-C, et al. Prone positioning in severe acute respiratory distress syndrome. N Engl J Med 2013;368(23):2159–68.

57. Gattinoni L, Busana M, Giosa L, et al. Prone positioning in acute respiratory distress syndrome. Semin Respir Crit Care Med 2019;40(01):094–100.

58. Guérin C, Beuret P, Constantin JM, et al. A prospective international observational prevalence study on prone positioning of ARDS patients: the APRONET (ARDS Prone Position Network) study. Intensive Care Med 2018;44(1):22–37.

59. Ehrmann S, Li J, Ibarra-Estrada M, et al. Awake prone positioning for COVID-19 acute hypoxaemic respiratory failure: a randomised, controlled, multinational, open-label meta-trial. Lancet Respir Med 2021. https://doi.org/10.1016/S2213-2600(21)00356-8. Published online August 20.

60. Papazian L, Forel J-M, Gacouin A, et al. Neuromuscular blockers in early acute respiratory distress syndrome. N Engl J Med 2010;363(12):1107–16.

61. Slutsky AS, Villar J. Early paralytic agents for ARDS? Yes, No, and sometimes. N Engl J Med 2019;380(21):2061–3.

62. Marik PE, Kaufman D. The effects of neuromuscular paralysis on systemic and splanchnic oxygen utilization in mechanically ventilated patients. Chest 1996;109(4):1038–42.

63. Fanelli V, Morita Y, Cappello P, et al. Neuromuscular blocking agent cisatracurium attenuates lung injury by inhibition of nicotinic acetylcholine receptor-α1. Anesthesiology 2016;124(1):132–40.

64. Early neuromuscular blockade in the acute respiratory distress syndrome. N Engl J Med 2019;380(21):1997–2008.

65. Alhazzani W, Belley-Cote E, Møller MH, et al. Neuromuscular blockade in patients with ARDS: a rapid practice guideline. Intensive Care Med 2020;46(11):1977–86.

66. Goligher EC, Fan E, Herridge MS, et al. Evolution of diaphragm thickness during mechanical ventilation. impact of inspiratory effort. Am J Respir Crit Care Med 2015;192(9):1080–8.

67. Goligher EC, Dres M, Fan E, et al. Mechanical ventilation-induced diaphragm atrophy strongly impacts clinical outcomes. Am J Respir Crit Care Med 2018;197(2):204–13.

68. Goligher EC, Brochard LJ, Reid WD, et al. Diaphragmatic myotrauma: a mediator of prolonged ventilation and poor patient outcomes in acute respiratory failure. Lancet Respir Med 2019;7(1):90–8.

69. Brochard L, Slutsky A, Pesenti A. Mechanical ventilation to minimize progression of lung injury in acute respiratory failure. Am J Respir Crit Care Med 2017;195(4):438–42.

70. Bellani G, Grasselli G, Teggia-Droghi M, et al. Do spontaneous and mechanical breathing have similar effects on average transpulmonary and alveolar pressure? a clinical crossover study. Crit Care Lond Engl 2016;20(1):142.

71. Dianti J, Bertoni M, Goligher EC. Monitoring patient–ventilator interaction by an end-expiratory occlusion maneuver. Intensive Care Med 2020;1–4. https://doi.org/10.1007/s00134-020-06167-3. Published online July 4.

72. Yoshida T, Nakahashi S, Nakamura MAM, et al. Volume-controlled ventilation does not prevent injurious inflation during spontaneous effort. Am J Respir Crit Care Med 2017;196(5):590–601.

73. Yoshida T, Torsani V, Gomes S, et al. Spontaneous effort causes occult pendelluft during mechanical ventilation. Am J Respir Crit Care Med 2013;188(12):1420–7.

74. Georgopoulos D, Prinianakis G, Kondili E. Bedside waveforms interpretation as a tool to identify patient-ventilator asynchronies. Intensive Care Med 2006;32(1):34–47.

75. Bellani G, Grassi A, Sosio S, et al. Plateau and driving pressure in the presence of spontaneous breathing. Intensive Care Med 2019;45(1):97–8.

76. Telias I, Damiani F, Brochard L. The airway occlusion pressure (P0.1) to monitor respiratory drive during mechanical ventilation: increasing awareness of a not-so-new problem. Intensive Care Med 2018;44(9):1532–5.

77. Telias I, Junhasavasdikul D, Rittayamai N, et al. Airway occlusion pressure as an estimate of respiratory drive and inspiratory effort during assisted ventilation. Am J Respir Crit Care Med 2020;201(9):1086–98.

78. Telias I, Brochard L, Goligher EC. Is my patient's respiratory drive (too) high? Intensive Care Med 2018;44(11):1936–9.

79. Bertoni M, Telias I, Urner M, et al. A novel noninvasive method to detect excessively high respiratory effort and dynamic transpulmonary driving pressure during mechanical ventilation. Crit Care 2019;23(1):346.

Patient-Ventilator Synchrony

Kevin C. Doerschug, MD, MS, FCCP

KEYWORDS

- Mechanical ventilation • Respiratory failure • Dysychrony • Asynchrony

KEY POINTS

- Patient-ventilator asynchrony develops when a patient's respiratory drive is not met with sufficient output from the ventilator.
- Patient-ventilator asynchrony causes injurious ventilation and can contribute to patient self-induced lung injury.
- Ventilator waveforms provide valuable information with which to diagnose patient-ventilator asynchrony.

INTRODUCTION

Mechanical ventilation of critically ill patients can be delivered precisely to a patient made passive through deep sedation or neuromuscular blockade. However, sedation and paralysis place patients at risk of atrophy of the diaphragm,[1,2] persistent neuromuscular weakness, prolonged ventilation,[3] and death.[4] In contrast, assist (or support) modes allow for patient-ventilator interactions, which, if synchronized, help preserve respiratory muscle function and generally require less sedation. Many critically ill patients, however, possess an elevated respiratory drive. If that drive is not met with sufficient output from mechanical ventilation, patient-ventilator asynchrony ensues. ICU clinicians must be skilled in the recognition of asynchrony, identification of its causes, and management of the ventilator to reduce asynchrony.

CAUSES OF ASYNCHRONY
Patient Factors Contributing to Asynchrony

Critical illness results in many perturbations known to increase respiratory drive, and a thorough discussion of the modulation of respiratory drive is complex and beyond the scope of this review. Arterial gas content, especially partial pressure of carbon dioxide ($PaCO_2$), is often considered a main determinant of respiratory drive. Indeed, increasing $PaCO_2$ leads to increasing respiratory effort by the patient.[5] However, several patient factors relevant to critical illness contribute to a persistently elevated respiratory drive and patient-ventilator asynchrony even when blood gases are normalized. Inflammation stimulates respiratory drive even in the absence of fever.[6] Pain, metabolic acidosis, pulmonary deadspace,[7] and altered chemoreceptor responses[8] also alter respiratory drive and are highly relevant to critical illness. Importantly, providers should be careful to not consider asynchrony as a sign of discomfort, as this thought process may lead to increases in comfort measures (ie, sedation and analgesia) rather than adjustment of the ventilator to match an unconscious drive to breathe more.

Ventilator Factors Contributing to Asynchrony

Although respiratory drive is usually increased in critical illness, factors of mechanical ventilation also contribute to ventilator output that is insufficient for a patient's respiratory drive. Lung-protective ventilation with tidal volumes of 6 to 8 cc/kg ideal body weight improves outcomes in patients with[9] and without acute respiratory distress syndrome (ARDS).[10] However, a decrease in tidal volume increases respiratory drive[11] and

Department of Internal Medicine, University of Iowa Carver College of Medicine, 200 Hawkins Drive, Iowa City, IA 52246, USA
E-mail address: kevin-doerschug@uiowa.edu

Clin Chest Med 43 (2022) 511–518
https://doi.org/10.1016/j.ccm.2022.05.005
0272-5231/22/© 2022 Published by Elsevier Inc.

asynchrony,[12] presumably mediated through lung stretch receptor reflexes.[13] Additionally, insufficient positive end-expiratory pressure (PEEP) may increase asynchrony and lung injury.[14]

HARMFUL EFFECTS OF ASYNCHRONY

Asynchrony leads to several, sometimes clinically subtle, undesired effects. At a basic level, asynchrony is an increased work of breathing with the potential for depletion of energy stores and production of lactic acid within respiratory muscles. Excessive work of breathing may lead to diaphragm dysfunction, atrophy, and an increased risk of death.[4] Asynchrony resulting in stacked breaths before exhalation of the first breath leads to a likely injurious tidal volume approaching 10 cc/kg.[15] Excessively negative pleural pressures create transpulmonary pressures that are not reflected by inspiratory pressures delivered by the ventilator, but result in injurious tidal volumes. However, even normal tidal volumes generated from excessive spontaneous efforts result in occult pendelluft, or regional overdistension, of the already injured lung.[16,17] Through these mechanisms, patient-ventilator asynchrony may precede patient decompensation,[18] contribute to failed liberation trials,[19] result in prolonged mechanical ventilation,[20] and contribute to patient mortality.[21]

CLASSIFICATION OF ASYNCHRONY

Patient-ventilator asynchronies can be classified by when they occur during the respiratory cycle. Asynchronies may occur during breath initiation (trigger asynchrony), during breath delivery (flow asynchrony), and the transition from inspiratory phase to expiratory phase (cycle asynchrony).

Trigger Asynchrony

Ineffective trigger asynchrony is defined as a patient inspiratory effort that does not trigger a breath supported by the ventilator. A spontaneous breath during mechanical ventilation is triggered when the diaphragm decreases pleural pressure below the trigger threshold of the ventilator, which is measured at the airway opening. Weak inspiratory strength (eg, neuromuscular weakness) or effort (sedation) may not lower pleural pressure sufficiently and thus fail to trigger the ventilator. Alternatively, intrinsic PEEP increases alveolar pressure, and normal respiratory muscles may fail to induce the larger drop in pleural pressure necessary to reach the trigger threshold. Accordingly, trigger asynchrony is present in nearly all patients with COPD,[22] but is commonly seen in

patients without obstructive lung disease; it can occur in any mode. Importantly, trigger asynchrony is associated with prolonged liberation from mechanical ventilation.[23] Ineffective trigger may be recognized by a deflection of the pressure-time curve without an accompanying increase in volume. More subtly, the expiratory flow may demonstrate an upward deflection from the normally decaying flow pattern.(Fig. 1). It is logical that failed triggers are often preceded by factors that increase intrinsic PEEP such as breaths that are relatively larger or with shorter respiratory cycle and expiratory times.[24]

Autotriggering occurs when an assisted (not controlled) breath is triggered and delivered by the ventilator without patient effort, and often indicates circuit leaks or hyperdynamic cardiac impulses.[25]

Reverse triggering is defined as entrainment of diaphragmatic muscles of a deeply sedated patient, whereby the patient is triggered to initiate an assisted breath by a controlled breath delivered by the ventilator.[26]

Flow Asynchrony

After a breath is triggered, the ventilator delivers a breath to the targeted pressure or flow. Flow asynchrony develops when the flow delivered by the ventilator is inadequate for the patient's needs, leading to increased patient inspiratory effort.[27] Most critically ill patients have elevated respiratory drive, thus their needs for inspiratory flow may differ significantly from healthy individuals. Flow asynchrony is recognized by a downward deflection in the pressure-time waveforms in flow-targeted (eg, volume-assist control, Fig. 2) and pressure-targeted modes (Fig. 3), reflecting the increasingly negative pleural pressure generated by the actively breathing patient. Breath-by-breath variations of the pressure-time waveforms are indicative of variable patient effort and thus signal flow asynchronies.

Cycle Asynchrony

The mechanical ventilator switches from inspiration to expiration in most ventilator modes according to a set inspiratory time. Cycle asynchrony ensues when this machine inspiratory time does not match the patient's neural inspiratory time. Observers of the flow-time curves will recognize cycle asynchrony by the upper (less negative) deflection in early expirations, indicating ongoing patient inspiratory effort (Fig. 4). The most obvious form of cycle asynchrony occurs when patient inspiratory effort is sufficient to generate a second stacked breath early in the expiratory phase.

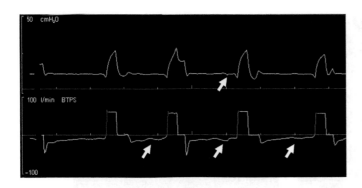

Fig. 1. Trigger asynchrony. Ineffective trigger is depicted in the pressure- (*upper*) and flow (*lower*)-vs-time waveforms. Arrows denote fluctuations in the waveform indicating patient effort that do not trigger a breath from the ventilator.

Stacked breaths are common during ventilation with lung-protective tidal volumes that require short set inspiratory times.[15] However, stacked breaths paradoxically result in tidal volumes approaching 10 cc/kg ideal body weight and are likely injurious rather than protective.

Pressure support modes of ventilation do not have a set inspiratory time, but instead terminate breaths once flow decays below a threshold set as a percentage of peak inspiratory flow. Airway resistance caused by obstructive lung disease may lead to a slower decay of inspiratory flow, which in turn prolongs inspiration and potentially increases tidal volume. If the inspiratory time of the ventilator is prolonged beyond neural inspiratory time, the patient may initiate active exhalation and thus have increased work or breathing.

MONITORING PATIENT-VENTILATOR SYNCHRONY
Waveforms

Given the previously stated harms of patient-ventilator asynchronies, providers must be able to recognize asynchrony. Fortunately, asynchrony can be detected and monitored through various methods. Practiced clinicians habitually evaluate not just numerical data from mechanical ventilators but also scrupulously inspect ventilator graphical waveforms in search of signs of asynchrony.[28] This method has the advantage of being noninvasive, requiring no additional resources, and universally available in modern ventilators. Consistent initial ventilator settings (eg, inspiratory flow 60 L/min in constant flow pattern) are helpful to establish a visual normal waveform, facilitating recognition of abnormal waveforms. Importantly, identification of patient-ventilator asynchrony via waveform analysis can be successfully performed by practitioners of varied professions with specific training.[29]

Esophageal Manometry

Measures of respiratory effort may provide hints toward occult asynchrony. Esophageal manometry can detect increasingly negative pleural pressure from diaphragmatic activity, and thus identify

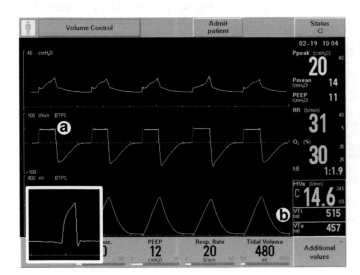

Fig. 2. Flow asynchrony in volume-assist-control mode. A pressure-time (*upper*) tracing during constant-flow targeted ventilation depicts downward deflection from the usual scalloped curve (*inset lower left*) as well as breath-to-breath variation indicate inadequate inspiratory flow. Note (a) that a visual estimate of flow (*middle tracing*) is less than 50 L/min (actual flow 46 L/min, not shown), and (b) the inspiratory tidal volume is larger than target tidal volume.

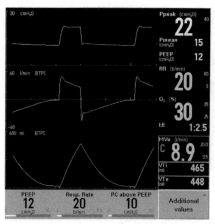 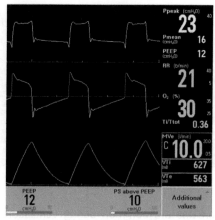

Fig. 3. Flow asynchrony in pressure-targeted modes. Passive ventilation with pressure-control mode of (*left*) demonstrates typical pressure-time tracings (*upper tracing*) including a plateau at the targeted pressure and a tidal volume deemed protective. Pressure support ventilation (*right*) with the same pressures as previous but with spontaneous respirations demonstrates concavity rather than plateau of the pressure-time waveform during inspiration, and results in larger tidal volumes that may not be protective.

when patient effort increases.[30] Enthusiasm for the use of esophageal manometry is dampened by its cost and the need for further education in order to interpret its data, as well as a lack of data to demonstrate a change in clinical outcomes. Unfortunately pleural pressure is not uniform throughout the thorax, and this heterogeneity is increased during spontaneous breathing. Thus esophageal manometry may not accurately reflect regional pleural pressure changes, leading to overdistension in the dependent, injured lung during spontaneous breathing.[16]

P0.1

The drop in airway pressure against a closed airway during the initial 100 milliseconds of a spontaneous breath, or P0.1, accurately estimates

respiratory drive.[31] Most modern ventilators provide measures of P0.1, although some estimate this without airway occlusion; these estimated values are reasonable estimates, as they correlate with electrical activity of the diaphragm and esophageal pressure-time constants.[32] Elevated P0.1 during a spontaneous breathing trial may predict failure as well as the potential for acute decompensation.[18] This noninvasive and readily available measure of respiratory drive may provide important clues of increased respiratory effort, prompting further investigation for occult asynchrony.

Expiratory Occlusion Pressure

While P0.1, measured during inspiration, estimates respiratory drive, it does not fully represent the

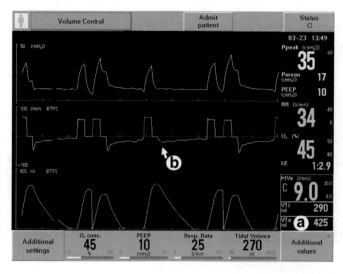

Fig. 4. Cycle asynchrony. Pressure- (*upper*), flow- (*middle*), and volume- (*lower*) time tracings all show stacked breaths, or delivery of a second breath before the prior breath is exhaled. Note the exhaled tidal volume (a) of the stacked breaths is 1.6 times the target tidal volume. More subtly, the expiratory flow tracing depicts an upward deflection (less expiratory flow, [b]) followed by a downward deflection (more expiratory flow) representing an active attempt to inhale prior to more passive exhalation. Both findings are examples of cycle asynchrony.

stress on the lung created by the combined effects of mechanical ventilation and respiratory effort. In contrast, the deflection of airway pressure during an applied end-expiratory occlusion maneuver (P_{occl}) represents the magnitude of patient effort. Noninvasive P_{occ} correlates with more invasive measures of respiratory effort from esophageal manometry,[33] and can accurately detect transpulmonary pressures greater than 20 cm H_2O.[34]

Inspiratory Hold

The peak pressure delivered by a ventilator is the sum of (1) PEEP, (2) the pressure to distend the lung to a given a given tidal volume (P_{elast}), and (3) the pressure to overcome the resistance of flow (P_{res}). Peak pressure in a passive patient will be higher than P_{plat}. Compared with a passive patient on identical pressure-cycled ventilator settings, an actively breathing patient will have larger transpulmonary pressures and thus larger tidal volumes and higher P_{plat}. Because of patient effort, P_{res} may not be fully estimated by P_{peak}, and an inspiratory hold may reveal a P_{plat} that is actually higher than P_{peak} (**Fig. 5**).[35] Accordingly, the true driving pressure (Pplat -PEEP) may be not be protective.[36] The direction and magnitude of the change in P_{plat} from P_{peak} during an inspiratory hold correlate with work of breathing measured by esophageal manometry.[37] Thus in pressure-cycled modes, an inspiratory hold that reveals P_{plat} higher than P_{peak} signifies an unmet respiratory drive and patient-ventilator asynchrony.

MITIGATION OF ASYNCHRONY
Overdrive

As asynchrony represents a respiratory drive that exceeds that delivered by the ventilator, increases in minute ventilation via increases in tidal volume or respiratory rate—ventilator overdrive—may serve to both increase delivery and suppress respiratory drive. Overdrive decreases $Paco_2$, potentially well below normal values, suppressing the work of breathing.[5] Overdrive does have limitations, however. An increased respiratory rate risks decreased expiratory time and the potential for dynamic hyperinflation (intrinsic PEEP). Increases in tidal volume risk injurious overdistension, although even the ARMA trial of lung-protective ventilation allowed tidal volumes up to 8 cc/kg IBW if asynchrony cannot otherwise be avoided. Certainly additional strategies to mitigate asynchrony should be attempted before resorting to increasing tidal volume. Other strategies are more specific to the type of asynchrony encountered.

Sufficient Flow

The elevated respiratory drives of most critically ill patients demand an inspiratory flow near 60 L/min; flows less than 50 L/min are rarely tolerated.[27] The shortened inspiratory time created by inspiratory flow greater than 60 L/min risks cycle asynchrony. Further increases in flow can lead to reflex tachypnea.[38] In flow-targeted modes, a constant flow, rather than decelerating flow, will assure flow is sufficient throughout inspiration, and facilitate easier recognition of abnormal patterns, but the choice and optimization of flow profiles remain poorly studied.

Increased Inspiratory Time

Cycle asynchrony typically arises when the set inspiratory time is less than that of the patient's neurologic inspiratory time. Increasing ventilator

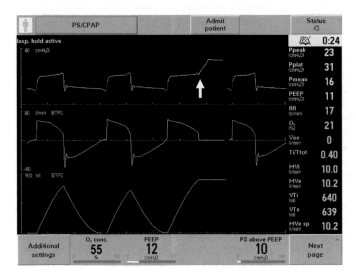

Fig. 5. Occult driving pressure in pressure support. Spontaneous respirations with pressure-support (pressure-targeted) mode with an inspiratory pressure of 10 cm H_2O more than PEEP of 12 cm H_2O results in tidal volumes over 600 mL. The pressure-time (*top*) tracing demonstrates concavity rather than constant pressure during inspiration, indicating flow asynchrony. An inspiratory hold (*arrow*) following the third breath reveals a plateau of 31 cm H_2O. The calculated actual driving pressure of 19 cm H_2O is much higher than the set pressure support of 10 cm H_2O, and demonstrates that patient-ventilator asynchrony may contribute to injurious ventilation.

set inspiratory times to approach that of the patient will therefore reduce the risk of cycle asynchrony. Inserting an inspiratory pause will increase the inspiratory time without decreasing flow, thereby avoiding flow asynchrony. This method reduces stacked breaths more effectively than sedation.[39]

Adjust Cycle-Off During Pressure Support

When inspiratory flow in pressure support mode is sustained longer than the patient's neural inspiratory time, increasing the percent cycle-off threshold (cycle-off at higher flow) will decrease the delivered inspiratory time to approach that of the patient and improve synchrony. This subsequently reduces tidal volume, intrinsic PEEP, and patient inspiratory effort.[40]

Increase Positive End-Expiratory Pressure

Effective triggering occurs when airway opening pressure is sufficiently lowered below PEEP. In obstructed patients with ineffective triggering caused by intrinsic PEEP, a higher applied PEEP (compared with lower PEEP) reduces the needed change in pleural pressure. Compared with low PEEP, a higher PEEP reduces the needed change in pleural pressure and minimizes ineffective triggering in patients with obstructive lung disease. High PEEP produces a more homogeneous distribution of pleural pressures during ARDS, which reduces inspiratory effort, tidal volume, and lung injury in patients.[14,41]

Neurally Adjusted and Proportional Assist Ventilatory Modes

Neurally adjusted ventilatory assist (NAVA) and proportional assist ventilation (PAV) are 2 modes that specifically recognize patient effort and thus improve synchrony in spontaneously breathing patients. Neither mode sets pressure, volume, flow, or inspiratory time. Instead, all of these variables change in response to the patient's ventilatory demand. NAVA is controlled an electromyographic electrode (placed via specialized nasogastric tube) and adjusts each breath according to diaphragmatic activity. The clinician can adjust the degree of assistance by altering the amount of inspiratory pressure applied per millivolt of EMG signal. NAVA decreases asynchrony,[42] and duration of mechanical ventilation may not affect survival.[43]

PAV measures work of breathing and adjusts the ventilator output to unload a proportion the work of breathing from the patient; the clinician sets the proportion (percent) unloaded by the ventilator. Compared with pressure support ventilation, PAV reduces cycle asynchrony,[44,45] albeit with longer inspiratory times and potentially larger tidal volumes.[44] Data demonstrating improved patient outcomes are lacking.

Both NAVA and PAV offer clinicians an opportunity to assess patient effort with the potential to reduce asynchrony. To this end, these modes have been successful. The current body of evidence does not demonstrate an effect of NAVA or PAV on patient-centered outcomes, although trials have been limited. The critical care community awaits further data of larger trials, perhaps including patient populations at high risk of asynchrony and powered to detect these important outcomes.

Techniques to Avoid

Over-reliance on blood gas analysis
Attempts to normalize blood gases, in particular $Paco_2$, often result in a minute ventilation that is insufficient for a critically ill patient's elevated respiratory drive. Rather, pH values between 7.2 and 7.55 have little physiologic consequence and are best tolerated by the clinician as needed to achieve patient-ventilator synchrony.

Excessive and ineffective sedation
Many clinicians consider increasing sedation as the first line of defense against asynchrony. However, prolonged deep sedation is associated with increased incidence of ICU delirium and long-term neuromuscular and cognitive symptoms. Importantly, increasing sedative/analgesic medications is actually less effective than optimizing ventilator settings at mitigating asynchrony.[39] In the setting of evolving drug shortages, sedation may be less available; thus clinicians are forced to focus on optimum ventilator management to mitigate asynchrony. With a high risk profile and inadequate effectiveness, it is suggested that sedation not be the first approach to address asynchrony regardless of drug availability.

Change of ventilator modes
Lung-protective ventilation using tidal volume 6 cc/kg ideal body weight with flow-targeted modes may lead to more asynchrony than larger tidal volumes. Similarly, a change to pressure support mode will likely improve synchrony but at the expense of increasing tidal volumes that may no longer be considered protective.[39] Further, the set pressures during pressure support ventilation may be deceptively reassuring, as they may not accurately represent transpulmonary pressures during excessive spontaneous effort. Attempts to decrease pressure support are often countered by increased patient effort and therefore little

change in injurious tidal volume. For these reasons, clinicians should search for mitigation strategies while maintaining lung-protective tidal volumes in flow-targeted ventilation.

SUMMARY

Patient-ventilator asynchrony develops when the output from mechanical ventilation does not match a patient's respiratory drive. Asynchrony contributes to increased work of breathing, diaphragm dysfunction, injurious overdistension of the lung, and is associated with adverse patient outcomes. Clinicians must be skilled at recognizing patient-ventilator asynchrony through scrupulous analysis of ventilator graphics. Ventilator adjustments mitigate asynchrony more effectively than sedation.

CLINICS CARE POINTS

- Patient-ventilator asynchrony contributes to excess work of breathing, diaphragm dysfunction, lung injury, and mortality in critically ill patients
- With specific training, clinicians can accurately identify patient-ventilator asynchronies
- Ventilator adjustments are more effective than sedation to decrease patient-ventilator asynchronies

DISCLOSURE

K.C. Doerschug has no relevant conflicts to disclose.

REFERENCES

1. Hudson MB, Smuder AJ, Nelson WB, et al. Both high level pressure support ventilation and controlled mechanical ventilation induce diaphragm dysfunction and atrophy. Crit Care Med 2012;40(4):1254–60.
2. Levine S, Nguyen T, Taylor N, et al. Rapid disuse atrophy of diaphragm fibers in mechanically ventilated humans. N Engl J Med 2008;358(13):1327–35.
3. Kress JP, Pohlman AS, O'Connor MF, et al. Daily interruption of sedative infusions in critically ill patients undergoing mechanical ventilation. N Engl J Med 2000;342(20):1471–7.
4. Goligher EC, Dres M, Fan E, et al. Mechanical ventilation-induced diaphragm atrophy strongly impacts clinical outcomes. Am J Respir Crit Care Med 2018;197(2):204–13.
5. Mauri T, Grasselli G, Suriano G, et al. Control of respiratory drive and effort in extracorporeal membrane oxygenation patients recovering from severe acute respiratory distress syndrome. Anesthesiology 2016;125(1):159–67.
6. Preas HL 2nd, Jubran A, Vandivier RW, et al. Effect of endotoxin on ventilation and breath variability: role of cyclooxygenase pathway. Am J Respir Crit Care Med 2001;164(4):620–6.
7. Nuckton TJ, Alonso JA, Kallet RH, et al. Pulmonary dead-space fraction as a risk factor for death in the acute respiratory distress syndrome. N Engl J Med 2002;346(17):1281–6.
8. Jacono FJ, Peng YJ, Nethery D, et al. Acute lung injury augments hypoxic ventilatory response in the absence of systemic hypoxemia. J Appl Physiol 2006;101(6):1795–802.
9. Acute Respiratory Distress Syndrome Network, Brower RG, Matthay MA, et al. Ventilation with lower tidal volumes as compared with traditional tidal volumes for acute lung injury and the acute respiratory distress syndrome. N Engl J Med 2000;342(18):1301–8.
10. Serpa Neto A, Cardoso SO, Manetta JA, et al. Association between use of lung-protective ventilation with lower tidal volumes and clinical outcomes among patients without acute respiratory distress syndrome: a meta-analysis. JAMA 2012;308(16):1651–9.
11. Kallet RH, Campbell AR, Dicker RA, et al. Effects of tidal volume on work of breathing during lung-protective ventilation in patients with acute lung injury and acute respiratory distress syndrome. Crit Care Med 2006;34(1):8–14.
12. Figueroa-Casas JB, Montoya R. Effect of tidal volume size and its delivery mode on patient-ventilator dyssynchrony. Ann Am Thorac Soc 2016;13(12):2207–14.
13. Hamilton RD, Winning AJ, Horner RL, et al. The effect of lung inflation on breathing in man during wakefulness and sleep. Respir Physiol 1988;73(2):145–54.
14. Yoshida T, Roldan R, Beraldo MA, et al. Spontaneous effort during mechanical ventilation: maximal injury with less positive end-expiratory pressure. Crit Care Med 2016;44(8):e678–88.
15. Pohlman MC, McCallister KE, Schweickert WD, et al. Excessive tidal volume from breath stacking during lung-protective ventilation for acute lung injury. Crit Care Med 2008;36(11):3019–23.
16. Yoshida T, Torsani V, Gomes S, et al. Spontaneous effort causes occult pendelluft during mechanical ventilation. Am J Respir Crit Care Med 2013;188(12):1420–7.
17. Yoshida T, Nakahashi S, Nakamura MAM, et al. Volume-controlled ventilation does not prevent injurious

inflation during spontaneous effort. Am J Respir Crit Care Med 2017;196(5):590–601.

18. Esnault P, Cardinale M, Hraiech S, et al. High respiratory drive and excessive respiratory efforts predict relapse of respiratory failure in critically Ill patients with COVID-19. Am J Respir Crit Care Med 2020; 202(8):1173–8.

19. Martos-Benítez FD, Domínguez-Valdés Y, Burgos-Aragüez D, et al. Outcomes of ventilatory asynchrony in patients with inspiratory effort. Rev Bras Ter Intensiva 2020;32(2):284–94.

20. Thille AW, Rodriguez P, Cabello B, et al. Patient-ventilator asynchrony during assisted mechanical ventilation. Intensive Care Med 2006;32(10):1515–22.

21. Blanch L, Villagra A, Sales B, et al. Asynchronies during mechanical ventilation are associated with mortality. Intensive Care Med 2015;41(4):633–41.

22. MacIntyre NR, Cheng KC, McConnell R. Applied PEEP during pressure support reduces the inspiratory threshold load of intrinsic PEEP. Chest 1997;111(1): 188–93.

23. Chao DC, Scheinhorn DJ, Stearn-Hassenpflug M. Patient-ventilator trigger asynchrony in prolonged mechanical ventilation. Chest 1997;112(6):1592–9.

24. Leung P, Jubran A, Tobin MJ. Comparison of assisted ventilator modes on triggering, patient effort, and dyspnea. Am J Respir Crit Care Med 1997;155(6):1940–8.

25. Imanaka H, Nishimura M, Takeuchi M, et al. Autotriggering caused by cardiogenic oscillation during flow-triggered mechanical ventilation. Crit Care Med 2000;28(2):402–7.

26. Akoumianaki E, Lyazidi A, Rey N, et al. Mechanical ventilation-induced reverse-triggered breaths: a frequently unrecognized form of neuromechanical coupling. Chest 2013;143(4):927–38.

27. Tobin MJ. Physiologic basis of mechanical ventilation. Ann Am Thorac Soc 2018;15(Suppl_1):S49–52.

28. Georgopoulos D, Prinianakis G, Kondili E. Bedside waveforms interpretation as a tool to identify patient-ventilator asynchronies. Intensive Care Med 2006;32(1):34–47.

29. Ramirez II, Arellano DH, Adasme RS, et al. Ability of ICU health-care professionals to identify patient-ventilator asynchrony using waveform analysis. Respir Care 2017;62(2):144–9.

30. Mauri T, Yoshida T, Bellani G, et al. Esophageal and transpulmonary pressure in the clinical setting: meaning, usefulness and perspectives. Intensive Care Med 2016;42(9):1360–73.

31. Whitelaw WA, Derenne JP, Milic-Emili J. Occlusion pressure as a measure of respiratory center output in conscious man. Respir Physiol 1975;23(2):181–99.

32. Telias I, Junhasavasdikul D, Rittayamai N, et al. Airway occlusion pressure as an estimate of respiratory drive and inspiratory effort during assisted ventilation. Am J Respir Crit Care Med 2020; 201(9):1086–98.

33. Bertoni M, Spadaro S, Goligher EC. Monitoring patient respiratory effort during mechanical ventilation: lung and diaphragm-protective ventilation. Crit Care 2020;24(1):106.

34. Bertoni M, Telias I, Urner M, et al. A novel non-invasive method to detect excessively high respiratory effort and dynamic transpulmonary driving pressure during mechanical ventilation. Crit Care 2019;23(1):346.

35. Sajjad H, Schmidt GA, Brower RG, et al. Can the plateau be higher than the peak pressure? Ann Am Thorac Soc 2018;15(6):754–9.

36. Amato MB, Meade MO, Slutsky AS, et al. Driving pressure and survival in the acute respiratory distress syndrome. N Engl J Med 2015;372(8): 747–55.

37. Kyogoku M, Shimatani T, Hotz JC, et al. Direction and magnitude of change in plateau from peak pressure during inspiratory holds can identify the degree of spontaneous effort and elastic workload in ventilated patients. Crit Care Med 2020;49(3): 517–26.

38. Puddy A, Younes M. Effect of inspiratory flow rate on respiratory output in normal subjects. Am Rev Respir Dis 1992;146(3):787–9.

39. Chanques G, Kress JP, Pohlman A, et al. Impact of ventilator adjustment and sedation-analgesia practices on severe asynchrony in patients ventilated in assist-control mode. Crit Care Med 2013;41(9): 2177–87.

40. Chiumello D, Polli F, Tallarini F, et al. Effect of different cycling-off criteria and positive end-expiratory pressure during pressure support ventilation in patients with chronic obstructive pulmonary disease. Crit Care Med 2007;35(11):2547–52.

41. Morais CCA, Koyama Y, Yoshida T, et al. High positive end-expiratory pressure renders spontaneous effort noninjurious. Am J Respir Crit Care Med 2018;197(10):1285–96.

42. Di Mussi R, Spadaro S, Mirabella L, et al. Impact of prolonged assisted ventilation on diaphragmatic efficiency: NAVA versus PSV. Crit Care 2016;20:1.

43. Kacmarek RM, Villar J, Parrilla D, et al. Neurally adjusted ventilatory assist in acute respiratory failure: a randomized controlled trial. Intensive Care Med 2020;46(12):2327–37.

44. Costa R, Spinazzola G, Cipriani F, et al. A physiologic comparison of proportional assist ventilation with load-adjustable gain factors (PAV+) versus pressure support ventilation (PSV). Intensive Care Med 2011;37(9):1494–500.

45. Vasconcelos RS, Sales RP, Melo LHP, et al. Influences of duration of inspiratory effort, respiratory mechanics, and ventilator type on asynchrony with pressure support and proportional assist ventilation. Respir Care 2017;62(5):550–7.

Extracorporeal Life Support in Respiratory Failure

Briana Short, MD*, Kristin M. Burkart, MD, MSc

KEYWORDS

- Extracorporeal membrane oxygenation (ECMO) • Extracorporeal life support (ECLS)
- Respiratory failure

KEY POINTS

- Extracorporeal life support (ECLS) is used in different types of respiratory failure including acute respiratory distress syndrome (ARDS), acute decompensated pulmonary hypertension, bridge to lung transplantation, and primary graft dysfunction after lung transplantation.
- ECLS in ARDS supports gas exchange which allows for low-volume low-pressure ventilation with the goal to reduce the risk of ventilator-induced lung injury.
- ECLS should be considered in severe ARDS when conventional management strategies fail to provide adequate and safe oxygenation or in the setting of elevated airway pressures and severe respiratory acidosis.
- Future directions in ECLS research aim to identify optimal management strategies while supported by ECLS, including optimal mechanical ventilation settings, role of prone positioning, weaning ECLS support, and long-term outcomes.

INTRODUCTION

Extracorporeal life support (ECLS) has an established role in the treatment of acute respiratory failure. First used in the 1970s,[1] its use has increased, and indications have broadened over the last few decades. Its initial growth was driven by advances in technology and improved safety profiles. Then, two separate events occurred in 2009[2]: the 2009 influenza A (H1N1) pandemic[3] and the publication of the extracorporeal membrane oxygenation (ECMO) conventional ventilatory support vs extracorporeal membrane oxygenation for severe adult respiratory failure (CESAR trial).[4] A decade after these events, data support the move of ECLS from salvage mode to standard of care in patients with very severe acute respiratory distress syndrome (ARDS).[5,6]

This review examines recently published studies and discusses current indications for ECLS in adults with respiratory failure. Finally, we explore future directions in patient care and research.

Extracorporeal Life Support Terminology

ECLS encompasses several modalities to provide support of the lungs or heart. ECLS includes ECMO and extracorporeal carbon dioxide removal ($ECCO_2R$). ECMO supports blood oxygenation and carbon dioxide removal, whereas $ECCO_2R$ only supports carbon dioxide removal. Both ECMO and $ECCO_2R$ have been studied in acute respiratory failure. The two major ECMO modalities are venovenous (VV) ECMO and venoarterial (VA) ECMO. VV-ECMO supports respiratory gas exchange, and VA-ECMO provides circulatory support.[6,7] Details of ECLS circuits,

Division of Pulmonary, Allergy, and Critical Care Medicine, Department of Medicine, Columbia University College of Physicians & Surgeons, 622 West 168th Street, PH 8 East, Room 101, New York, NY 10032, USA
* Corresponding author. Division of Pulmonary, Allergy, and Critical Care Medicine, Department of Medicine, Columbia University College of Physicians & Surgeons, 622 West 168th Street, PH 8 East, Room 101, New York, NY 10032, USA.
E-mail address: bs2886@cumc.columbia.edu

Clin Chest Med 43 (2022) 519–528
https://doi.org/10.1016/j.ccm.2022.05.006
0272-5231/22/© 2022 Elsevier Inc. All rights reserved.

configurations, and gas exchange membranes have been described.[6,8]

Rationale for Extracorporeal Life Support in Respiratory Failure

Early use of ECMO for respiratory failure focused on improving oxygenation with the goal to avoid tissue hypoxia. Historically, it was most often deployed as a salvage mode to support refractory hypoxemia. Over the last 20 years, it has become evident that ventilator-induced lung injury (VILI) is a significant driver of mortality[9] and that ventilator strategies to mitigate VILI decrease mortality in patients with ARDS.[10] Furthermore, secondary analyses of the Acute Respiratory Distress Syndrome Network trial[10] suggests a safe upper limit for plateau pressure may not exist thus shifting the role of ECLS in hypoxemic respiratory failure toward supporting gas exchange with the goal to facilitate low-volume low-pressure ventilation and reduce the risk of VILI.[9]

Extracorporeal Life Support in Respiratory Failure

Interest in ECLS for adults with respiratory failure increased in 2009 during H1N1 pandemic[3] and with the publication of CESAR.[4] In the CESAR trial, patients with severe ARDS transferred to a single ECMO center were more likely to survive compared with those who received conventional treatment (63% vs 47%, $P = 0.03$); however, only 76% of transferred patients received ECMO and lung-protective ventilation was not mandated in the conventional arm.[4] Despite limitations in the evidence base, use of ECMO for ARDS significantly increased after 2009.[11]

Evidence for the Use of Extracorporeal Membrane Oxygenation in Acute Respiratory Distress Syndrome

The ECMO to Rescue Lung Injury in Severe ARDS (EOLIA) trial, an international multicenter randomized controlled trial (RCT) of ECMO in patients with very severe ARDS, was published in 2018.[12] Eligible patients (**Fig. 1**) were randomized to conventional low tidal volume (V_T) ventilation or VV-ECMO with lower tidal volumes and lower airway pressures than current standards (V_T decreased to maintain plateau pressure ≤ 24 cm H_2O with positive-end expiratory pressure [PEEP] ≥ 10 cm H_2O; corresponding driving pressure ≤ 14 cm H_2O).

There was a large, albeit not statistically significant, decrease in mortality in the ECMO arm (35% vs 46%, $P = 0.09$). Two deaths were attributed to ECMO and the ECMO group had significantly higher rates of severe thrombocytopenia (27% vs 16%) and bleeding requiring transfusion (46% vs. 28%) without statistically significant differences in ischemic or hemorrhagic strokes.

A post hoc Bayesian analysis of EOLIA found a high probability that ECMO had a 60-day mortality benefit in patients with severe ARDS.[13] Likewise, a meta-analysis pooling mortality data from 429 patients enrolled in CESAR or EOLIA found a significantly lower 60-day mortality in the ECMO group compared with the control group (34% vs 47%; $P = 0.008$),[14] and an individualized patient data meta-analysis in severe ARDS also found improved 90-day mortality in patients receiving ECMO compared with conventional management (36% vs 48%; $P = 0.013$).[15] Taken all together, these data strongly suggest a mortality benefit with ECMO in patients with severe ARDS.

Extracorporeal Membrane Oxygenation in Coronavirus Disease 2019-Related Acute Respiratory Distress Syndrome

The role of ECMO for coronavirus disease 2019 (COVID-19)-related ARDS evolved throughout the pandemic. Early reports of high mortality rates with ECMO (84%–94%) deterred some from recommending its use,[16,17] whereas subsequent studies reported more favorable outcomes with mortality rates similar to EOLIA.[18,19] One of the largest studies found an in-hospital 90-day mortality of 37.4% among 1035 ECMO-supported patients with COVID-19.[18] More recently, higher mortality rates have been reported[20,21] with one study reporting an in-hospital mortality of 73% among 768 ECMO-supported patients with COVID-19-related ARDS.[20]

Although the benefit of ECMO in COVID-19-related ARDS remains unclear, several society guidelines recommend ECMO to support patients with severe COVID-19-related ARDS who meet EOLIA eligibility criteria.[22–24] Throughout the pandemic, the overall use of ECMO has grown as COVID-19 is now the leading cause of ARDS globally.[25]

Extracorporeal Life Support During a Public Health Crisis

As critically ill patients with COVID-19 overwhelmed hospitals[26] experts tempered enthusiasm for the role of ECMO early in the pandemic.[27] Efficacy of ECMO in COVID-19-related ARDS was unknown, and ECMO is a resource-consumptive technology requiring highly trained staff, lower nurse-to-patient ratios, and more space per patient.[27,28] At a time when hospitals experienced critical shortages in staff and

---

Invasive mechanical ventilation < 7 d

**Mechanical Ventilation Optimization Requirements
(prior to randomization):**
- $FiO_2 \geq 0.80$
- PEEP ≥ 10 cm H_2O,
- V_T of 6 mL/kg of predicted body wt

Met one of the following criteria:
- PaO2:FiO_2 <50 for >3h , or
- PaO2:FiO_2 <80 for >6h or
- pH <7.25 with $PaCO_2 \geq 60$ mm Hg for ≥ 6 h (respiratory rate 35 breaths per min, adjust ventilator settings to keep plateau pressure ≤ 32 cmH_2O)

**Prone positioning and neuromuscular blockade were
encouraged prior to randomization**

Fig. 1. Eligibility criteria for EOLIA: Criteria used to consider ECMO in severe ARDS. ARDS, acute respiratory distress syndrome; cmH_2O, centimeters of water; FiO_2, fraction of inspired oxygen; mm Hg, milliliter of mercury; $Paco_2$, partial pressure of carbon dioxide; PaO_2, partial pressure of oxygen; PEEP, positive-end expiratory pressures; VILI, ventilator-induced lung injury; VT, tidal volume.

space,[22,26] a call for ECMO was met with a call for pause and discussion around the ethics of resource allocation.[29,30]

The role of ECMO during public health crises extends beyond COVID-19, but the principles remain the same. Ultimately, the decision to ration ECMO in a public health crisis should be based on ethical principles and grounded within triage guidelines based on these principles.[29]

Best Practice Ventilation Strategies in Extracorporeal Life Support-Supported Acute Respiratory Distress Syndrome

In ARDS, VV-ECMO allows for ultra-protective ventilation ($V_T \leq 4$ mL/kg of predicted body weight [PBW] and plateau pressure ≤ 24 cm H_2O), which may further decrease the risk of VILI compared with standard lung-protective ventilation (V_T of 6 mL/kg of PBW and plateau pressure ≤ 30 cm H_2O).[31–33] Optimal ventilation strategies during ECMO are unknown; however, data from EOLIA and other studies have informed best practice recommendations (**Fig. 2**) for ventilator strategies.[34]

Key Take-Home Points on Extracorporeal Membrane Oxygenation for Severe Acute Respiratory Distress Syndrome

- ECMO may improve mortality in patients with severe ARDS.
- In patients with severe ARDS refractory to conventional management strategies (lung-protective ventilation, PEEP titration, deep sedation, prone positioning, and consideration of neuromuscular blockade), ECMO should be considered.

- In ECMO-supported patients, initiate ultra-protective ventilation strategies to minimize risk of VILI, a major cause of mortality in ARDS.

Extracorporeal Life Support in Non-Acute Respiratory Distress Syndrome Respiratory Failure

The role of ECLS to support respiratory failure in patients without ARDS (**Box 1**) is not well studied. RCTs supporting the use of ECMO for these are unlikely, as there is either lack of clinical equipoise or the event is uncommon thereby limiting the ability to rigorously study.

Outside of ARDS, BTT,[35,37] and VA-ECMO for decompensated PH with right heart failure[45] have the most data.

Extracorporeal Membrane Oxygenation in Bridge to Lung Transplantation

Long wait times on transplant lists increase the risk of patients developing respiratory failure requiring mechanical support with invasive mechanical ventilation, ECMO, or both. ECMO as BTT may reduce the need for invasive mechanical ventilation and thus avoid known ventilator-associated complications. Furthermore, ECMO as BTT mitigates deconditioning by allowing patients to actively participate in physical therapy; thereby maintaining transplant eligibility—even with prolonged wait times.[35–37]

The goal of ECLS in BTT is not simply survival to lung transplant. Instead, it is to decrease wait-list mortality rates while achieving favorable long-term survival. In 2019, two centers published similar long-term survival outcomes in BTT

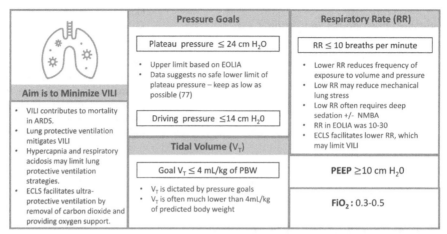

	Pressure Goals	Respiratory Rate (RR)
Aim is to Minimize VILI • VILI contributes to mortality in ARDS. • Lung protective ventilation mitigates VILI • Hypercapnia and respiratory acidosis may limit lung protective ventilation strategies. • ECLS facilitates ultra-protective ventilation by removal of carbon dioxide and providing oxygen support.	Plateau pressure ≤ 24 cm H₂O • Upper limit based on EOLIA • Data suggests no safe lower limit of plateau pressure – keep as low as possible (77) Driving pressure ≤14 cm H₂O	RR ≤ 10 breaths per minute • Lower RR reduces frequency of exposure to volume and pressure • Low RR may reduce mechanical lung stress • Low RR often requires deep sedation +/- NMBA • RR in EOLIA was 10-30 • ECLS facilitates lower RR, which may limit VILI
	Tidal Volume (V_T)	
	Goal V_T ≤ 4 mL/kg of PBW • V_T is dictated by pressure goals • V_T is often much lower than 4mL/kg of predicted body weight	**PEEP** ≥10 cm H₂0
		FiO₂: 0.3-0.5

Fig. 2. Ventilator strategies for ECLS-supported ARDS: Best practice recommendations. Figure depicting recommended ventilator strategies for patients with ARDS requiring ECLS. Refer to text for reference citations. ARDS, acute respiratory distress syndrome; cmH₂O, centimeters of water; ECLS, extracorporeal life support; ECMO, extracorporeal membrane oxygenation; FiO₂, fraction of inspired oxygen; mL/Kg, milliliters per kilogram; NMBA, neuromuscular blockade; PBW, predicted body weight; PEEP, positive-end expiratory pressures; RR, respiratory rate.

recipients compared with non-BTT recipients.[35,37] In the largest series, 121 adult patients were placed on ECMO as BTT from 2009 to 2018. Of the 121 patients, 70 (59%) were successfully transplanted, and 64 (91%) of the transplant recipients survived to hospital discharge with an 83% 3-year survival rate, which was not significantly different than propensity-matched, non-BTT transplant recipients. Ambulation was the only independent predictor of successful BTT (OR 7.6, 95% CI 2.16–26.6; $P = 0.002$).[37]

Extracorporeal Membrane Oxygenation in Acute Decompensated Pulmonary Hypertension

VA-ECMO has been successfully used to support decompensated PH with right-sided heart failure

---

Box 1
Potential indications for extracorporeal membrane oxygenation in non-acute respiratory distress syndrome respiratory failure

• Bridge to lung transplantation (BTT)[35–37]

• Primary graft dysfunction after lung transplantation[38]

• Decompensated pulmonary hypertension (PH)[36,39,40]

• Status asthmaticus[41,42]

• Massive acute pulmonary embolism[43,44]

---

as a BTT and a bridge to recovery.[40,46] Recently, a single-center cohort study reported outcomes of 98 patients with decompensated PH placed on ECMO[47] for BTT (55%) and non-BTT indications (45%). In this cohort, patients had severely elevated right ventricular systolic pressures (73 mm Hg; interquartile range (IQR) 58–100 mm Hg) and were not expected to live without ECMO support. The overall survival to hospital discharge was 54%. These findings suggest a role for ECLS in patients with decompensated PH at centers with PH and ECMO expertise.[47]

Extracorporeal Carbon Dioxide Removal in Hypoxemic Respiratory Failure

The use of ultra-protective ventilation in ARDS, to further limit VILI, may be limited by hypercapnia and severe acidosis. It was theorized that ECCO₂-R, through carbon dioxide removal, would facilitate ultra-protective ventilation, reduce VILI,[48,49] and improve survival in ARDS. The Strategy of UltraProtective Lung Ventilation With Extracorporeal CO2 Removal for New-Onset Moderate to severe ARDS (SUPERNOVA) trial demonstrated feasibility of ECCO₂R to allow lower volume and lower pressure ventilation strategies (V_T 4 mL/kg of PBW and plateau pressure ≤ 25 cm H₂O) in patients with moderate ARDS (Pao₂:Fio₂ ratio of 100–200 mm Hg with PEEP≥5 cm H₂O).[50]

In the recent pRotective vEntilation With VenovenouS Lung assisT in Respiratory Failure (REST) Randomized Clinical Trial, 412 patients with acute hypoxemic respiratory failure (Pao₂:Fio₂ ratio <

150 mm Hg with PEEP $\geq$ 5 cm H2O) were randomized to $ECCO_2R$ with lower tidal volume ventilation (goal $V_T \leq$ 3 mL/kg of PBW) or standard care with conventional lung-protective ventilation (recommended V_T of 6 mL/kg of PBW). $ECCO_2R$ was deployed for at least 24 hours and no more than 7 days.

This multicenter, randomized, pragmatic clinical trial found no difference in 90-day mortality between the $ECCO_2R$ and standard care groups (41.5% vs 39.5%, P = 0.68). Of note, there were significantly fewer ventilator-free days in the $ECCO_2R$ group compared with the standard care group (7.1 vs. 9.2, P = 0.02), and serious adverse events were more common in the $ECCO_2R$ group compared with the standard care group (31% vs 9%, respectively), including intracranial hemorrhages (9 vs 0). The trial was stopped early due to futility.[51]

Although SUPERNOVA demonstrated feasibility of $ECCO_2R$ to allow for ultra-protective ventilation, REST failed to demonstrate a 90-day mortality benefit. The results from the REST pragmatic clinical trial do not support the use of $ECCO_2R$ for hypoxemic respiratory failure.

Future Directions in Patient Care and Research

The role for ECMO in severe ARDS refractory to conventional strategies has been established; thus, future trials investigating survival in ECMO-supported severe ARDS are unlikely. Instead, ECLS research efforts on optimal management strategies of patients during ECLS and long-term outcomes of ECMO-supported ARDS survivors are needed. Moreover, future research should work to identify patients who will most likely benefit from ECLS support. Ongoing technological advances in the field will not be discussed in this review but have a central role in this technology-centered field.

Key Research Area: Management Strategies During Extracorporeal Life Support

Optimal ventilation strategies
With the focus of ECLS in respiratory failure shifting toward limiting VILI, there is a notable paucity of data on optimal ventilator strategies (Fig. 3). In fact, no prospective trials have studied the optimal ventilation strategy to mitigate VILI and improve outcomes. Patients enrolled in EOLIA[12] for elevated airway pressures and severe respiratory acidosis had the greatest reduction in mortality suggesting a mortality benefit from decreased VILI with ultra-protective ventilation.

Future trials are needed to delineate optimal ventilator settings to mitigate VILI and improve

outcomes in ECMO-supported ARDS. Specifically, different intensities of low-volume low-pressure ventilation and different respiratory frequencies (ultra-protective vs "near-apneic" ventilation) have been proposed as potential strategies to more effectively limit VILI.[52,53]

Research on the impact of spontaneous breathing and extubation while on ECMO and specific goals for gas exchange during ECMO-supported respiratory failure is also needed.[34]

Prone positioning
The role of prone positioning in ECMO-supported ARDS is not well studied. There is strong data for improved mortality with prone positioning in ARDS[54] but it is unknown if the same benefits extend to patients supported by ECMO with ultra-protective ventilation. A small study suggested benefit,[55] and in a recent retrospective multicenter cohort study, prone positioning was associated with lower hospital mortality compared with propensity-matched supine ECMO-supported patients (30% vs 53%; P = 0.024).[56] An RCT comparing prone position to supine position, in ECMO-supported patients with severe ARDS, is currently enrolling PRONing to Facilitate Weaning From ECMO in Patients With Refractory Acute Respiratory Distress Syndrome (PRO-NECMO).[57] Results from this trial will inform the role of prone positioning in ECMO-supported ARDS.

Weaning form mechanical support
Recently, two small studies investigated weaning strategies for VV-ECMO.[58,59] Gannon and colleagues[58] studied a proactive, systematic, and standardized approach to weaning ECMO, similar to standardized approaches to weaning mechanical ventilation, whereas Al Fares and colleagues[59] sought to identify parameters associated with safe weaning from VV-ECMO. Future studies should measure survival in addition to successful decannulation, as most often patients remain on invasive mechanical ventilation and are critically ill.

Adjunctive therapies: anticoagulation, sedation, and mobilization
Blood circulation through a foreign membrane increases the hypercoagulable state of patients requiring ECMO.[60] Antithrombotic agents are frequently used to decrease the risk of clot formation, yet anticoagulation protocols are center-specific.[60] Consensus across centers on anticoagulant type, therapeutic goal, and monitoring are lacking;[61] however, small feasibility studies have shown safety in using thromboelastography and anti-Xa compared with activated partial thromboplastin time.[62,63] Future research on anticoagulation

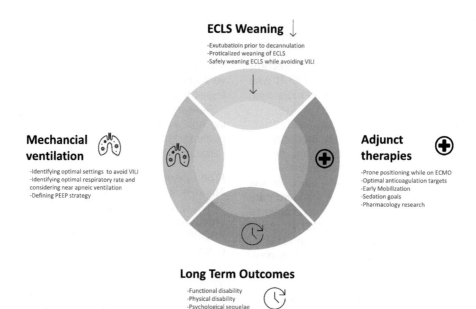

Fig. 3. Future directions. Figure depicting future directions in research and patient care for ECLS. ECLS, extracorporeal life support; ECMO, extracorporeal membrane oxygenation; PEEP, positive-end expiratory pressures; VILI, ventilator-induced lung injury.

methods as well as developing materials to reduce the hypercoagulable effect of ECLS are needed.[64]

It has been shown that reducing sedation and increasing mobilization mitigates intensive care unit acquired weakness and delirium.[65] Mobilization is frequently delayed and moderate to deep sedation is regularly targeted in patients requiring ECMO.[66] Although sedation is often needed at the initiation of ECLS support, the goal is to minimize sedation similar to patients not requiring ECLS.[67] A recent retrospective study demonstrated feasibility and safety of mobilization while on ECMO.[68] Future research is needed to investigate risks and benefits of early mobilization and decreased sedation.

Key Research Area: Long-Term Outcomes

Long-term outcomes for ECMO-supported ARDS survivors have not been well studied. A recent, relatively small meta-analysis[69] reported greater decrements in health-related quality of life in ARDS survivors managed with ECMO compared with survivors of mechanical ventilation, and interestingly, ECMO survivors had significantly less depression and anxiety compared with those managed with mechanical ventilation.

Short-term survival alone should not be considered an adequate outcome measure for the use of ECMO in ARDS. Functional disability and psychological sequelae have been shown to persist 5 years after surviving ARDS.[70] Prospective systematic evaluation of long-term outcomes in survivors of

ECMO-supported ARDS is necessary and should mirror similar work done in survivors of ARDS.[70]

Key Research Area: Extracorporeal Carbon Dioxide Removal in chronic obstrutive pulmonary disease (COPD)

Use of $ECCO_2R$ in patients with an acute COPD exacerbation, who are failing noninvasive positive pressure ventilation, may avoid the need for invasive mechanical ventilation.[71] Likewise, its use in patients who are already intubated may facilitate early liberation from invasive mechanical ventilation.[72,73] Thus far, studies have not shown survival advantages or reduced ventilator-free days and have been associated with high rates of ECLS-related complications.[71,73] Currently, $ECCO_2R$ for the management of COPD exacerbations should be restricted to research studies.

The Vent-Avoid trial is an ongoing multicenter, international RCT is investigating $ECCO_2R$ as an alternative or adjunct to mechanical ventilation in COPD exacerbations requiring respiratory support. The primary outcome is ventilator-free days.[74]

Research Challenges for the Future

Acute respiratory failure requiring ECLS is a relatively uncommon event making research in this field challenging but not unsurmountable. Using study designs with predictive enrichment strategies that identify populations most likely to benefit from ECLS might be necessary.[75] Furthermore, coordinated efforts between high-volume ECLS centers are essential, and research networks, such as the international ECMO Network (ECMO-Net; www.internationalecmonetwork.org) and large registries, such as the Extracorporeal Life Support Organization (www.elso.org) are critical if research on ECLS for acute respiratory failure is going to be successful.[76]

SUMMARY

ECLS in acute respiratory failure is most widely accepted for severe ARDS; however, its role has evolved over time to include several other indications, most commonly BTT and acute decompensated PH. An essential element of ECLS-supported ARDS management is to reduce VILI, with the goal to improve survival and long-term outcomes. Future research efforts should focus on optimal management strategies while on ECLS, long-term outcomes, and technological advancements.

CLINICS CARE POINTS

- Extracorporeal life support (ECLS) use in severe acute respiratory distress syndrome (ARDS) should be considered when conventional management strategies fail to provide adequate and safe oxygenation or in the setting of elevated airway pressures and severe respiratory acidosis.

- ECLS in ARDS allows for ultra-low lung-protective ventilation, thereby reducing the risk of ventilator induced lung injury, a significant contributor to mortality in ARDS.

- Potential indications for ECLS in acute respiratory failure include bridge to lung transplantation, decompensated pulmonary hypertension, status asthmaticus, primary graft dysfunction after lung transplant, and massive pulmonary embolism.

- Future directions in ECLS research and patient care include identifying optimal management strategies while supported by ECLS including optimal mechanical ventilation, role of prone positioning, weaning ECLS support, and strategies for mobilization, sedation, and anticoagulation.

- Future research efforts need to include survival and long-term outcomes.

DISCLOSURE

None.

REFERENCES

1. Hill JD, O'Brien TG, Murray JJ, et al. Prolonged extracorporeal oxygenation for acute post-traumatic respiratory failure (shock-lung syndrome). Use of the Bramson membrane lung. N Engl J Med 1972;286:629–34.
2. Brodie D. The evolution of extracorporeal membrane oxygenation for adult respiratory failure. Ann Am Thorac Soc 2018;15:S57–60.
3. Australia, New Zealand Extracorporeal Membrane Oxygenation Influenza I, Davies A, Jones D, et al. Extracorporeal membrane oxygenation for 2009 influenza A(H1N1) acute respiratory distress syndrome. JAMA 2009;302:1888–95.
4. Peek GJ, Mugford M, Tiruvoipati R, et al. Efficacy and economic assessment of conventional ventilatory support versus extracorporeal membrane oxygenation for severe adult respiratory failure (CESAR): a multicentre randomised controlled trial. Lancet 2009;374:1351–63.
5. Abrams D, Ferguson ND, Brochard L, et al. ECMO for ARDS: from salvage to standard of care? Lancet Respir Med 2019;7:108–10.
6. Brodie D, Slutsky AS, Combes A. Extracorporeal life support for adults with respiratory failure and related indications: a review. JAMA 2019;322:557–68.
7. Conrad SA, Broman LM, Taccone FS, et al. The extracorporeal life support organization maastricht treaty for nomenclature in extracorporeal life support. a position paper of the extracorporeal life support organization. Am J Respir Crit Care Med 2018;198:447–51.
8. Combes A, Schmidt M, Hodgson CL, et al. Extracorporeal life support for adults with acute respiratory distress syndrome. Intensive Care Med 2020;46:2464–76.
9. Slutsky AS, Ranieri VM. Ventilator-induced lung injury. N Engl J Med 2013;369:2126–36.
10. Acute Respiratory Distress Syndrome N, Brower RG, Matthay MA, et al. Ventilation with lower tidal volumes as compared with traditional tidal volumes for acute lung injury and the acute respiratory distress syndrome. N Engl J Med 2000;342:1301–8.
11. Fan E, Gattinoni L, Combes A, et al. Venovenous extracorporeal membrane oxygenation for acute respiratory failure : a clinical review from an international group of experts. Intensive Care Med 2016;42:712–24.
12. Combes A, Hajage D, Capellier G, et al. Extracorporeal membrane oxygenation for severe acute respiratory distress syndrome. N Engl J Med 2018;378:1965–75.

13. Goligher EC, Tomlinson G, Hajage D, et al. Extracor-poreal membrane oxygenation for severe acute res-piratory distress syndrome and posterior probability of mortality benefit in a post hoc bayesian analysis of a randomized clinical trial. JAMA 2018;320:2251–9.

14. Munshi L, Walkey A, Goligher E, et al. Venovenous extracorporeal membrane oxygenation for acute respiratory distress syndrome: a systematic review and meta-analysis. Lancet Respir Med 2019;7: 163–72.

15. Combes A, Peek GJ, Hajage D, et al. ECMO for se-vere ARDS: systematic review and individual patient data meta-analysis. Intensive Care Med 2020;46: 2048–57.

16. Namendys-Silva SA. ECMO for ARDS due to COVID-19. Heart Lung 2020;49:348–9.

17. Henry BM, Lippi G. Poor survival with extracorporeal membrane oxygenation in acute respiratory distress syndrome (ARDS) due to coronavirus disease 2019 (COVID-19): pooled analysis of early reports. J Crit Care 2020;58:27–8.

18. Barbaro RP, MacLaren G, Boonstra PS, et al, Extra-corporeal Life Support O. Extracorporeal membrane oxygenation support in COVID-19: an international cohort study of the Extracorporeal Life Support Or-ganization registry. Lancet 2020;396:1071–8.

19. Ramanathan K, Shekar K, Ling RR, et al. Extracorpo-real membrane oxygenation for COVID-19: a sys-tematic review and meta-analysis. Crit Care 2021; 25:211.

20. Karagiannidis C, Strassmann S, Merten M, et al. High in-hospital mortality in COVID patients receiving ECMO in Germany - a critical analysis. Am J Respir Crit Care Med 2021;204(8):991–4.

21. Lorusso R, Combes A, Coco VL, et al. ECMO for COVID-19 patients in Europe and Israel. Intensive Care Med 2021;47:344–8.

22. Badulak J, Antonini MV, Stead CM, et al. Extracorpo-real membrane oxygenation for COVID-19: updated 2021 guidelines from the extracorporeal life support organization. ASAIO J 2021;67:485–95.

23. Alhazzani W, Evans L, Alshamsi F, et al. Surviving sepsis campaign guidelines on the management of adults with coronavirus disease 2019 (COVID-19) in the ICU: first update. Crit Care Med 2021;49: e219–34.

24. World Health Organization. COVID-19 clinical man-agement: living guidance, 25 January 2021. World Health Organization; 2021. p. 1–116.

25. de Chambrun P, Brodie D, Combes A. Appraising the real-life need for extracorporeal membrane oxygenation during the COVID-19 pandemic. Am J Respir Crit Care Med 2021;204:2–4.

26. Anderson BR, Ivascu NS, Brodie D, et al. Breaking silos: the team-based approach to coronavirus dis-ease 2019 pandemic staffing. Crit Care Explor 2020;2:e0265.

27. MacLaren G, Fisher D, Brodie D. Preparing for the most critically ill patients with COVID-19: the poten-tial role of extracorporeal membrane oxygenation. JAMA 2020;323:1245–6.

28. Ramanathan K, Antognini D, Combes A, et al. Plan-ning and provision of ECMO services for severe ARDS during the COVID-19 pandemic and other outbreaks of emerging infectious diseases. Lancet Respir Med 2020;8:518–26.

29. Abrams D, Lorusso R, Vincent JL, et al. ECMO dur-ing the COVID-19 pandemic: when is it unjustified? Crit Care 2020;24:507.

30. Supady A, Badulak J, Evans L, et al. Should we ration extracorporeal membrane oxygenation during the COVID-19 pandemic? Lancet Respir Med 2021; 9:326–8.

31. Fan E, Brodie D, Slutsky AS. Acute respiratory distress syndrome: advances in diagnosis and treat-ment. JAMA 2018;319:698–710.

32. Rozencwajg S, Guihot A, Franchineau G, et al. Ultra-protective ventilation reduces biotrauma in patients on venovenous extracorporeal membrane oxygena-tion for severe acute respiratory distress syndrome. Crit Care Med 2019;47:1505–12.

33. Terragni PP, Del Sorbo L, Mascia L, et al. Tidal vol-ume lower than 6 ml/kg enhances lung protection: role of extracorporeal carbon dioxide removal. Anesthesiology 2009;111:826–35.

34. Abrams D, Schmidt M, Pham T, et al. Mechanical ventilation for acute respiratory distress syndrome during extracorporeal life support. Research and practice. Am J Respir Crit Care Med 2020;201: 514–25.

35. Benazzo A, Schwarz S, Frommlet F, et al. Twenty-year experience with extracorporeal life support as bridge to lung transplantation. J Thorac Cardiovasc Surg 2019;157:2515–2525 e2510.

36. de Perrot M, Granton JT, McRae K, et al. Impact of extracorporeal life support on outcome in patients with idiopathic pulmonary arterial hypertension awaiting lung transplantation. J Heart Lung Trans-plant 2011;30:997–1002.

37. Tipograf Y, Salna M, Minko E, et al. Outcomes of extracorporeal membrane oxygenation as a bridge to lung transplantation. Ann Thorac Surg 2019;107: 1456–63.

38. Hartwig MG, Walczak R, Lin SS, et al. Improved sur-vival but marginal allograft function in patients treated with extracorporeal membrane oxygenation after lung transplantation. Ann Thorac Surg 2012; 93:366–71.

39. Abrams DC, Brodie D, Rosenzweig EB, et al. Upper-body extracorporeal membrane oxygenation as a strategy in decompensated pulmonary arterial hy-pertension. Pulm Circ 2013;3:432–5.

40. Rosenzweig EB, Brodie D, Abrams DC, et al. Extra-corporeal membrane oxygenation as a novel

bridging strategy for acute right heart failure in group 1 pulmonary arterial hypertension. ASAIO J 2014;60:129–33.

41. Brenner K, Abrams DC, Agerstrand CL, et al. Extracorporeal carbon dioxide removal for refractory status asthmaticus: experience in distinct exacerbation phenotypes. Perfusion 2014;29:26–8.

42. Bromberger BJ, Agerstrand C, Abrams D, et al. Extracorporeal carbon dioxide removal in the treatment of status asthmaticus. Crit Care Med 2020;48:e1226–31.

43. Meneveau N, Guillon B, Planquette B, et al. Outcomes after extracorporeal membrane oxygenation for the treatment of high-risk pulmonary embolism: a multicentre series of 52 cases. Eur Heart J 2018;39:4196–204.

44. Kmiec L, Philipp A, Floerchinger B, et al. Extracorporeal membrane oxygenation for massive pulmonary embolism as bridge to therapy. ASAIO J 2020;66:146–52.

45. Ali JM, Vuylsteke A, Fowles JA, et al. Transfer of patients with cardiogenic shock using veno-arterial extracorporeal membrane oxygenation. J Cardiothorac Vasc Anesth 2020;34:374–82.

46. Javidfar J, Brodie D, Sonett J, et al. Venovenous extracorporeal membrane oxygenation using a single cannula in patients with pulmonary hypertension and atrial septal defects. J Thorac Cardiovasc Surg 2012;143:982–4.

47. Rosenzweig EB, Gannon WD, Madahar P, et al. Extracorporeal life support bridge for pulmonary hypertension: a high-volume single-center experience. J Heart Lung Transplant 2019;38:1275–85.

48. Boyle AJ, Sklar MC, McNamee JJ, et al. Extracorporeal carbon dioxide removal for lowering the risk of mechanical ventilation: research questions and clinical potential for the future. Lancet Respir Med 2018;6:874–84.

49. Combes A, Tonetti T, Fanelli V, et al. Efficacy and safety of lower versus higher CO2 extraction devices to allow ultraprotective ventilation: secondary analysis of the SUPERNOVA study. Thorax 2019;74:1179–81.

50. Combes A, Fanelli V, Pham T, et al. European Society of Intensive Care Medicine Trials G, the "Strategy of Ultra-Protective lung ventilation with Extracorporeal CORfN-OmtsAi. Feasibility and safety of extracorporeal CO2 removal to enhance protective ventilation in acute respiratory distress syndrome: the SUPERNOVA study. Intensive Care Med 2019;45:592–600.

51. McNamee JJ, Gillies MA, Barrett NA, et al. Effect of lower tidal volume ventilation facilitated by extracorporeal carbon dioxide removal vs standard care ventilation on 90-day mortality in patients with acute hypoxemic respiratory failure: the rest randomized clinical trial. JAMA 2021;326(11):1013–23.

52. Zakhary B, Fan E, Slutsky A. Should patients with acute respiratory distress syndrome on venovenous extracorporeal membrane oxygenation have ventilatory support reduced to the lowest tolerable settings? Yes. Crit Care Med 2019;47:1143–6.

53. Shekar K, Brodie D. Should patients with acute respiratory distress syndrome on venovenous extracorporeal membrane oxygenation have ventilatory support reduced to the lowest tolerable settings? No. Crit Care Med 2019;47:1147–9.

54. Guerin C, Papazian L, Reignier J, et al. Investigators of the A, Proseva t. Effect of driving pressure on mortality in ARDS patients during lung protective mechanical ventilation in two randomized controlled trials. Crit Care 2016;20:384.

55. Guervilly C, Prud'homme E, Pauly V, et al. Prone positioning and extracorporeal membrane oxygenation for severe acute respiratory distress syndrome: time for a randomized trial? Intensive Care Med 2019;45:1040–2.

56. Giani M, Martucci G, Madotto F, et al. Prone positioning during venovenous extracorporeal membrane oxygenation in acute respiratory distress syndrome. a multicenter cohort study and propensity-matched analysis. Ann Am Thorac Soc 2021;18:495–501.

57. PRONing to facilitate weaning from ECMO in Patients with refractory acute respiratory distress syndrome (PRONECMO). Available at: https://clinicaltrials.gov/ct2/show/NCT04607551. Accessed August 28, 2021.

58. Gannon WD, Stokes JW, Bloom S, et al. Safety and feasibility of a protocolized daily assessment of readiness for liberation from venovenous extracorporeal membrane oxygenation. Chest 2021;160(5):1693–703.

59. Al-Fares AA, Ferguson ND, Ma J, et al. Achieving safe liberation during weaning from VV-ECMO in patients with severe ARDS: the role of tidal volume and inspiratory effort. Chest 2021;160(5):1704–13.

60. ELSO anticoagulation guidelines. 2014. Available at: https://www.elso.org/Portals/0/Files/elsoanticoagulationguideline8-2014-table-contents.pdf. Accessed August 28, 2021.

61. Protti A, Iapichino GE, Di Nardo M, et al. Anticoagulation management and antithrombin supplementation practice during veno-venous extracorporeal membrane oxygenation: a worldwide survey. Anesthesiology 2020;132:562–70.

62. Aubron C, McQuilten Z, Bailey M, et al, endorsed by the International EN. Low-dose versus therapeutic anticoagulation in patients on extracorporeal membrane oxygenation: a pilot randomized trial. Crit Care Med 2019;47:e563–71.

63. Panigada M, Lapichino GE, Brioni M, et al. Thromboelastography-based anticoagulation management during extracorporeal membrane oxyge

nation: a safety and feasibility pilot study. Ann Intensive Care 2018;8:7.

64. Willers A, Arens J, Mariani S, et al. New trends, advantages and disadvantages in anticoagulation and coating methods used in extracorporeal life support devices. Membranes (Basel) 2021;11(8):617.

65. Devlin JW, Skrobik Y, Gelinas C, et al. Clinical practice guidelines for the prevention and management of pain, agitation/sedation, delirium, immobility, and sleep disruption in adult patients in the ICU. Crit Care Med 2018;46:e825–73.

66. Marhong JD, DeBacker J, Viau-Lapointe J, et al. Sedation and mobilization during venovenous extracorporeal membrane oxygenation for acute respiratory failure: an international survey. Crit Care Med 2017;45:1893–9.

67. Extracorporeal Life Support Organization. General guidelines for all ECLS casees. 2017. Available at: https://www.elso.org/Portals/0/ELSO%20Guidelines%20General%20All%20ECLS%20Version%201_4.pdf. Accessed July 28, 2021.

68. Abrams D, Madahar P, Eckhardt CM, et al. Early mobilization during ECMO for cardiopulmonary failure in adults: factors associated with intensity of treatment. Ann Am Thorac Soc 2021;19(1):90–8.

69. Wilcox ME, Jaramillo-Rocha V, Hodgson C, et al. Long-term quality of life after extracorporeal membrane oxygenation in ARDS survivors: systematic review and meta-analysis. J Intensive Care Med 2020;35:233–43.

70. Herridge MS, Tansey CM, Matte A, et al, Canadian critical care trials G. Functional disability 5 years after acute respiratory distress syndrome. N Engl J Med 2011;364:1293–304.

71. Braune S, Sieweke A, Brettner F, et al. The feasibility and safety of extracorporeal carbon dioxide removal to avoid intubation in patients with COPD unresponsive to noninvasive ventilation for acute hypercapnic respiratory failure (ECLAIR study): multicentre case-control study. Intensive Care Med 2016;42:1437–44.

72. Abrams DC, Brenner K, Burkart KM, et al. Pilot study of extracorporeal carbon dioxide removal to facilitate extubation and ambulation in exacerbations of chronic obstructive pulmonary disease. Ann Am Thorac Soc 2013;10:307–14.

73. Del Sorbo L, Pisani L, Filippini C, et al. Extracorporeal Co2 removal in hypercapnic patients at risk of noninvasive ventilation failure: a matched cohort study with historical control. Crit Care Med 2015;43:120–7.

74. Extracorporeal CO2 removal with the hemolung RAS for mechanical ventilation avoidance during acute exacerbation of COPD (VENT-AVOID). Available at: https://clinicaltrials.gov/ct2/show/NCT03255057. Accessed August 27, 2021.

75. Goligher EC, Amato MBP, Slutsky AS. Applying precision medicine to trial design using physiology. extracorporeal co2 removal for acute respiratory distress syndrome. Am J Respir Crit Care Med 2017;196:558–68.

76. Brodie D, Vincent JL, Brochard LJ, et al. Research in extracorporeal life support: a call to action. Chest 2018;153:788–91.

COVID-19 and the Transformation of Intensive Care Unit Telemedicine

Eric W. Cucchi, MS, PA-C[a], Scott E. Kopec, MD[b], Craig M. Lilly, MD[c],*

KEYWORDS

• Telemedicine • Telehealth • Tele-ICU • Digital health • Digital medicine • Critical care • COVID-19

KEY POINTS

- ICU telemedicine center critical care specialists played an important role in the expansion of critical care services during the COVID-19 pandemic.
- Off-hours oversight of noncritical care prescribing providers allowed a sudden and substantial transformation of the existing hospital workforce to serve critically ill patients without delay for training those who did not care for the critically ill before the pandemic.
- Bedside providers used the telemedicine system to increase their efficiency and combat the effects of COVID-19 isolation.
- New models of reimbursement for ICU telemedicine services and monitoring and more efficient telemedicine tools became available during the pandemic.

INTRODUCTION

COVID-19, caused by the SARS-COV-2 RNA virus,[1,2] reshaped our everyday way of life.[3] At the time of writing, there have been more than 100 million cases worldwide and more than 3 million deaths[4] despite recommendations from the Center for Disease Control (CDC) to stay 6 feet apart, avoid crowds, avoid poorly ventilated indoor spaces,[5] and limit travel.[6] The COVID-19 pandemic has infiltrated so deeply into our society that it has changed the very way we communicate with one another. According to the US Bureau of Labor Statistics, between 25% and 35% of the US workforce was working remotely between May and August 2020.[7] The change in communication strategies seen in the public sector has also impacted how health care is delivered, and support for the critically ill has been no exception.

Expanding Access to Critical Care Specialist-Directed Management Using Telemedicine

It has been accepted by medical professionals since the time of Machiavelli that early recognition and prompt action for battlefield injuries and medical conditions, including hectic fever (sepsis), allow the application of treatments and techniques that become less effective if delayed.[8] The concept of time windows for interventions is now well-recognized and has shaped life-saving early recognition programs for thrombotic disorders including myocardial infarction and stroke. The value of ICU telemedicine specialist support for

[a] Digital Medicine Program, UMass Memorial Medical Center, University of Massachusetts Medical School, Graduate School of Nursing, University of Massachusetts, 281 Lincoln Street, Worcester, MA 01605, USA; [b] Internal Medicine Residency Program, University of Massachusetts Medical School, 55 Lake Avenue North, Worcester, MA 01655, USA; [c] Medicine, Surgery, and Anesthesiology, University of Massachusetts Medical School, 55 Lake Ave. North, Worcester, MA 01605, USA
* Corresponding author.
E-mail address: Craig.Lilly@umassmed.edu

Clin Chest Med 43 (2022) 529–538
https://doi.org/10.1016/j.ccm.2022.05.007
0272-5231/22/© 2022 Elsevier Inc. All rights reserved.

less common, high mortality-risk conditions is highlighted by the following case example.

A 45-year-old asthmatic mother of 4 presented to an otolaryngologist with progressive nasal occlusion. For many years she had noted episodes of wheezing and nasal congestion after exposure to ibuprofen and reported no other medical conditions. Examination of her nasal mucosa revealed bilateral near occlusion with nasal polyps. After testing negative for COVID-19 nucleic acid secretion she underwent removal of the polyps from her left nare. The next morning, she noted worsening left facial pain and swelling. She presented the following evening to the Emergency Department of her local hospital with a temperature of 101° F, a 0.25 cm blister on her upper lip, and hoarseness. Laboratory evaluation revealed a WBC of 12×10^9/L, lactate level of 8 mmol/L, and a clear chest radiograph with an elevated L hemidiaphragm. Blood cultures were obtained, piperacillin-tazobactam and vancomycin administered, and 25 mL/Kg isotonic crystalloid was administered when sinus tachycardia and hypotension were identified.

Hoarseness was evaluated by a covering otolaryngologist who noted nasal and pharyngeal soft tissue edema and recommended transfer to an operating room for airway assessment and control. Laryngoscopy revealed edema that extended to her vocal cords and endotracheal intubation was performed. Norepinephrine was administered for hypotension. Examination of the operative site was unremarkable and debridement was deemed not to be indicated. After the operation, the patient was transported to her local hospital ICU whereby central and arterial lines were inserted and CT scans of the neck, head, and chest were ordered by an ICU nurse practitioner. Scans demonstrated small pockets of air adjacent to the platysma muscle and were interpreted as not demonstrating convincing evidence of necrotizing fasciitis. Vasopressin and phenylephrine were prescribed for progressive hypotension. The ICU nurse practitioner contacted the otolaryngologist who was unable to offer an off-hours source control procedure. The laboratory reported that blood cultures were growing gram-positive cocci in chains and clusters and the patient was noted to be oliguric and progressively acidemic. On the arrival of the morning shift physician's assistant the blood culture isolate had been identified as beta-hemolytic *Streptococcus*; the otolaryngologist was contacted and recommended the evacuation of the patient to an academic medical center for a source control procedure. On arrival at the academic medical center, the patient was rushed to an operating theater and pronounced dead of a

cardiac arrest that occurred during the resection of necrotic neck tissue. Necrotizing fasciitis was confirmed at autopsy.

It is notable that the ICU telemedicine program that would have provided critical care specialist oversight to the affiliate practitioners was terminated several years prior when its financial support was redirected to a lucrative specialty surgery program.

DISCUSSION
Intensive Care Unit Telemedicine Support Models: the Emergent Expansion of Our Critical Care Workforce During the COVID-19 Pandemic

The COVID-19 pandemic provided insights into how the traditional critical care consultative and hub-and-spoke models of critical care support performed during the first influx and were modified and made sustainable for the second influx of patients with COVID-19. The recognition of evolving respiratory failure and controlled, elective, protocol-adherent rather than reactive, emergent, less-controlled care was a central change.

Telemedicine support models are best compared by their key activation, reporting, and efficiency of care delivery characteristics that affect their ability to support the rapid expansion of service delivery. The ability of the hub-and-spoke model to connect new "spokes" to existing infrastructure was leveraged during the pandemic to increase critical care capacity (**Fig. 1**). The consultative model is activated when the clinical skill, availability, and priorities of a bedside provider allow the recognition of evolving physiologic instability and specialist assistance is needed. In practice, the costs of this determination include time, effort, and vigilance by bedside providers who, when in crisis, have compelling competing demands for their time and energy. The extent to which recognition, prioritization, and costs of intervention inhibit the activation of ICU telemedicine services is larger than most clinicians suspect. It has been reported that only 1 in 50 emergent tele-ICU interventions are initiated by a bedside provider before a telemedicine clinician had determined that an emergent intervention was required.[9] The case presented above provides a clear example of the safety advantages of automated event warning systems that are independent of bedside provider judgment and vigilance.

The hub-and-spoke model of tele-ICU support differs from the consultative model in several aspects that affect the efficiency of service delivery (**Fig. 2**). The hub-and-spoke model monitors patients with advanced analyses of monitor-

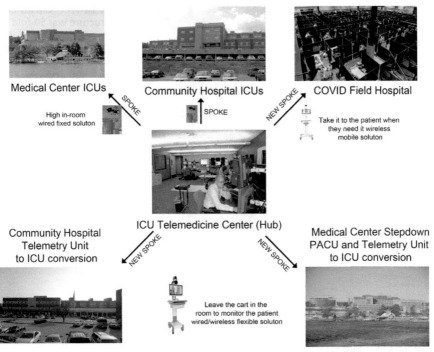

Fig. 1. The expansion of existing tele-ICU infrastructure by adding spokes to established ICU telemedicine centers to expand the medical center and community hospital ICU capacity and provide safe care at field hospital sites that did not exist before the pandemic. During the COVID-19 pandemic, the hub-and-spoke model deployed telemedicine carts with monitoring capability to direct off-site critical care clinicians to at-risk patients, often before physiologic instability and organ failure had occurred. This allowed an approximate 15% increase in bed ICU capacity by conversion of telemetry beds and intensivist support of care by bedside staff who did not work in an ICU before the pandemic. This was conducted without additional telemedicine center staffing.

generated vital sign signals that identify nearly all, and predict some, episodes of hemodynamic instability or respiratory failure. The ability of these predictions to direct critical care specialist reviews to patients who can benefit allows for better and more timely matching of patient need with specialist services than the consultative model. The ability to exchange health information from electronic records and to interact with patients, family members, and bedside caregivers using real-time, audiovisual links[10,11] allow the delivery of care by off-site specialists over wide geographic areas using a leveraged workforce service delivery model (see **Fig. 1**).

Indeed, it has been estimated that the integration of tele-communication and information systems allows a 10- or more-fold increase in access to ICU specialist care. A specialist that would cover a 15-bed ICU can provide direction using physician extenders for the patients of 150 telemedicine-monitored ICU beds.[12] The higher negative predictive value of telemedicine system alerts than biomedical monitor alarms more efficiently targets specialist attention to patients with evolving hemodynamic instability and respiratory failure than

central monitor station alarms and traditional care models. The hub-and-spoke monitoring model also uses electronic detection that allows an off-site support center to encourage adherence to evidence-based ICU best practices. In addition to improved best practice adherence, a large multicenter study of ICU telemedicine processes and outcomes associated with critical care specialist case review in the first hours after ICU admission[13] and less than 3-min response times to alerts for physiologic instability with more improved outcomes after an ICU telemedicine intervention.[12]

In the case of our 45 year old with life-threatening septic shock from a surgical site infection, critical care specialist case review from the Emergency Department likely would not have produced early surgical debridement but would have facilitated transfer before she was moribund. In addition, a workflow-integrated specialist case review would have enabled a critical care specialist-to-otolaryngologist discussion regarding a diagnosis of necrotizing fasciitis and the role of timely source control.

This event occurred despite the fact that her local hospital used a Leapfrog[14] compliant

2-Step Hub and Spoke Connection

Step 1. Automated   or in room   Step 2. Consultant reviews
case identification   button notification   clinical summary and
                                              uses established connections
                                                while reviewing EHR

6-Step Consultation Connection

Step 1. Recogniton of   Step 2. Request for   Step 3. Available
     instability   consultation   consultant is notifiied

Step 4. Transport and   Step 5. Consultant   Step 6. Consultant securely
connect mobile device   connects to   connects to and reviews
                         mobile cart   EHR

Fig. 2. Lateral expansion of existing infrastructure was 50-fold more effective than the deployment of the consultative model. This is due, in part, to the more efficient 2-step activation characteristics of the hub-and-spoke infrastructure (*top*) compared with the 6-step activation process for arranging telemedicine intensivist consultations (*bottom*). Expansion of the consultative model also requires the resolution of crediting, privileging, privacy, connectivity, and security barriers before being deployed.

consultative model of critical care delivery. After-hours critical care specialist involvement was at the discretion of FCCS-certified prescribers who briefed the specialist about the events of the night only after transfer to the referral center.

The Role of the Tele-Intensive Care Unit Critical Care Specialist in a Leveraged Workforce Environment

One strategy for increasing access to ICU care is to use telemedicine critical care specialist oversight of physician extenders and physicians who have not met critical care specialty board training requirements to provide intensivist curated critical care. Providing critical care training and ICU telemedicine oversight of physician extenders, including nurse practitioners and physician assistants, is associated with lower societal critical care costs and reduced usage of postacute care among Medicare beneficiaries.[15]

Comparative Effectiveness of Intensive Care Unit Telemedicine Center and Specialist Network Consultative Models of Intensive Care Unit Workforce Expansion During the Pandemic

The "Network of Networks" model, in which resources of under-used centers are diverted to centers that are overwhelmed, played a much smaller role than the lateral growth of existing ICU telemedicine centers during the pandemic. The within-network hub-and-spoke model leveraged existing licensed, privileged and credentialed, critical care providers and used telemedicine cart technologies to increase ICU bed capacity by 15% to 20% (approximately 1500 nonfederal ICU beds).[16,17] ICU telemedicine center professionals supported bedside nurses, physicians, physician assistants, and nurse practitioners who cared for patients in telemetry-equipped spaces that did not house critically ill patients before the pandemic (see **Fig. 1**). In addition, when elective surgical volume decreased during the pandemic, telemedicine critical care specialists were able to help ICU staff who had not routinely cared for acute hypoxemic respiratory failure before the pandemic to support patients with COVID-19 associated critical illness. The outcomes of the patients managed in these transformed and monitored spaces did not differ significantly from those of patients housed in pre-epidemic respiratory ICU beds. The in-hospital mortality among 547 patients admitted to a pre-pandemic ICU bed of 22% was not significantly different than the rate of 26% observed for 223 surge space ICU admitted patients (chi-square test; $P = .24$). In the context of the national emergency, this expansion from 250,000 to 280,000 monitored patient hours per day was accomplished nearly completely without increasing the ICU telemedicine center workforce. The large geographic scope of the pandemic effectively prevented ICU telemedicine centers from serving patients beyond their system because all centers experienced nearly simultaneous overwhelming local demand.

In addition to increasing medical center COVID-19 capacity, the hub-and-spoke model allowed patients with high-acuity COVID-19 to be cared for in community hospital ICU beds that were vacant when elective surgical volume declined during the pandemic. The critical care specialists of supporting telemedicine centers were able to apply validated, standardized protocols for severe hypoxemia, implement ventilation strategies not routinely before the pandemic, and implement and supervise rescue protocols such as prone ventilation.

A recent report from the National Emergency Critical Care Telemedicine Network allows comparison of the timeliness and effectiveness of expansion of hub-and-spoke model centers with a volunteer consultative model of tele-critical care.[18] A cadre of 248 remote experts provided advice to 260 bedside caregivers, equating to190 hours of clinician interactions and a maximum of 4560 hours of patient stay coverage per day. From a service point of view, the comparative effectiveness of the consultative model to the hub-and-spoke model is 4560/280,000 or 1.6%. Comparison of effectiveness from a workforce size perspective reveals that the consultative model required 248 trained and credentialed specialists to cover 190 patients, or 1.3 specialists per patient served. The hub-and-spoke model used 78 critical care specialists to serve 11,825 patients, or 1 specialist to 150 patients covered. Hub-and-spoke was several-fold more efficient than the consultative model. The time to credentialing for the consultative model was 28 days while hub-and-spoke specialists were credentialed at the time of pandemic onset.

The more favorable service characteristics of hub-and-spoke account for the fact that lateral expansion of telemedicine center support was the dominant form of ICU telemedicine support used during the pandemic (see **Fig. 2**). It is notable that none of the medical centers experiencing a surge of patients with COVID-19 elected to use the services of the National Emergency Critical Care Telemedicine Network.[18]

Key limitations of both models include the availability of functional telecommunication equipment, bedside monitoring equipment, and access to electronic health records. ICU telemedicine centers with established connectivity, network security clearances, and technical support resources were better positioned than volunteer network consultants to provide additional network-connected telemedicine equipment and nursing and pharmacy support services. ICU telemedicine centers were able to add spokes to their hubs by rapidly connecting new devices to their established networks (see **Fig. 1**).

In addition, ICU telemedicine center health informatics professionals connected off-the-shelf telecommunications equipment when it was available and transformed EHR documentation carts into both mobile (wireless) and fixed (wired) ICU telemedicine carts when preassembled carts were no longer available (**Fig. 3**). One specialist could assemble a telemedicine cart every 4 hours. The ability to securely connect these devices to an existing network allowed rapid deployment and testing. Patients were more reliably monitored and rescue interventions were more rapidly made using grid-powered, wired carts than by battery-powered, wireless devices that were powered upon demand. This ability to use the widely available essential components listed in **Fig. 3** to create and connect ICU telemedicine equipment, not existing prepandemic, allowed a rapid 10% to 25% increase in ICU bed capacity by transforming telemetry beds (see **Fig. 1**). This approach also allowed support and oversight of nurses that were not caring for ICU patients before the pandemic by experienced, telemedicine center nurses who had CCRN-E training[19] as well as tele-pharmacist review of orders.[20]

Telemedicine Center Support for Hospital Overflow Patients with COVID-19

In addition to critically ill patients with COVID-19, many hospitals were flooded with patients with noncritically ill COVID-19 pneumonia who were at high risk for respiratory failure. During the height of the pandemic, it became necessary to monitor lower-risk patients in non–telemetry-equipped hospital locations and in field hospitals. Because monitor feed data were not available for these patients, telemedicine center personnel could not use automated detection methods. As an alternative, they used daily visual inspection of hospital vital sign flowsheet data to perform binary risk stratification. Patients with an oxygen prescription of 4 L/min or an increment of 2 or more liters/min in the prior 12 hours, an increase from baseline to a persistent respiratory rate (RR) greater than 25/min, or a notation indicating respiratory distress were classified as high risk. All others were

ICU Telemedicine Cart Component Parts

Pan-Tilt-Zoom Camera and wireless antena

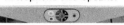

Microphone and Speaker

Telemedicine Help Button

Power Supply, Network and Sound Cards

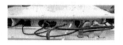

Cabels and connections

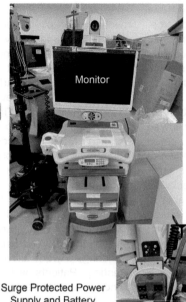

Monitor

Surge Protected Power Supply and Battery

Fig. 3. When off-the-shelf devices were no longer available, telemedicine team information systems professionals continued to expand ICU capacity by cobbling together the camera, microphone, speaker, help button, power supply, sound and network cards, cables, connections, power supply, battery, and antenna (for wireless carts) into a functional telemedicine cart from spare or parts that were commercially available or could be scavenged from out of service devices or carts originally designed for EHR documentation or other nontelemedicine uses. One skilled professional was able to build a cart every 4 hours.

classified as low-risk for hypoxemic respiratory failure in the subsequent 24 hours. Telemedicine clinicians contacted the bedside providers of high-risk patients and offered ICU transfer for life support.

High-risk and low-risk patients were demographically similar, but high-risk patients had higher oxygen flow rate prescriptions and creatinine levels. Telemedicine center risk stratification had 91% sensitivity and 90% specificity for detecting hypoxemic respiratory failure during the subsequent 24 hours. The negative predictive value (NPV) was 0.991 and the positive predictive value (PPV) was 0.348. None of the low-risk patients who did not have care limitations required rescue. The 3 rapid response events among 127 risk-stratified patients with COVID-19 were significantly fewer than the 42 events observed among 265 COVID-19 negative, unscreened, adult inpatients who were hospitalized during the study period ($P < .001$). The in-hospital mortality of high-risk patients who elected rescue was significantly lower than that of those who declined ICU transfer for life support (22% vs 65%, $P < .001$).

Bedside Provider Usage of Telemedicine System Resources

Early in the COVID-19 pandemic in the setting of national and local patient volume surges[21] there

were limits to the amount of personal protective equipment (PPE) available at the bedside.[22] The specter of running out of PPE generated interest in using tele-ICU system resources to reduce room entry events to limit the consumption of PPE. Bedside providers were enthusiastic about their use of audio–video tools and the number of telemedicine interactions by bedside providers dramatically increased near the time they were granted camera access (**Fig. 4**). As the use of the ICU telemedicine became part of bedside provider practice, aggregate bedside camera usage exceeded tele-ICU team usage, and there was an increase in the number of bedside nurse requests for assistance from off-site team members (see **Fig. 4**).

Telemedicine System Support for Severe Hypoxemic Respiratory Failure Procedures

The management of COVID-19 associated, refractory, severe hypoxemia with prone ventilation spurred the development of protocol-driven proning teams. The position of the camera and microphone high in the room allowed monitoring members of the team to assure protocol adherence and patient safety. This method of monitoring was perceived by proning team members to be safer and more efficient than in-room monitoring. Telemedicine care delivery became standard ICU work.

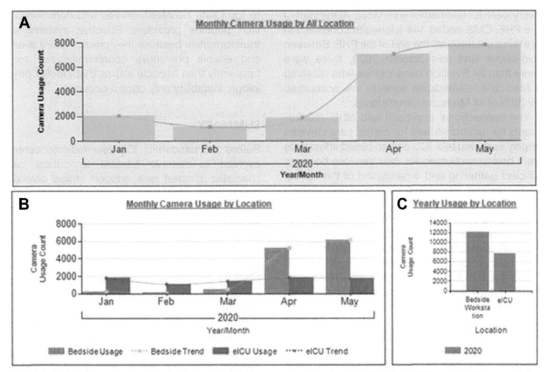

Fig. 4. Wired ICU in room camera usage episodes increased at the time of COVID-19 ICU caseload increased during the pandemic (A). The increase in camera usage by off-site usage (B; *red bars*) was in proportion to the ICU telemedicine-supported ICU bed expansion. A more than 10-fold increase in camera usage by bedside providers occurred at the time that access was granted (B; *blue bars*). Camera usage by bedside ICU providers exceeded, in aggregate, telemedicine provider usage (C).

Intensive Care Unit Telemedicine Support for Patients in COVID-19 Isolation

Unintended consequences of COVID-19 visitation policies were barriers to patient–family interaction and emotional support. These well-intentioned measures resulted in isolation and loneliness with their adverse effects on mood and well-being.[23] The importance of physical proximity of family and friends, deeply needed at the time of an unplanned critical care crisis, became even more evident. Moreover, visitation policies disrupted interactions of providers with families and medical decision makers that had formerly fostered trusting relationships. Telecommunication connections were used to provide emotional support by connecting patients to their loved one's mobile devices and allowing them to interact with support center nurses and intensivists. ICU telemedicine systems were also used to support family-inclusive ICU rounding.

COVID-19 Intensive Care Unit Telemedicine Service Reimbursement

Before 2020, Centers for Medicare and Medicaid Services provided reimbursement for some telehealth service transactions on a limited basis.[24] The January 27, 2020 declaration of a Public Health Emergency (PHE) for 2019 Novel Coronavirus (2019-nCoV)[25] enacted Social Security Act (SSA) Section 1135 authority to waive reimbursement requirements during a national emergency.[26] CMS allowed temporary changes in transactional restrictions after the declaration of PHE, the SSA 1135 waiver, and the Coronavirus Preparedness and Response Supplemental Appropriations Act.[27,28] The changes made by CMS rules combined with the many provisions to states laws mandating that commercial payors[29] restore access to health care by reimbursing telemedicine-based transactions.

There is increasing evidence that these policy changes dramatically increased the volume of telemedicine transactions. Koonin and colleagues found that, in the first quarter of 2020, the number of telehealth visits increased by 50% compared with the same period of 2019.[30] The Centers for Medicare and Medicaid Services (CMS) also reported that the volume of telemedicine transactions increased. Before the PHE, there were 15,000 Medicare fee-for-service beneficiary claims every week for telemedicine services. At the start of the PHE, CMS added 144 telehealth codes which are reimbursable until the end of the PHE. Between mid-March and mid-October 2020, there were more than 24.5 million beneficiaries who received a Medicare telemedicine service; this accounted for 38% of all Medicare beneficiaries.[31]

The transactional approach and other requirements for reimbursement for critical care services largely excluded tele-ICU center-based specialists from being reimbursed for their services because efficient gathering and organization of the clinical facts required for critical care decision making were performed by team members other than the critical care specialist. Accordingly, the most efficient specialists in our critical care workforce were not paid for their services because they could not meet inappropriately lengthy time requirements for transactional critical care CPT codes. Increased efficiency and access to the specialist care that beneficiaries demand are convincing drivers for the development of telemedicine service reimbursement strategies that are appropriate for leveraged workforce-delivered services. The practical obstacles to expanding services using transactional reimbursement were well-appreciated by the leaders of the Department of Veterans Affairs who are expanding ICU telemedicine services for the federal hospital system by funding regional programs for the services that they provide using a subscription model.

A subscriptional reimbursement approach on a per monitored bed day-basis is an attractive option for expanding ICU telemedicine in nonfederal hospital systems because it delivers the right combination of critical care specialist, subspecialty nursing, pharmacy, and technical support personnel as a package. Bundling these services over large geographic areas better aligns service provider available with the need for critical care services than the current transaction-based system. The financial benefits of ICU workforce leveraging have been shown to exceed the costs of privileging and credentialing off-site providers.[32,33] Importantly, this model removes the lack of locally available personnel as a barrier to the delivery of critical care services.

Predictive Analytics for Early Intervention

Hub-and-spoke centers with continuously available personnel are able to leverage increasingly sophisticated event prediction and early warning software to target evaluation and management services. This software is designed to reduce time-to-event recognition and increase the amount of preevent time off-site specialists have

to formulate countermeasures and communicate with bedside providers. Effective systems are transformative because they predict future events and enable preventive countermeasures more frequently than bedside alarms that identify physiologic instability only once it occurs.

SUMMARY

Before the pandemic, ICU telemedicine centers evolved to remove barriers to critical care specialist-directed care, support critical care delivery by providers who are not critical care specialists and respond promptly to alerts for evolving physiologic instability. These activities have been associated with improved hospital and ICU mortality and length of stay in before-and-after tele-ICU studies,[9,34,35] encourage higher rates of adherence to ICU best practices,[9,13] increase access to critical care services, and generate favorable financial outcomes.[32] Their ability to provide a leveraged workforce solution allowed lateral growth and expansion of services to help broker the influx of patients with acute hypoxemic respiratory failure during the COVID-19 pandemic. Health care systems with ICU telemedicine centers were able to more rapidly and robustly expand their delivery of high-quality critical care evaluation and management services than those deploying consultative telemedicine models.

The pandemic also encouraged the use of ICU telemedicine tools by bedside providers to reduce room entry events that consumed PPE, combat COVID-19 isolation and loneliness, and supervise prone ventilation teams. The pandemic brought new methods for reimbursing ICU telemedicine monitoring and service delivery and encouraged the development of improved predictive analytics.

CLINICS CARE POINTS

- COVID-19 associated rapid increases in critical care volume encouraged the lateral growth of hub-and-spoke tele-ICU programs.

- ICU telemedicine critical care specialists supported a safe and rapid expansion of the delivery of effective critical care services by noncritical care providers during the pandemic.

- ICU telemedicine tools were incorporated by rapid response and prone ventilation teams, but also by patients and families, more readily than before the pandemic.

- The value of telemedicine support is more widely accepted by patients, families, and providers and novel reimbursement strategies are making ICU telemedicine the standard of care in the federal hospital system.

ACKNOWLEDGMENTS

The authors recognize the contributions of Greg Wongkam who detailed and photographed the creation of the ICU telemedicine carts from the component parts, Natasha Dudiki MD, for her invaluable assistance with collecting and collating manual detection of respiratory failure data, and Gurudev Lotun for the data integration and assembly of the ICU mortality database.

DISCLOSURE

E.W. Cucchi, S.E. Kopec, and C.M. Lilly have no potential financial conflicts of interest related to the content of this article.

REFERENCES

1. The species Severe acute respiratory syndrome-related coronavirus: classifying 2019-nCoV and naming it SARS-CoV-2. Nat Microbiol 2020;5(4):536–44.
2. Gawande A. Why doctors hate their computers. In: Remnick D, editor. The New Yorker. New York: Conde Nast; 2018. p. 1–24.
3. Grundy BL, Crawford P, Jones PK, et al. Telemedicine in critical care: an experiment in health care delivery. JACEP 1977;6(10):439–44.
4. Coronavirus.jhu.edu. Johns hopkins university & medicine coronavirus resource center. In. Global deaths. 2021.
5. Control CoD. Things you need to know. 2021. Available at: https://www.cdc.gov/coronavirus/2019-ncov/your-health/need-to-know.html. Accessed February 9, 2021.
6. Control CoD. Travel. Centers of Disease control. 2021. Available at: https://www.cdc.gov/coronavirus/2019-ncov/your-health/need-to-know.html. Accessed February 9,2021.
7. Statistics UBoL. TED: the economic daily. 2020. Available at: https://www.bls.gov/opub/ted/2020/one-quarter-of-the-employed-teleworked-in-august-2020-because-of-covid-19-pandemic.htm#:~:text=About%201%20in%204%20people,month%20these%20data%20were%20collected. Accessed February 9, 2021.
8. Machiavelli N, Constantine P. The essential writings of Machiavelli. New York: Modern Library; 2007.
9. Lilly CM, Cody S, Zhao H, et al. Hospital mortality, length of stay, and preventable complications among critically ill patients before and after tele-ICU reengineering of critical care processes. JAMA 2011;305(21):2175–83.
10. Grundy BL, Jones PK, Lovitt A. Telemedicine in critical care: problems in design, implementation, and assessment. Crit Care Med 1982;10(7):471–5.
11. Kumar S, Merchant S Fau - Reynolds R, Reynolds R. Tele-ICU: efficacy and cost-effectiveness of remotely managing critical care. (1559-4122 (Electronic)).
12. Lilly CM, Zubrow MT, Kempner KM, et al. Critical care telemedicine: evolution and state of the art. Crit Care Med 2014;42(11):2429–36.
13. Lilly CM, McLaughlin JM, Zhao H, et al. A multicenter study of ICU telemedicine reengineering of adult critical care. Chest 2014;145(3):500–7.
14. Logani S, Green A, Gasperino J. Benefits of high-intensity intensive care unit physician staffing under the affordable care Act. Crit Care Res Pract 2011;2011:170814.
15. Trombley MJ, Hassol A, Lloyd JT, et al. The impact of enhanced critical care training and 24/7 (Tele-ICU) support on medicare spending and postdischarge utilization patterns. Health Serv Res 2018;53(4):2099–117.
16. Halpern NA, Tan KS, DeWitt M, et al. Intensivists in U.S. Acute care hospitals. Crit Care Med 2019;47(4):517–25.
17. Association AH. Hospital size and geographic distribution. American Hospital Assocaition. Available at: https://www.ahadata.com/aha-hospital-statistics, 2011. Accessed October 2, 2011.
18. Pamplin JC, Scott BK, Quinn MT, et al. Technology and disasters: the evolution of the national emergency tele-critical care network. Crit Care Med 2021;49(7):1007–14.
19. Davis TM, Barden C, Olff C, et al. Professional accountability in the tele-ICU: the CCRN-E. Crit Care Nurs Q 2012;35(4):353–6.
20. Forni A, Skehan N, Hartman CA, et al. Evaluation of the impact of a tele-ICU pharmacist on the management of sedation in critically ill mechanically ventilated patients. Ann Pharmacother 2010;44(3):432–8.
21. Evaluation IfHMa. COVID-19 projections hospital resource use. Institute for Health Metrics and Evaluation; 2021. Available at: https://covid19.healthdata.org/global?view=total-deaths&tab=trend. Accessed February 19, 2021.
22. Livingston E, Desai A, Berkwits M. Sourcing personal protective equipment during the COVID-19 pandemic. JAMA 2020;323(19):1912–4.
23. Cutitta F. What's important: the institutionalization of loneliness: my 100 Days in the hospital with COVID-19. J Bone Joint Surg Am 2020;102(18):1569–71.

24. Services CfMaM. Information on Medicare tele-health. Washington DC: Centers for Medicare and Medicaid Services; 2018.

25. II AMA. Determination that a public health emergency exists. US department of health and human services, office of the assistant secretary of preparedness and response. 2020. Available at: https://www.phe.gov/emergency/news/healthactions/phe/Pages/2019-nCoV.aspx. Accessed April 2, 2021.

26. Congress TUS. The Social Security Act. In:1935.

27. Services TCoMaM. Medicare telemedicine health care provider fact sheet. In: Services DoHaH, editor. CMS.gov/Newsroom: CMS; 2020.

28. Congress US. Coronavirus Preparedness and Response. Supplemental Appropriations Act. In: Congress US, ed. H.R.6074 Public Law No: 116-123 (03/06/2020)2020.

29. Boards FoSM. U.S. States and Territories Modifying Requirements for Telehealth in Response to COVID-19(Out-of-state physicians; preexisting provider-patient relationships; audio-only requirements; etc.). Euless, TX: Federation of State Medical Boards; 2021. p. 21.

30. Koonin LM, Hoots B, Tsang CA, et al. Trends in the use of telehealth during the emergence of the COVID-19 pandemic - United States, january-march 2020. MMWR Morb Mortal Wkly Rep 2020; 69(43):1595–9.

31. Services CfMaM. Trump administration finalizes permanent expansion of medicare telehealth services and improved payments for time doctors spend with patients. 2020. Available at: https://www.cms.gov/newsroom/press-releases/trump-administration-finalizes-permanent-expansion-medicare-telehealth-services-and-improved-payment. Accessed April 2, 2021.

32. Lilly CM, Motzkus C, Rincon T, et al. ICU telemedicine program financial outcomes. Chest 2017; 151(2):286–97.

33. Lilly CM, Motzkus CA. ICU telemedicine: financial analyses of a complex intervention. Crit Care Med 2017;45(9):1558–61.

34. Wilcox ME, Adhikari NK. The effect of telemedicine in critically ill patients: systematic review and meta-analysis. Crit Care 2012;16(4):R127.

35. Young LB, Chan PS, Lu X, et al. Impact of telemedicine intensive care unit coverage on patient outcomes: a systematic review and meta-analysis. Arch Intern Med 2011;171(6):498–506.

Patient-Centered and Family-Centered Care in the Intensive Care Unit

Katharine E. Secunda, MD[a], Jacqueline M. Kruser, MD, MS[b],*

KEYWORDS

- Patient-centered care • Family-centered care • Behavior and behavior mechanisms • Respect
- Palliative care • Professional–patient relationship • Humanization

KEY POINTS

- Patient-centered and family-centered care (PFCC) is challenging to operationalize in the intensive care unit (ICU) environment.
- The foundation of PFCC is respect for the dignity and humanity of all persons.
- PFCC practices include affirmation of patients' personhood, patient-centered and family-centered communication, and interventions to improve family presence, support, and participation in care.
- Optimal PFCC requires continued efforts to address health-care disparities, encourage authentic patient and family engagement, and humanize the ICU environment for patients, families, and health-care professionals.

INTRODUCTION

Patient-centered and family-centered care (PFCC) is widely recognized as integral to health-care delivery.[1–3] Broadly defined, PFCC is organized around the needs, values, and preferences of patients and their families. In theory, this concept is obvious and easy to endorse. Yet, a growing body of evidence suggests PFCC is challenging to operationalize, particularly in the technical environment of the intensive care unit (ICU).

The ICU system is primarily designed to rapidly deliver life-sustaining technology. ICU clinicians are trained to save lives by making decisions quickly and with incomplete information. Through this fundamental nature of the ICU, an imperative to use life-sustaining technology arises that is described by medical social scientists as "giving the best care that is technically possible; the only legitimate and explicitly recognized constraint is the state of the art."[4] Although technological advances have indisputably reduced mortality in critical illness, there is growing recognition that a singular focus on technology can displace human dimensions of care.[5] As **Fig. 1** illustrates and sociologist Nancy Kentish-Barnes describes, "in the ICU, the patient becomes a body whose organs must be maintained, and this body in turn disappears behind the machines."[6]

Additionally, critically ill patients are often unable to communicate, which creates challenges for the ICU team to ascertain and uphold patients' individual values, goals, and preferences. Only 1 of 3 American adults has created an advance directive (AD) describing their preferences about life-sustaining treatment.[7] Even when ADs are established, multiple barriers limit their utility, including instability of adults' end-of-life preferences[8,9] and lack of access to AD documents when needed.[10] Furthermore, when surrogate decision makers are making treatment decisions on behalf of a critically ill patient, they often struggle to accurately represent the patients' preferences.[11]

[a] Department of Medicine, Division of Pulmonary and Critical Care, University of Pennsylvania; [b] Department of Medicine, Division of Allergy, Pulmonary, and Critical Care, University of Wisconsin School of Medicine and Public Health, 600 Highland Avenue, Madison, WI 53792, USA
* Corresponding author.
E-mail address: jkruser@wisc.edu

Clin Chest Med 43 (2022) 539–550
https://doi.org/10.1016/j.ccm.2022.05.008

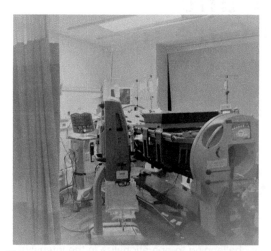

Fig. 1. ICU patient in a bed to facilitate prone positioning, surrounded by multiple sources of life-sustaining treatment.

In this article, we will discuss the history and terminology of PFCC, describe interventions to promote PFCC, and highlight limitations to the current model and future directions.

HISTORY AND TERMINOLOGY

The Picker Institute introduced the concept of "patient-centered care" in 1993 as a response to growing concerns about disease-centered or clinician-centered care.[12] This concept included 5 dimensions: (1) respect for patients' values, preferences, and expressed needs; (2) coordination and integration of care; (3) information, communication, and education; (4) physical comfort; (5) emotional support; and (6) involvement of family and friends."[12] In 2001, the Institute of Medicine advocated for patient-centered care that is "respectful of and responsive to individual patient preferences, needs, and values and ensures that patient values guide all clinical decisions."[1]

Family-centered care—an approach to health care that is respectful of and responsive to families' needs and values—was initially introduced in the context of pediatrics[13] but is now recognized across populations and care settings.[2] Family is defined by the patient as those who provide support and with whom the patient has a significant relationship. Given that patients in the ICU are often too ill to communicate, families are asked to participate in complex medical decision-making. Families also face significant caregiving burden for survivors of critical illness.[14] Up to one-half of family members of critically ill patients experience psychological symptoms during and after the critical illness.[15,16] Family-centered care

in the ICU recognizes the importance of the family to a patient's recovery, provides support for families for decision-making, caregiving and bereavement, and attempts to reduce future suffering for family members after critical illness.

Several fields and concepts inform and overlap with PFCC. Palliative care medicine is oriented around improving quality of life for patients with serious illness and families by attending to physical, psychosocial, and spiritual needs.[17] The concept of dignity-conserving care emerged from palliative medicine but applies across the spectrum of health care and emphasizes patients' personhood.[18] The related model of human-centered care arose from the recognition that patients in the ICU are susceptible to dehumanization, the process by which individuals are seen as having lost their positive human qualities.[19] To counter this tendency, human-centered care honors the dignity of all persons; it additionally identifies health-care professionals as potential beneficiaries of humanized care settings that may mitigate burnout.[20,21] Finally, patient and family engagement (PFE) is considered a key pillar in quality improvement and patient safety initiatives.[22] PFE describes a set of behaviors, organizational policies, and values that foster the inclusion of patients and families as active participants on health-care teams and in health-care systems. What unites each of these concepts is the value of human dignity and the notion that the fundamental purpose of health care is respecting the dignity and value of patients and their families.

MEASURING AND QUANTIFYING THE PROBLEM

There is an expanding body of literature dedicated to measuring PFCC. Gazarian and colleagues propose a practical definition of dignity and respect, suggesting that dignity represents the inherent worth of all human beings, and respect represents the behavioral or social norms that appropriately honor and acknowledge such dignity.[23] Respectful ICU care requires (1) recognition of fundamental human needs (ie, physical, emotional, and psychological safety), (2) acknowledgment of patients as unique individuals, and (3) attention to the critical status and vulnerability of patients and families in the ICU.[19,23–25] Specific behaviors of respectful care are well described[25–27]; concrete examples are shown in **Table 1**.[19]

Approximately 30% of ICU patients and families report experiencing disrespect during their ICU stay.[28,29] Disrespectful care can damage patient–clinician relationships, lead to long-lasting adverse

Table 1
Examples of respectful and disrespectful behaviors

Situation	Disrespectful Approach	Respectful Approach
Entering the patient's room	Enter without warning or acknowledgment	Knock before entering
Approaching a patient's bed	Neglect to introduce oneself	"Hello, I'm Dr. Schmidt. I'm a physician in training"
During emotionally charged encounters (eg, during ACLS or family meeting)	Multiple unintroduced staff, only partly involved	Appropriate staff present; those who are present are introduced and involved
Addressing a patient	"Bud" or "Dear" or similarly colloquial term	"Mr./Ms. Jones, what do you prefer that I call you?" (If know, use preferred name)
Necessary physical examination in conscious patient	Wordlessly performing the examination	"May I examine your abdomen?"
Necessary physical examination in unconscious patient	Wordlessly performing the examination	"I'll be examining your abdomen"
Discussion of "code status"	"If your heart stops, should we try to restart it?"	A personalized approach that considers the contexts and trajectories of illness from the patient's perspective
Rounding	Patients and families excluded from rounds	Patients and families included in rounds
Referring to patients	Room 502 or "the heart"	"Jill in 502" or "Steve with heart failure"
General protection of modesty/privacy	Private parts of body exposed; drapes left open	Only necessary parts of body exposed; drapes closed
Response to patient's needs, including pain	Slow response times	Timely response
Attention during encounter	Reading texts on cell phone; reviewing material for another patient	Attending directly to the given patient and family

Definition of abbreviation: ACLS, advanced cardiac life support.
Reprinted with permission of the American Thoracic Society.
Copyright © 2021 American Thoracic Society. all rights reserved.
Samuel M. Brown, Elie Azoulay, Dominique Benoit, Terri Payne Butler, Patricia Folcarelli, Gail Geller, Ronen Rozenblum, Ken Sands, Lauge Sokol-Hessner, Daniel Talmor, Kathleen Turner, and Michael D. Howell; The American Journal of Respiratory and Critical Care Medicine (Volume 197, Issue 11), pp. 1389-1395.
The American Journal of Respiratory and Critical Care Medicine is an official journal of the American Thoracic Society.

effects on physical and psychological health,[30,31] and may even be associated with risk of physical harm to patients.[30,32–34] A multicenter survey demonstrated that more than one-third of ICUs had a poor "climate of mutual respect."[35] A climate in which disrespect and dehumanization is widely accepted may ingrain such behaviors into the wider ICU team and contribute to deficiencies in patient care.[36–38] At the same time, high rates of burnout experienced by ICU clinicians may be linked to witnessing or participating in (sometimes unintentional) acts of dehumanization and disrespect.[21]

Most patient satisfaction surveys include a dimension related to respect.[39] The Hospital Consumer Assessment of Healthcare Providers and Systems survey is a global assessment of patient satisfaction but does contain dimensions related to respect.[40] The family satisfaction in the ICU survey measures satisfaction with care and decision-making, constructs that overlap with acts of respect.[41,42] However, surveys assessing patient and family satisfaction may suffer from ceiling effects, wherein responses are skewed favorably, making it difficult to distinguish meaningful change in PFCC.[43] Geller and colleagues developed a specific tool to measure ICU patient and family experiences of respect.[28] This tool evaluates clinician behaviors such as greetings and introductions, bedside manner, listening and sharing information, attending to modesty, honoring patients' preferences, and responding to patients' needs/requests. These behaviors are simple, yet powerful and pragmatic to protect against dehumanization.

Respect is increasingly recognized as a system-level outcome; as such, measurement of respectful behaviors in the ICU requires assessment of unit-level structures. CORE-ICU is a clinician-reported measure of overall environment and climate of respect in the ICU.[44] The ethical climate of the ICU, defined as the organizational practices and conditions that affect the way difficult patient care problems are discussed and resolved, is also crucial to optimal ICU functioning.[45] The Ethical Decision-Making Climate Questionnaire measures latent factors affecting the decision-making climate in the ICU within 3 domains: interdisciplinary collaboration and communication, physician leadership, and ethical environment.[35] Several investigators propose treating acts of disrespect as patient safety events and recommend using existing quality and safety frameworks (such as root cause analysis) to audit such incidents.[46,47]

INTERVENTIONS TO PROMOTE PATIENT-CENTERED AND FAMILY-CENTERED CARE
Personhood and Humanization

PFCC requires acknowledging patients as unique individuals. Several interventions emphasize eliciting information about patients that refocuses attention on personhood, guards against dehumanization, and promotes deeper connections among patients, families, and clinicians. Chochinov and colleagues developed the single question Patient Dignity Question[18]: "What do I need to know about you as a person to give you the best care possible?" Another questionnaire documenting personal attributes called "This is Me" (TIME) has been well-received by patients, and clinicians reported TIME enhanced their respect and compassion for patients.[48] "About me" boards (**Fig. 2**) display important information about the patient's background, personality, interests, and preferences. Such tools may deepen patient–clinician relationships, enhance interdisciplinary communication, and motivate patients and families.[49–52] Clinicians describe a deeper sense of meaning and job satisfaction after implementation of a "Get to know me" tool.[52]

ICU diaries are another intervention to affirm personhood and support patients and families. ICU diaries are written records of the ICU stay maintained by family members and clinicians and may allow patients to reconstruct their illness narrative, combat frightening memories, and regain a sense of reality.[53–56] ICU diaries have been shown to mitigate the development of post-traumatic stress disorder (PTSD) symptoms, anxiety, and depression in ICU patients and reduce psychological symptoms for family members.[53,55,57] Family members value ICU diaries because they help families to understand medical information, communicate with clinicians, and humanize the relationship with the patient and ICU team.[58]

Family Presence and Participation

Active partnership with patients' families in the ICU is critical to PFCC. Family presence includes unrestricted visitation,[59] participation in daily work rounds with the ICU team,[60] and the invitation to remain present during CPR and procedures.[61] Family presence in the ICU is associated with decreased anxiety, shorter length of stay, and higher patient and family satisfaction with care.[2,62] Family presence has also been shown to decrease the risk for delirium.[63,64] Family members' active participation in patient care activities fosters PFCC. Qualitative studies demonstrate that family members value their role as a care provider for their loved ones in the ICU.[65,66] Family members who partnered with nurses to deliver patient care such as bathing or massage perceived increased respect, collaboration, and support.[67] Family participation in patient care rituals has been associated with reduced symptoms of PTSD 90 days after patient death or discharge.[68]

The COVID-19 pandemic has resulted in deimplementation of many family-centered care practices and has been associated with worse PFCC.[69,70] Bereaved family members report not only poor communication and inadequate support during their loved ones' ICU stay[71] but also feelings of abandonment, powerlessness, and unreality, as well as disruptions in typical end-of-life rituals, which can lead to complicated grief.[72,73] Limited family presence is linked to poor clinical outcomes. Visitation restrictions resulted in delayed decisions to limit treatments before death and lengthened ICU stays,[74] and lack of family presence was associated with a higher risk of delirium for ICU patients with COVID-19.[63] Prohibiting family presence has also negatively affected health-care workers.

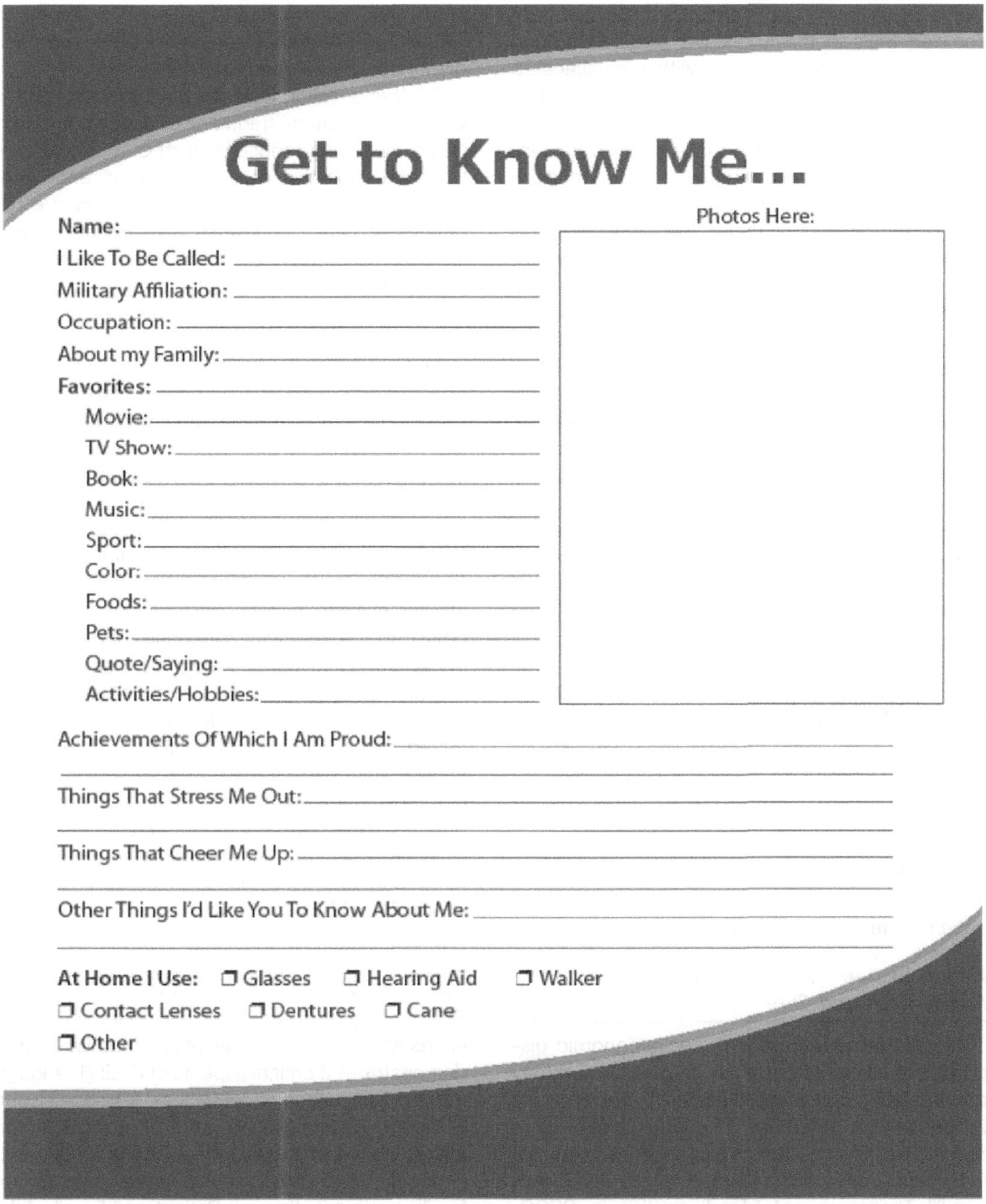

Get to Know Me...

Name: _____

I Like To Be Called: _____

Military Affiliation: _____

Occupation: _____

About my Family: _____

Favorites: _____

    Movie: _____

    TV Show: _____

    Book: _____

    Music: _____

    Sport: _____

    Color: _____

    Foods: _____

    Pets: _____

    Quote/Saying: _____

    Activities/Hobbies: _____

Photos Here:

Achievements Of Which I Am Proud: _____

Things That Stress Me Out: _____

Things That Cheer Me Up: _____

Other Things I'd Like You To Know About Me: _____

At Home I Use: ❐ Glasses   ❐ Hearing Aid   ❐ Walker
❐ Contact Lenses   ❐ Dentures   ❐ Cane
❐ Other

Fig. 2. ICU Diary "Get to Know Me" page. (*From* K Taylor A Blair, Sarah D Eccleston, Hannah M Binder, Mary S McCarthy; Journal of Patient Experience (Volume 4, Issue 1), pp. 4-9; copyright © 2017 by SAGE Publications, Inc.; with permission.)

Clinicians reported moral distress related to changing visitation policies and restrictions.[75,76] Health-care workers had to facilitate virtual "good byes" between families and dying patients, placing them more clearly in the face of suffering.[77] These experiences add to the high burden of burnout in critical care providers.

Communication

A key tenant of PFCC is that patients' values, goals, and preferences guide medical decision-making. Because family members are often surrogate decision-makers, routine, structured communication with attention to surrogates' informational needs is widely recommended.[2,78] Several randomized trials in the ICU have centered around communication interventions within multifaceted family support interventions.[79–81] In a recent trial of a comprehensive family support intervention in the ICU, surrogate decision-makers in the intervention group reported higher quality of communication and degree of patient-centeredness and family-centeredness, although there was no difference in surrogates' symptoms of anxiety or depression 6 months after ICU discharge.[81] The ICU length of stay was lower among patients who died in the hospital in the intervention group. A recent meta-analysis of protocolized family support interventions demonstrated improved communication, enhanced shared decision-making with family, and reduced ICU length of stay.[82] Improvements in communication with patients who cannot speak are also paramount to facilitate participation in decision-making and expression of their needs. Strategies to augment patients' ability to communicate include the use of communication boards and speaking valves and leak speech for ventilated patients.[83]

THE FUTURE OF PATIENT-CENTERED AND FAMILY-CENTERED CARE

Significant progress has been made in recent years in the promotion of PFCC in the ICU. Yet, further attention is needed in 3 areas: disparities in health-care delivery, patient and family engagement (PFE), and intentional efforts to humanize the ICU workplace environment for the betterment of patients, families, and staff.

Health Disparities and Patient-Centered and Family-Centered Care

There are racial, ethnic, and socioeconomic disparities in the most common causes of morbidity and mortality in the United States.[84] Disparities in incidence and outcomes of critical illness occur before, during, and after critical illness and involve individual, community, and hospital-level factors.[85] There are notable disparities in PFCC-focused practices such as serious illness communication and end-of-life care.[86–88] African Americans and individuals with limited English proficiency (LEP) experience worse communication quality[89,90] are less likely to have ADs and more likely to receive high-intensity care before death and die in the ICU.[87,91–93] Disparities in end-of-life care are mediated by multiple factors, including inconsistent access, provider biases, health-care literacy, and patient and family preferences.[94] Importantly, more research is needed to understand whether differences in end-of-life

care reflect differences in patients' and families' values and preferences or whether they represent disparities in health-care delivery.[95]

By being responsive to preferences, needs, values, and cultural traditions of patients and families, PFCC may reduce inequities in critical care. Specialty palliative care consultation and better serious illness communication may improve disparities in care.[96] Palliative care consultation in seriously ill African Americans is associated with higher satisfaction with care, increased documentation of treatment preferences, and higher rates of home death and hospice referrals.[97,98] A commitment to culturally competent communication may also mitigate disparities. Errors in medical interpretation are more frequent and more likely of clinical consequence when nonprofessional interpreters are used compared with professional interpreters.[99] Implementation of protocols for scheduling interpreters and tracking adherence increases interpreter presence on family-centered rounds for families with LEP.[100] Hospitals must stratify clinical, quality, and patient experience data by race, ethnicity, language, and socioeconomic status to better recognize disparities and identify opportunities for improvement. Health systems should provide clinicians with evidence-based racial and cultural sensitivity training and implicit and explicit bias training.[101] Studies of communication or family support interventions often exclude people with LEP. We urgently need to include patients and families with diverse cultures and languages in such studies to better inform PFCC best practices.

Meaningful Patient and Family Engagement

PFE centers health-care delivery around the experiences and priorities of patients and families. **Fig. 3** demonstrates 3 critical aspects of PFE: (1) engagement occurs along a continuum, (2) engagement occurs at different levels, and (3) multiple factors affect the willingness and ability of patients to engage. Health-care systems engage patients and families primarily through Patient and Family Advisory Councils (PFACs), organizations of current and former patients, family members, and caregivers that work with clinicians and hospital leadership to improve patient and family experience, advise on patient care practices, organizational policies and procedures, and recommend how to better measure and evaluate PFE.[102,103] True PFE avoids tokenism, which exists when the unequal power relations among patients, families, and clinicians within the health-care system cause patients and families to have a circumscribed role in these processes.[104,105] Organizations should empower

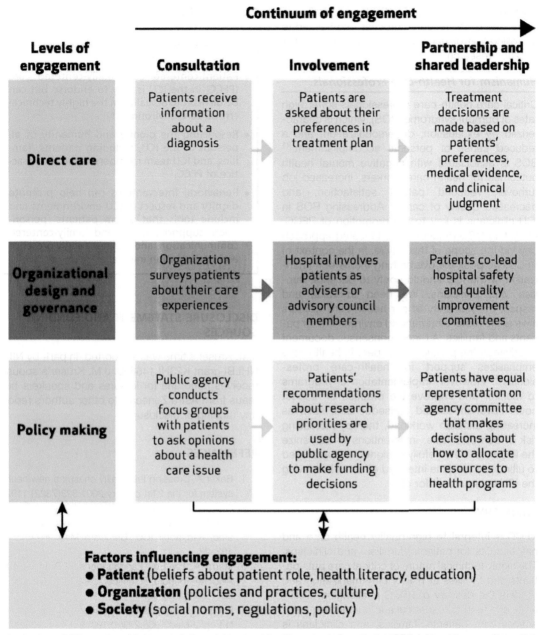

Fig. 3. A multidimensional framework for patient and family engagement in health and health care. (*From* Kristin L. Carman, Pam Dardess, Maureen Maurer, Shoshanna Sofaer, Karen Adams, Christine Bechtel, and Jennifer Sweeney; Health Affairs (Volume 32, Issue 2), pp. 223-231; copyright © 2013 by Project Hope.)

PFACs to pursue meaningful projects, integrate patient and family advisors into governance bodies, ensure involvement in community health activities, and promote recruitment and sustained engagement of diverse patient and family representatives.

Similarly, patient engagement in research requires moving beyond simple participation to active partnership in research.[106] The benefits of PFE in the research process are myriad. Lived experiences of patients and families can inform research questions and priorities, identify patient-centered and family-centered outcomes, and guide researchers to improve enrollment and consent processes. The Patient-Centered Outcomes Research Institute champions involvement of patients and families in every step of the research process and has led to a proliferation of patient, family, and community-engaged research.[107]

Humanism for Health-care Professionals

Critical care health-care professionals suffer high rates of burnout syndrome (BOS), which is characterized by exhaustion, depersonalization, and a reduced sense of personal accomplishment.[21] BOS is associated with negative mental health outcomes for health-care workers, increased job turnover, reduced patient satisfaction, and decreased quality of care.[21] Addressing BOS in ICU clinicians is key to the promotion of PFCC. Mitigating BOS requires a multifaceted approach beyond the scope of this article. In the context of PFCC, we posit the overarching theme of humanization of the ICU should apply to patients, families, *and* clinicians. We need to value and respect the humanity of our health-care workers if we are to foster a humanized environment for patients and families. A recent consensus document to advance the practice of respect in health-care emphasizes support for health-care professionals.[46] However, implementation of programs to monitor and improve the practice of respect could have unintended consequences, such as increasing clinician workload, thereby increasing risk of burnout. Thus, interventions to humanize the ICU must be carefully designed and assessed to ultimately yield the intended effect of improving the ICU environment for all.

SUMMARY

PFCC is integral to high-quality health care and has benefits for patients, families, and clinicians. The highly technical nature of critical care puts patients and families at risk of dehumanization and renders the delivery of PFCC challenging. Deliberate attention to respectful and humanizing interactions with patients, families, and clinicians is essential for successful PFCC in the ICU. Current PFCC efforts focus on patients' personhood, patient-centered and family-centered communication, and interventions to improve family presence, support, and participation. It is imperative that we study how health-care disparities influence PFCC and, furthermore, explore how PFCC can promote health equity. Optimal PFCC requires authentic engagement with patients and families of diverse backgrounds and experiences to inform quality improvement and research initiatives. Finally, we must work together to create a humanistic ICU environment not just for our patients but for ourselves.

CLINICS CARE POINTS

- Patient-centered and family-centered care (PFCC) in the ICU is easy to endorse but can be difficult to actualize in the highly technical critical care environment.
- Respecting the dignity and humanity of all persons in the ICU, including patients, families, and ICU team members, is the core practice of PFCC.
- Behavioral interventions can help promote dignity and respect in ICU environments and include tools that affirm patients' personhood, support patient- and family-centered communication, and increase family presence and participation in care.

DISCLOSURE STATEMENT AND FUNDING SOURCES

J.M. Kruser's time was supported, in part, by NIH/NHLBI grant K23HL146890. J.M. Kruser's spouse receives honoraria for lectures and speakers bureaus from Astra Zeneca. No other authors report any funding or disclosures.

REFERENCES

1. Baker A. Crossing the quality chasm: a new health system for the 21st century 2001;323(7322):1192.
2. Davidson JE, Aslakson RA, Long AC, et al. Guidelines for family-centered care in the neonatal, pediatric, and adult ICU. Crit Care Med 2017;45(1):103–28.
3. Marra A, Ely EW, Pandharipande PP, et al. The ABCDEF bundle in critical care. Crit Care Clin 2017;33(2):225–43.
4. Fuchs VR. The growing demand for medical care. N Engl J Med 1968;279(4):190–5.
5. Todres L, Galvin KT, Holloway I. The humanization of healthcare: a value framework for qualitative research. Int J Qual Stud Health Well-being 2009;4(2):68–77.
6. Kentish-Barnes N. La mort à l'hôpital. Paris: Seuil; 2008.
7. Yadav KN, Gabler NB, Cooney E, et al. Approximately one in three US adults completes any type of advance directive for end-of-life care. Health Aff (Project Hope) 2017;36(7):1244–51.
8. Auriemma CL, Nguyen CA, Bronheim R, et al. Stability of end-of-life preferences: a systematic review of the evidence. JAMA Intern Med 2014;174(7):1085–92.

9. Kim YS, Escobar GJ, Halpern SD, et al. The natural history of changes in preferences for life-sustaining treatments and implications for inpatient mortality in younger and older hospitalized adults. J Am Geriatr Soc 2016;64(5):981–9.

10. Morrison RS, Olson E, Mertz KR, et al. The inaccessibility of advance directives on transfer from ambulatory to acute care settings. JAMA 1995; 274(6):478–82.

11. Shalowitz DI, Garrett-Mayer E, Wendler D. The accuracy of surrogate decision makers: a systematic review. Arch Intern Med 2006;166(5):493–7.

12. Gerteis ME-LS, Daley J, Delbanco T. Through the patient's eyes: understanding and promoting patient-centered care. 1sttioned. San Francisco (CA): Jossey-Bass; 1993.

13. Kuo DZ, Houtrow AJ, Arango P, et al. Family-centered care: current applications and future directions in pediatric health care. Matern child Health J 2012;16(2):297–305.

14. Desai SV, Law TJ, Needham DM. Long-term complications of critical care. Crit Care Med 2011; 39(2):371–9.

15. Azoulay E, Pochard F, Kentish-Barnes N, et al. Risk of post-traumatic stress symptoms in family members of intensive care unit patients. Am J Respir Crit Care Med 2005;171(9):987–94.

16. Davidson JE, Jones C, Bienvenu OJ. Family response to critical illness: postintensive care syndrome-family. Crit Care Med 2012;40(2):618–24.

17. WHO definition of palliative care. Available at: https://www.who.int/cancer/palliative/definition/en/. Accessed March 28, 2021.

18. Chochinov HM, McClement S, Hack T, et al. Eliciting personhood within clinical practice: effects on patients, families, and health care providers. J Pain Symptom Manag 2015;49(6):974–80.e2.

19. Brown SM, Azoulay E, Benoit D, et al. The practice of respect in the ICU. Am J Respir Crit Care Med 2018;197(11):1389–95.

20. Velasco Bueno JM, La Calle GH. Humanizing intensive care: from theory to practice. Crit Care Nurs Clin North Am 2020;32(2):135–47.

21. Moss M, Good VS, Gozal D, et al. A critical care societies collaborative statement: burnout syndrome in critical care health-care professionals. A call for action. Am J Respir Crit Care Med 2016;194(1): 106–13.

22. Carman KL, Dardess P, Maurer M, et al. Patient and family engagement: a framework for understanding the elements and developing interventions and policies. Health Aff (Project Hope) 2013;32(2):223–31.

23. Gazarian PK, Morrison CR, Lehmann LS, et al. Patients' and care partners' perspectives on dignity and respect during acute care hospitalization. J Patient Saf 2017.

24. Aboumatar H, Forbes L, Branyon E, et al. Understanding treatment with respect and dignity in the intensive care unit. Narrative Inq Bioeth 2015; 5(1a):55a–67a.

25. Bidabadi FS, Yazdannik A, Zargham-Boroujeni A. Patient's dignity in intensive care unit: A Critical ethnography. Nurs Ethics 2019;26(3):738–52.

26. Carrese J, Forbes L, Branyon E, et al. Observations of respect and dignity in the intensive care unit. Narrative Inq Bioeth 2015;5(1a):43a–53a.

27. Gazarian PK, Morrison CRC, Lehmann LS, et al. Patients' and care partners' perspectives on dignity and respect during acute care hospitalization. J Patient Saf 2021;17(5):392–7.

28. Geller G, Branyon ED, Forbes LK, et al. ICU-RESPECT: an index to assess patient and family experiences of respect in the intensive care unit. J Crit Care 2016;36:54–9.

29. Law AC, Roche S, Reichheld A, et al. Failures in the respectful care of critically ill patients. Joint Comm J Qual Patient Saf 2019;45(4):276–84.

30. Entwistle VA. Hurtful comments are harmful comments: respectful communication is not just an optional extra in healthcare. Health Expect 2008; 11(4):319–20.

31. Sokol-Hessner L, Folcarelli PH, Sands KE. Emotional harm from disrespect: the neglected preventable harm. BMJ Qual Saf 2015;24(9): 550–3.

32. Cooper WO, Guillamondegui O, Hines OJ, et al. Use of unsolicited patient observations to identify surgeons with increased risk for postoperative complications. JAMA Surg 2017;152(6):522–9.

33. Hernan AL, Giles SJ, Fuller J, et al. Patient and carer identified factors which contribute to safety incidents in primary care: a qualitative study. BMJ Qual Saf 2015;24(9):583.

34. Rosenstein AH, O'Daniel M. A survey of the impact of disruptive behaviors and communication defects on patient safety. Joint Comm J Qual Patient Saf 2008;34(8):464–71.

35. Van den Bulcke B, Piers R, Jensen HI, et al. Ethical decision-making climate in the ICU: theoretical framework and validation of a self-assessment tool. BMJ Qual Saf 2018;27(10):781–9.

36. Foulk T, Woolum A, Erez A. Catching rudeness is like catching a cold: the contagion effects of low-intensity negative behaviors. J Appl Psychol 2016;101(1):50–67.

37. Woolum A, Foulk T, Lanaj K, et al. Rude color glasses: the contaminating effects of witnessed morning rudeness on perceptions and behaviors throughout the workday. J Appl Psychol 2017; 102(12):1658–72.

38. Riskin A, Erez A, Foulk TA, et al. The impact of rudeness on medical team performance: a randomized trial. Pediatrics 2015;136(3):487–95.

39. Handley SC, Bell S, Nembhard IM. A systematic review of surveys for measuring patient-centered care in the hospital setting. Med Care 2021;59(3): 228–37.

40. Goldstein E, Farquhar M, Crofton C, et al. Measuring hospital care from the patients' perspective: an overview of the CAHPS Hospital Survey development process. Health Serv Res 2005;40(6 Pt 2):1977–95.

41. Heyland DK, Tranmer JE. Measuring family satisfaction with care in the intensive care unit: the development of a questionnaire and preliminary results. J Crit Care 2001;16(4):142–9.

42. Wall RJ, Engelberg RA, Downey L, et al. Refinement, scoring, and validation of the family satisfaction in the intensive care unit (FS-ICU) survey. Crit Care Med 2007;35(1):271–9.

43. Moret L, Nguyen JM, Pillet N, et al. Improvement of psychometric properties of a scale measuring inpatient satisfaction with care: a better response rate and a reduction of the ceiling effect. BMC Health Serv Res 2007;7:197.

44. Beach MC, Topazian R, Chan KS, et al. Climate of respect evaluation in ICUs: development of an instrument (ICU-CORE). Crit Care Med 2018;46(6): e502–7.

45. Hamric AB, Blackhall LJ. Nurse-physician perspectives on the care of dying patients in intensive care units: collaboration, moral distress, and ethical climate. Crit Care Med 2007;35(2):422–9.

46. Sokol-Hessner L, Folcarelli PH, Annas CL, et al. A road map for advancing the practice of respect in health care: the results of an interdisciplinary modified delphi consensus study. Joint Comm J Qual Patient Saf 2018;44(8):463–76.

47. Sokol-Hessner L, Kane GJ, Annas CL, et al. Development of a framework to describe patient and family harm from disrespect and promote improvements in quality and safety: a scoping review. Int J Qual Health Care 2019;31(9):657–68.

48. Pan JL, Chochinov H, Thompson G, et al. The TIME Questionnaire: a tool for eliciting personhood and enhancing dignity in nursing homes. Geriatr Nurs (NY) 2016;37(4):273–7.

49. Billings JA, Keeley A, Bauman J, et al. Merging cultures: palliative care specialists in the medical intensive care unit. Crit Care Med 2006;34(11 Suppl):S388–93.

50. Blair KTA, Eccleston SD, Binder HM, et al. Improving the patient experience by implementing an ICU diary for those at risk of post-intensive care syndrome. J Patient experience 2017;4(1):4–9.

51. Gajic O, Anderson BD. Get to know me" board. Crit Care explorations 2019;1(8):e0030.

52. Hoad N, Swinton M, Takaoka A, et al. Fostering humanism: a mixed methods evaluation of the Footprints Project in critical care. BMJ open 2019; 9(11):e029810.

53. Kredentser MS, Blouw M, Marten N, et al. Preventing posttraumatic stress in ICU survivors: a single-center pilot randomized controlled trial of ICU diaries and psychoeducation. Crit Care Med 2018;46(12):1914–22.

54. Parker AM, Sricharoenchai T, Raparla S, et al. Posttraumatic stress disorder in critical illness survivors: a metaanalysis. Crit Care Med 2015;43(5): 1121–9.

55. Jones C, Bäckman C, Capuzzo M, et al. Intensive care diaries reduce new onset post traumatic stress disorder following critical illness: a randomised, controlled trial. Crit Care (London, England) 2010;14(5):R168.

56. Egerod I, Christensen D, Schwartz-Nielsen KH, et al. Constructing the illness narrative: a grounded theory exploring patients' and relatives' use of intensive care diaries. Crit Care Med 2011;39(8): 1922–8.

57. Garrouste-Orgeas M, Coquet I, Périer A, et al. Impact of an intensive care unit diary on psychological distress in patients and relatives. Crit Care Med 2012;40(7):2033–40.

58. Garrouste-Orgeas M, Périer A, Mouricou P, et al. Writing in and reading ICU diaries: qualitative study of families' experience in the ICU. PLoS One 2014; 9(10):e110146.

59. Giannini A, Miccinesi G, Prandi E, et al. Partial liberalization of visiting policies and ICU staff: a before-and-after study. Intensive Care Med 2013;39(12): 2180–7.

60. Allen SR, Pascual J, Martin N, et al. A novel method of optimizing patient- and family-centered care in the ICU. J Trauma acute Care Surg 2017;82(3): 582–6.

61. Beesley SJ, Hopkins RO, Francis L, et al. Let them in: family presence during intensive care unit procedures. Ann Am Thorac Soc 2016;13(7):1155–9.

62. Kleinpell R, Heyland DK, Lipman J, et al. Patient and family engagement in the ICU: report from the task force of the World Federation of societies of intensive and critical care medicine. J Crit Care 2018;48:251–6.

63. Pun BT, Badenes R, Heras La Calle G, et al. Prevalence and risk factors for delirium in critically ill patients with COVID-19 (COVID-D): a multicentre cohort study. Lancet Respir Med 2021;9(3): 239–50.

64. Rosa RG, Tonietto TF, da Silva DB, et al. Effectiveness and safety of an Extended ICU visitation model for delirium prevention: a before and after study. Crit Care Med 2017;45(10):1660–7.

65. Davidson JE. Family-centered care: meeting the needs of patients' families and helping families

adapt to critical illness. Crit Care Nurse 2009;29(3): 28–34 [quiz: 35].

66. Engström A, Söderberg S. The experiences of partners of critically ill persons in an intensive care unit. Intensive Crit Care Nurs 2004;20(5):299–308 [quiz: 309–10].

67. Mitchell M, Chaboyer W, Burmeister E, et al. Positive effects of a nursing intervention on family-centered care in adult critical care. Am J Crit Care 2009;18(6):543–52 [quiz: 553].

68. Amass TH, Villa G, Omahony S, et al. Family care rituals in the ICU to reduce symptoms of post-traumatic stress disorder in family members—a multicenter, multinational, before-and-after intervention trial. Crit Care Med 2020;48(2):176–84.

69. Hart JL, Turnbull AE, Oppenheim IM, et al. Family-centered care during the COVID-19 Era. J Pain Symptom Manag 2020;60(2):e93–7.

70. Hart JL, Taylor SP. Family presence for critically ill patients during a pandemic. Chest 2021;160(2): 549–57.

71. Kentish-Barnes N, Cohen-Solal Z, Morin L, et al. Lived experiences of family members of patients with severe COVID-19 who died in intensive care units in France. JAMA Netw open 2021;4(6): e2113355.

72. Moore B. Dying during covid-19. Hastings Cent Rep 2020;50(3):13–5.

73. Morris SE, Moment A, Thomas JD. Caring for bereaved family members during the COVID-19 pandemic: before and after the death of a patient. J Pain Symptom Manag 2020;60(2):e70–4.

74. Azad TD, Al-Kawaz MN, Turnbull AE, et al. Coronavirus disease 2019 policy restricting family presence may have delayed end-of-life decisions for critically ill patients. Crit Care Med 2021;49(10): e1037–9.

75. Kanaris C. Moral distress in the intensive care unit during the pandemic: the burden of dying alone. Intensive Care Med 2021;47(1):141–3.

76. Cook DJ, Takaoka A, Hoad N, et al. Clinician perspectives on caring for dying patients during the pandemic : a mixed-methods study. Ann Intern Med 2021;174(4):493–500.

77. Rabow MW, Huang CS, White-Hammond GE, et al. Witnesses and Victims both: healthcare workers and grief in the time of COVID-19. J Pain Symptom Manag 2021;62(3):647–56.

78. Kon AA, Davidson JE, Morrison W, et al. Shared decision making in ICUs: an American college of critical care medicine and American thoracic society policy statement. Crit Care Med 2016;44(1): 188–201.

79. Carson SS, Cox CE, Wallenstein S, et al. Effect of palliative care-led meetings for families of patients with chronic critical illness: a randomized clinical trial. JAMA 2016;316(1):51–62.

80. Curtis JR, Treece PD, Nielsen EL, et al. Randomized trial of communication Facilitators to reduce family distress and intensity of end-of-life care. Am J Respir Crit Care Med 2016;193(2):154–62.

81. White DB, Angus DC, Shields AM, et al. A randomized trial of a family-support intervention in intensive care units. N Engl J Med 2018; 378(25):2365–75.

82. Lee HW, Park Y, Jang EJ, et al. Intensive care unit length of stay is reduced by protocolized family support intervention: a systematic review and meta-analysis. Intensive Care Med 2019;45(8): 1072–81.

83. Ten Hoorn S, Elbers PW, Girbes AR, et al. Communicating with conscious and mechanically ventilated critically ill patients: a systematic review. Crit Care (London, England) 2016;20(1):333.

84. Wong MD, Shapiro MF, Boscardin WJ, et al. Contribution of major diseases to disparities in mortality. N Engl J Med 2002;347(20):1585–92.

85. Soto GJ, Martin GS, Gong MN. Healthcare disparities in critical illness. Crit Care Med 2013;41(12): 2784–93.

86. Cole AP, Nguyen DD, Meirkhanov A, et al. Association of care at minority-serving vs non-minority-serving hospitals with use of palliative care among racial/ethnic minorities with metastatic cancer in the United States. JAMA Netw open 2019;2(2): e187633.

87. Chino F, Kamal AH, Leblanc TW, et al. Place of death for patients with cancer in the United States, 1999 through 2015: racial, age, and geographic disparities. Cancer 2018;124(22):4408–19.

88. Faigle R, Ziai WC, Urrutia VC, et al. Racial differences in palliative care use after stroke in majority-White, minority-serving, and racially integrated U.S. Hospitals. Crit Care Med 2017;45(12): 2046–54.

89. Shen MJ, Peterson EB, Costas-Muñiz R, et al. The effects of race and racial concordance on patient-physician communication: a systematic review of the literature. J racial ethnic Health disparities 2018;5(1):117–40.

90. Thornton JD, Pham K, Engelberg RA, et al. Families with limited English proficiency receive less information and support in interpreted intensive care unit family conferences. Crit Care Med 2009; 37(1):89–95.

91. Barnato AE, Anthony DL, Skinner J, et al. Racial and ethnic differences in preferences for end-of-life treatment. J Gen Intern Med 2009;24(6): 695–701.

92. Yarnell CJ, Fu L, Manuel D, et al. Association between immigrant status and end-of-life care in ontario, Canada. JAMA 2017;318(15):1479–88.

93. Barwise A, Jaramillo C, Novotny P, et al. Differences in code status and end-of-life decision

making in patients with limited English proficiency in the intensive care unit. Mayo Clin Proc 2018; 93(9):1271–81.

94. Bazargan M, Bazargan-Hejazi S. Disparities in palliative and hospice care and completion of advance care planning and directives among non-hispanic blacks: a scoping review of recent literature. Am J Hosp Palliat Care 2021;38(6): 688–718.

95. Kross EK, Rosenberg AR, Engelberg RA, et al. Postdoctoral research training in palliative care: Lessons Learned from a T32 program. J Pain Symptom Manag 2020;59(3):750–60.e8.

96. Starr LT, O'Connor NR, Meghani SH. Improved serious illness communication may help mitigate racial disparities in care among black Americans with COVID-19. J Gen Intern Med 2021;36(4): 1071–6.

97. Starr LT, Ulrich CM, Junker P, et al. Goals-of-Care consultation associated with increased hospice enrollment among propensity-matched cohorts of seriously ill African American and white patients. J Pain Symptom Manag 2020;60(4):801–10.

98. Sharma RK, Cameron KA, Chmiel JS, et al. Racial/ethnic differences in inpatient palliative care consultation for patients with advanced cancer. J Clin Oncol 2015;33(32):3802–8.

99. Flores G, Laws MB, Mayo SJ, et al. Errors in medical interpretation and their potential clinical consequences in pediatric encounters. Pediatrics 2003; 111(1):6–14.

100. Cheston CC, Alarcon LN, Martinez JF, et al. Evaluating the Feasibility of incorporating in-person interpreters on family-centered rounds: a QI initiative 2018;8(8):471–8.

101. Maina IW, Belton TD, Ginzberg S, et al. A decade of studying implicit racial/ethnic bias in healthcare providers using the implicit association test. Social Sci Med (1982) 2018;199:219–29.

102. Guide to patient and family engagement in hospital quality and safety. Available at: https://www.ahrq.gov/patient-safety/patients-families/engagingfamilies/guide.html. Accessed July 3, 2021.

103. Webster PD, Johnson BH. Developing and sustaining a patient and family advisory council. Institute for Family-Centered Care; 2000.

104. Majid U. The dimensions of tokenism in patient and family engagement: a concept analysis of the literature. J Patient experience 2020;7(6):1610–20.

105. Hahn DL, Hoffmann AE, Felzien M, et al. Tokenism in patient engagement. Fam Pract 2017;34(3): 290–5.

106. Fiest KM, Sept BG, Stelfox HT. Patients as researchers in adult critical care medicine. Fantasy or reality? Ann Am Thorac Soc 2020;17(9): 1047–51.

107. Selby JV, Forsythe L, Sox HC. Stakeholder-driven comparative effectiveness research: an update from PCORI. JAMA 2015;314(21):2235–6.

Survivorship After Critical Illness and Post-Intensive Care Syndrome

Leigh M. Cagino, MD, MSc[a],*, Katharine S. Seagly, PhD[b],
Jakob I. McSparron, MD[c]

KEYWORDS

• Survivorship • Post-intensive care unit syndrome • Recovery

KEY POINTS

• Intensive care unit (ICU) survivors encounter a wide range of challenges following ICU stay.
• Post-ICU syndrome is a term created to describe common sequelae in three major domains: physical, cognitive, and psychiatric.
• A comprehensive and individualized approach should guide the management of ICU survivors.

INTRODUCTION

Improvements in intensive care unit (ICU) care over the past decades have resulted in a significant increase in the number of ICU survivors. Many of these patients do not rapidly return to their premorbid baseline. Rather, their recovery continues throughout their hospitalizations and in the months and years following discharge.[1,2] To better define the obstacles faced by survivors, the term post-intensive care syndrome (PICS) was created with the goal of capturing long-term consequences and describing these new or worsening problems following a critical illness.[3] Descriptions of this clinical syndrome have focused on three overarching domains: physical, cognitive, and psychological; however, ICU survivors represent an extremely heterogeneous population of patients with varying presentations of signs and symptoms.[4,5] Although the term PICS includes the most common complications following critical illness, the plight of the ICU survivor is complex and unique to each individual.

Quantifying the number of patients affected by PICS is challenging given the variable diagnostic assessment methods in the literature. Existing data suggest that more than half of ICU survivors will experience at least one aspect of PICS.[6] Estimating 4.8 million ICU survivors each year in the United States alone demonstrates the magnitude of this syndrome.[7,8] Most studies addressing the occurrence of PICS have evaluated the incidence of each individual impairment as shown in **Table 1**. One multicenter cohort study demonstrated that 64% and 56% of ICU survivors experienced at least one impairment at 3 and 12 months, respectively.[6] More than 20% of patients have impairments in multiple domains at similar intervals.[6,9]

Clinical Manifestations

The three major domains of PICS (cognitive, physical, and psychological) provide a framework for symptom identification and description as shown in **Table 2**. However, these areas are closely linked and should not be viewed or treated in isolation. The interactions between physical function, psychological health, and cognition play a key role in

a Division of Pulmonary and Critical Care Medicine, University of Michigan, 2800 Plymouth Rd, NCRC-14 G100-01, Ann Arbor, MI 48109, USA; b Division of Rehabilitation Psychology and Neuropsychology, Department of Physical Medicine and Rehabilitation, University of Michigan, 325 E Eisenhower Parkway, Ann Arbor, MI 48108, USA; c Division of Pulmonary and Critical Care Medicine, University of Michigan, 1500 East Medical Center Drive, 3920F Taubman Center, Ann Arbor, MI 48109, USA
* Corresponding author.
E-mail address: caginol@med.umich.edu

Clin Chest Med 43 (2022) 551–561
https://doi.org/10.1016/j.ccm.2022.05.009
0272-5231/22/© 2022 Elsevier Inc. All rights reserved.

Table 1
Prevalence of post-intensive care syndrome domains at 3 and 12 months.

Prevalence of PICS Domains	3 months	12 months
Cognition (1–2): Attention Language Executive function Motor speed Visual-spatial abilities	40%	34%–55%
Psychological		
Anxiety (3)	48%	36%
Depression (4)	37%	42%
PTSD (5)	22%	24%
Physical		
ADLs (6)	32%	27%
ICU acquired weakness (7)	22%	14%

Notes: Rates based on different studies and scoring systems by (1) the Repeatable Battery for Assessment of Neuropsychological Status global cognition score,[19] (2) the telephone neuropsychological test battery,[20] (3) the Hospital Anxiety and Depression Scale,[28] (4) the Beck Depression Inventory-II,[49] (5) the PTSD Checklist–Civilian Version,[28] (6) the Katz Activities of Daily Living (ADL),[49] and (7) ICU acquired weakness as measured by multiple standardized clinical evaluations, 6-minute walk test and Medical Outcomes Short-Form 36 health-related quality of life survery.[43]

the survivorship experience and viewing symptoms through a holistic biopsychosocial lens is indicated to ensure all factors contributing to symptom experience are addressed and optimized where possible as outlined in **Fig. 1**[10] However, much of the current research evaluates risk factors for individual components of PICS as opposed to the whole syndrome. A recent systematic review and meta-analysis to identify risk factors of PICS found only one of 89 studies reported on the simultaneous presence of all three major domains PICS.[11] These impairments, in their varying presentations, have been associated with decreased health-related quality of life in the months and years following critical illness.[12–16]

Cognitive sequelae generally refer to changes in attention, memory, language, executive function, processing and motor speed, and visuospatial abilities.[3,17] One proposed mechanism for these changes is neurologic injury from acute systemic inflammatory dysregulation or impairments in cerebrovascular hemodynamics, though symptoms and outcomes are most likely multifactorial for most patients.[18] The degree of cognitive impairments can be severe for some. Pandharipande and colleagues[19] prospectively evaluated 821 ICU patients for changes in cognition and found that at 3 months post-ICU discharge, 40% of patients had global cognition scores 1.5 standard deviations below the population means and 26% had scores 2 standard deviations below the population means. These deficits were present in 34% and 24% of patients at 12 months, respectively.

Jackson and colleagues[20] followed 122 survivors of acute respiratory distressed syndrome (ARDS) and found that 55% had some form of cognitive impairment at six months.[20] These impairments can interfere with social and occupational functioning and are associated with decreased employment at 12 months following ICU discharge.[21]

It may be best to conceptualize etiology of long-term cognitive impact in the ICU survivor as various combinations of irreversible risk factors, pathophysiologic events, and modifiable risk factors that then produce an accumulated sum of risk for long-term cognitive impairment.[18,20] Risk factors for cognitive decline following ARDS include preexisting cognitive impairment, neurologic injury, delirium, mechanical ventilation, prolonged exposure to sedating medications, sepsis, systemic inflammation, and environmental factors in the ICU, which can occur in various combinations.[18–20,22–25] Long-term cognitive impairment occurs when a tipping point is reached for a particular patient, in which the accumulated sum of risk factors is too great for the patient's cognitive or brain reserve to compensate.

Psychological sequelae can include depression, anxiety, and posttraumatic stress. Wunsch and colleagues[26] performed a large cohort study of 24,179 critically ill patients from Denmark and found that those receiving mechanical ventilation had higher rates of new mental health diagnoses and use of psychotropic medications following discharge. These psychological sequelae can be

Table 2
Symptoms, prevention, and treatment of post-intensive care syndrome. Descriptions of the main symptoms, risk factor mitigation, and current management strategies within each post-intensive care syndrome domain

	Physical	Cognition	Psychological
Symptoms	Weakness Dyspnea Pain Impairment mobility	Memory difficulty Impaired executive function Decreased processing speed Impaired attention Language impairment	Anxiety Depression Posttraumatic stress

Prevention	ABCDEF Bundle
	  Assess, prevent, and manage pain
	  Both spontaneous awakening trials and
	    spontaneous breathing trials
	  Choice of analgesia and sedation
	  Delirium: assess, prevent, and manage
	  Early mobility and exercise
	  Family engagement and empowerment		

Treatment	Post-ICU Services
	  Physical therapy
	  Occupational therapy
	  Cognitive therapy
	  Nutrition
	  Pharmacy review
	Post-ICU Clinic
	  Peer support
	  Medication management
	  Coordination of follow-up care		

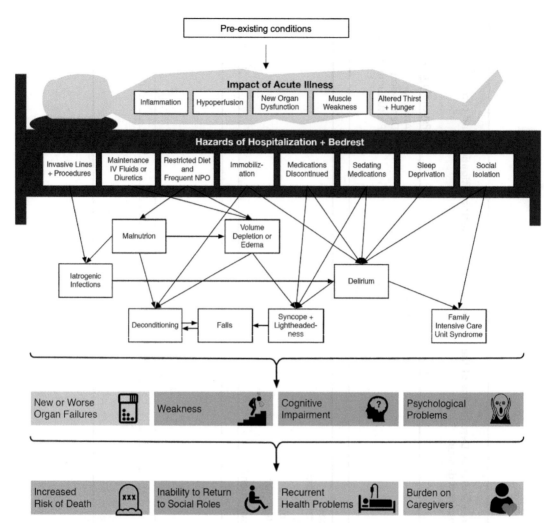

Fig. 1. Factors contributing to the survivorship experience. Outlines the various factors and impacts on both development of PICS and hardships faced by ICU survivor. (*Adapted from* Oxford Textbook of Medicine, permission pending.)

persistent; a large multicenter cohort study found increased rates of mental health diagnoses in survivors of ARDS up to 5 years following illness.[27] Anxiety is the most common psychological symptom following ICU stay with rates at 3 months following discharge at 46%, followed by depression at 40% and posttraumatic stress disorder (PTSD) at 22%; up to 18% may have three of these diagnoses.[28] A recent cohort study from Canada using provincial databases found that survivors of a critical illness also have an increased risk of suicide and self-harm. Prior diagnosis of anxiety, depression, and posttraumatic stress as well as invasive mechanical ventilation and renal replacement therapy were associated with this increase.[29]

Many risk factors for cognitive impairments also increase the risk for poor psychological adjustments following critical illness. As with pre-existing cognitive vulnerabilities, prior psychological vulnerabilities can predispose patients to worsening psychological comorbidities.[27] Depressive symptoms following critical illness have been associated with a variety of factors including younger age, alcohol dependence, female sex, and longer duration of mechanical ventilation and sedation, specifically benzodiazepine use.[30–34] Depressive symptoms associated have been linked to the inability to return home and higher needs and assistance in the 4 months following discharge.[35] Posttraumatic stress can be an especially debilitating complication for survivors. PTSD can be seen in patients with acute stress or delusional memories during their ICU stay, with many studies reporting an association between use of physical restraints and higher rates of

PTSD.[5,33,36] Posttraumatic stress symptoms can also occur with a delayed onset of up to 1 year in as many as 16% of patients.[37]

Physical impairments following critical illness encompass a variety of symptoms, including reduced strength of limb muscles, handgrip, and respiratory function.[38] The term ICU acquired weakness refers to neuromuscular dysfunction that has no plausible etiology other than critical illness. Manifestations of ICU-acquired weakness will generally include diffuse, symmetric weakness of all extremities, decreased tone, and deep tendon reflex.[39–41] Weakness is generally either a result of a neurogenic disturbance referred to as "critical illness neuropathy" or a myogenic disturbance referred to as "critical illness myopathy"; if felt that the impairment is a result of a combination the term "critical illness neuromyopathy" is used.[41,42] Although ICU-acquired weakness may improve within 12 months, weakness can be associated with impairments in physical function and health-related quality of life that may still be present at 24 months following discharge.[43] ICU-acquired weakness has been associated with increased hospital mortality.[44–47] Older age and baseline activity of daily living dependency have been consistently associated with the development of ICU acquired weakness.[47–50] Additional aspects of ICU stay including mechanical ventilation, sepsis, longer durations of ICU stay, and steroid use have had a correlation with the development of physical impairment.[51–55] In addition to ICU acquired weakness, joint contractures are seen regularly among ICU survivors. A single-center retrospective study found that 39% of patients have at least one joint contracture at the time of transfer out of ICU.[56]

There are many other symptoms experienced by ICU survivors outside the traditional three domains of PICS. Sleep disturbance is common among survivors with a recent systematic review showing a prevalence of abnormal sleep at 10% to 61% 6 months after hospital discharge.[57] Poor sleep following critical illness has been associated with worse cognitive function, depression, anxiety, and health-related quality of life.[57,58] In addition to overall sleep quality, a recent study of ARDS survivors found that during the first year following ICU discharge, more than two-thirds of survivors had clinically significant fatigue as measured by the Assessment of Chronic Illness Therapy Fatigue Scale.[59] Decreases in lung function based on pulmonary function tests are seen immediately following ICU stay for patients with ARDS; however, Herridge and colleagues[16] showed that in a prolonged follow-up study of ARDS survivors, pulmonary function test (PFTs) were normal to near normal at 5 years after discharge.[60] Dysphagia is also a common complication following an ICU stay, particularly in patients with prolonged mechanical ventilation, neurologic disease, and emergency admissions.[61] It is associated with increased inpatient costs, length of stay, and mortality.[62] Although not classically included in the PICS definition, these are all important sequalae for survivors and deserve continued attention in both clinical practice and literature on PICS.

Diagnosis and Management

It can be challenging to make the diagnosis of PICS given the heterogeneity of the presentation and evolution of symptoms following critical illness. Although PICS is related to critical illness, survivors generally present to noncritical care practitioners with symptoms and the importance of recognition by these providers is crucial for early intervention and appropriate therapy. Guidelines recommend screening for PICS 2 to 4 weeks following discharge in selected at-risk patients and serial assessment should occur with important health and life changes.[5] A list of validated tools and scoring systems used to evaluate PICS is listed in **Table 3**, although the appropriate diagnosis of PICS requires a thoughtful history and physical examination. This is important for all domains of PICS, although the physical examination is particularly important for the evaluation of ICU-acquired weakness where diagnosis includes a neurologic examination and motor assessment.[40] Electrophysiological assessments including both electromyography and single nerve conduction studies can be used for the diagnosis of ICU-acquired weakness, especially on unconscious or uncooperative patients; however, these tests are more invasive and require specialized training and are not required for routine diagnosis.[41,63]

Prevention of risk factors for PICS is important in its mitigation. This can take place from the beginning of ICU admission. Minimizing mechanical ventilation tidal volume, minimizing the duration of exposure to sedating medications, maintaining hemodynamic stability, and optimizing fluid balance may be useful medical interventions in the acute setting, while ensuring routine reorientation from all providers, frequent interaction with familiar voices, when possible, reduction of unhelpful stimuli that may cause agitation, and early intervention with a psychologist may be useful interventions.[64–67] Although measures such as improving sleep quality have been associated with decreased rates of delirium, use of antipsychotics for the treatment of delirium has not shown to be effective.[68,69]

Table 3
Validated scores and tests. Tests used for diagnosing and monitoring post-intensive care syndrome sequelae

Validated Scores and Tests		
Cognition		Montreal Cognitive Assessment[5–98]
Psychological	Depression/anxiety	Hospital Anxiety and Depression Scale, Patient Health Questionnaire, General Anxiety Disorder-7[99–101]
	Posttraumatic stress	Impact of Event Scale-Revised and Impact of Event of Scale-6[102]
Physical		6-min walk test Medical Research Council sum score[41] Hand grip strength/knee and ankle muscle strength[38,103,104]
Health-related Quality of Life		European Quality of Life-5D-5 L[5–105]

Engaging in physical and occupation therapy early in the hospital course is recommended.[66,70–74] A recent multivariate analysis of risk and protective factors for post-ICU cognitive impairment identified early active mobilization as a significant protective factor, indicating early rehabilitation optimizes cognitive outcomes in addition to physical well-being[75]

There has been much investigation into the use of ICU diaries during critical illness with mixed results. These diaries are completed by health care staff and families to help fill in the gaps in patients' memories during ICU stays. Although there is evidence to support their use in aiding patients in their psychological recovery and decreasing anxiety and depression, there is less evidence to support that diaries can help prevent posttraumatic stress symptoms.[76–80] Other attempts at reducing trauma during ICU stays may also show benefits. Regular bedside presence of family members, music, and animal therapy in the ICU can improve patient experience, although the effect of these interventions on the prevention of PICS is unclear.[81–84]

Follow-up care for the ICU survivor is crucial in their recovery. Much attention has been paid to the development of ICU recovery clinics. These clinics provide a comprehensive approach to addressing multiple domains that can affect patients. Post-ICU clinics can provide screening for physical, cognitive, and psychological concerns, coordination of care, medication reconciliation, and appropriate referral to needed therapies, interventions, and specialists.[85] These clinics are becoming more available throughout the world with a continued investigation regarding their impacts on recovery from PICS.[86–88] In addition to specialized post-ICU clinics, models within primary care follow-up focusing specifically on post-ICU care have also been developed. A randomized control trial from 2016 compared a primary care-based intervention on sepsis survivors versus usual care within primary care. This did not show a significant difference in health care-related quality of life, but the intervention was correlated with improvements of physical function and activities of daily living impairment.[89] Further evaluation into effective models for post-ICU follow-up is needed to better address the needs of survivors.

Long-Term Outcomes

The ICU survivor faces many obstacles other than the outlined domains of PICS. Once patients leave the ICU and eventually the hospital, they may face difficulties with readjusting to life at home. New functional impairments and new medical conditions place survivors at high rates of hospital readmission. A study evaluating rehospitalization for all survivors of critical illness found a readmission rate of 16% within 30 days of hospital discharge.[90] Looking at survivors of severe sepsis, readmission rate within 90 days was 42.6% with survivors spending more time in inpatient facilities in the year following severe sepsis hospitalization than the year prior.[91]

Given health impairments and increase in health care utilization, unemployment following the critical illness is common. A prospective cohort study by Norman and colleagues[21] showed a decrease in employment of 62% at 2 months and 49% at 12 months. Patients with more significant cognitive impairment and those with depression and anxiety were less likely to return to work[92]; however, those who are able to return to work have better health care-related quality of life.[88,93] Inability to return to work, along with medical bills and changes in insurance coverage can lead to financial toxicity which can also impede recovery.[94]

Survivors also face increased mortality following critical illness. An observational cohort of elderly

US Health and Retirement Study participants who were hospitalized because of acute hypoxic respiratory failure had a 24.4% increase in late mortality when compared with matched nonhospitalized adults.[95] Another retrospective cohort study by Wunch and colleagues[96] evaluating Medicare beneficiaries showed that ICU survivors had a higher 3-year mortality at 39.5% compared with 34.5% of hospitalized controls and 14.9% of general controls; patients who required mechanical ventilation had an even higher 3-year mortality rate at 57.6%.

Despite these difficulties associated with ICU survivorship, there has also been the identification of resilience and posttraumatic growth following critical illness.[97] In a mixed-methods study by Maley and colleagues,[98] resilience, as measured by the Connor–Davidson Resiliency 10-Item Scale, was normal in 63% of survivors and high in 9% of survivors and correlated with less self-reported symptoms of executive dysfunction, anxiety, and depression. Posttraumatic growth has been described in other populations such as patients with cancer and is tied to increased resilience.[99] Some smaller studies have identified posttraumatic growth as an important factor for optimizing well-being after critical illness, finding that it was associated with lower rates of depression. Patient appraisal factors, including their perceived impact on their acute respiratory distress and their sense of coping efficacy, were also important predictors for outcomes including depression, anxiety, and perceived health.[100] Although further investigation is needed on the role of resilience, positive self-appraisals, and posttraumatic growth in ICU survivors, it is the hope that with increased education and appropriate follow-up care, these traits can be promoted within the ICU survivor population.

COVID (SARS-CoV-2) Considerations

The recent COVID-19 pandemic has brought increased attention to the hardships of the ICU survivor and importance of screening for PICS, which is separate from the general "long-haul" post-COVID-19 symptoms that patients with non-critically ill cases of COVID-19 may face. Given that many of the severe cases of COVID-19 were cases of pneumonia and ARDS requiring ICU with prolonged mechanical ventilation and increased sedation, we would expect to see an emergence of PICS-related symptoms among this population.[101] Special attention and diligence in evaluating for PICS within critically ill survivors of COVID-19 will take on new importance.

SUMMARY

Improvements in critical care medicine have contributed to a marked increase in the number of patients who survive ICU admissions. Survivors of critical illness face numerous challenges following hospitalization. Recovery and rehabilitation are complex and must be individualized for each patient. PICS is a framework that may help providers identify deficits and provide support to patients and family members. Continued exploration into the difficulties, ICU survivors face is needed to identify strategies to prevent and manage long-term sequelae after critical illness.

DISCLOSURE

The authors have nothing to disclose.

REFERENCES

1. Angus DC, Carlet J, Brussels Roundtable P. Surviving intensive care: a report from the 2002 Brussels Roundtable. Intensive Care Med 2003;29(3):368–77.
2. Iwashyna TJ. Survivorship will be the defining challenge of critical care in the 21st century. Ann Intern Med 2010;153(3):204–5.
3. Needham DM, Davidson J, Cohen H, et al. Improving long-term outcomes after discharge from intensive care unit: report from a stakeholders' conference. Crit Care Med 2012;40(2):502–9.
4. Svenningsen H, Langhorn L, Agard AS, et al. Post-ICU symptoms, consequences, and follow-up: an integrative review. Nurs Crit Care 2017;22(4):212–20.
5. Mikkelsen ME, Still M, Anderson BJ, et al. Society of critical care medicine's international consensus conference on prediction and identification of long-term impairments after critical illness. Crit Care Med 2020;48(11):1670–9.
6. Marra A, Pandharipande PP, Girard TD, et al. Co-occurrence of post-intensive care syndrome problems among 406 survivors of critical illness. Crit Care Med 2018;46(9):1393–401.
7. Wunsch H, Angus DC, Harrison DA, et al. Variation in critical care services across North America and Western Europe. Crit Care Med 2008;36(10):2787–93.
8. Vincent JL, Marshall JC, Namendys-Silva SA, et al. Assessment of the worldwide burden of critical illness: the intensive care over nations (ICON) audit. Lancet Respir Med 2014;2(5):380–6.
9. Kawakami D, Fujitani S, Morimoto T, et al. Prevalence of post-intensive care syndrome among Japanese intensive care unit patients: a prospective, multicenter, observational J-PICS study. Crit Care 2021;25(1):69.

10. Brown SM, Bose S, Banner-Goodspeed V, et al. Approaches to addressing post-intensive care syndrome among intensive care unit survivors. a narrative review. Ann Am Thorac Soc 2019;16(8):947–56.

11. Lee M, Kang J, Jeong YJ. Risk factors for post-intensive care syndrome: a systematic review and meta-analysis. Aust Crit Care 2020;33(3):287–94.

12. Dowdy DW, Eid MP, Sedrakyan A, et al. Quality of life in adult survivors of critical illness: a systematic review of the literature. Intensive Care Med 2005; 31(5):611–20.

13. Jackson JC, Mitchell N, Hopkins RO. Cognitive functioning, mental health, and quality of life in ICU survivors: an overview. Psychiatr Clin North Am 2015;38(1):91–104.

14. Myhren H, Ekeberg O, Stokland O. Health-related quality of life and return to work after critical illness in general intensive care unit patients: a 1-year follow-up study. Crit Care Med 2010;38(7):1554–61.

15. Kapfhammer HP, Rothenhausler HB, Krauseneck T, et al. Posttraumatic stress disorder and health-related quality of life in long-term survivors of acute respiratory distress syndrome. Am J Psychiatry 2004;161(1):45–52.

16. Herridge MS, Tansey CM, Matte A, et al. Functional disability 5 years after acute respiratory distress syndrome. N Engl J Med 2011;364(14):1293–12304.

17. Jackson JC, Hart RP, Gordon SM, et al. Six-month neuropsychological outcome of medical intensive care unit patients. Crit Care Med 2003;31(4): 1226–34.

18. Sasannejad C, Ely EW, Lahiri S. Long-term cognitive impairment after acute respiratory distress syndrome: a review of clinical impact and pathophysiological mechanisms. Crit Care 2019;23(1):352.

19. Pandharipande PP, Girard TD, Jackson JC, et al. Long-term cognitive impairment after critical illness. N Engl J Med 2013;369(14):1306–16.

20. Mikkelsen ME, Christie JD, Lanken PN, et al. The adult respiratory distress syndrome cognitive outcomes study: long-term neuropsychological function in survivors of acute lung injury. Am J Respir Crit Care Med 2012;185(12):1307–15.

21. Norman BC, Jackson JC, Graves JA, et al. Employment outcomes after critical illness: an analysis of the bringing to light the risk factors and incidence of neuropsychological dysfunction in ICU survivors Cohort. Crit Care Med 2016;44(11):2003–9.

22. Hopkins RO, Weaver LK, Pope D, et al. Neuropsychological sequelae and impaired health status in survivors of severe acute respiratory distress syndrome. Am J Respir Crit Care Med 1999;160(1): 50–6.

23. Hopkins RO, Weaver LK, Collingridge D, et al. Two-year cognitive, emotional, and quality-of-life outcomes in acute respiratory distress syndrome. Am J Respir Crit Care Med 2005;171(4):340–7.

24. Davydow DS, Zatzick D, Hough CL, et al. In-hospital acute stress symptoms are associated with impairment in cognition 1 year after intensive care unit admission. Ann Am Thorac Soc 2013;10(5): 450–7.

25. Pisani MA, Redlich C, McNicoll L, et al. Underrecognition of preexisting cognitive impairment by physicians in older ICU patients. Chest 2003; 124(6):2267–74.

26. Wunsch H, Christiansen CF, Johansen MB, et al. Psychiatric diagnoses and psychoactive medication use among nonsurgical critically ill patients receiving mechanical ventilation. JAMA 2014; 311(11):1133–42.

27. Bienvenu OJ, Friedman LA, Colantuoni E, et al. Psychiatric symptoms after acute respiratory distress syndrome: a 5-year longitudinal study. Intensive Care Med 2018;44(1):38–47.

28. Hatch R, Young D, Barber V, et al. Anxiety, depression and post traumatic stress disorder after critical illness: a UK-wide prospective cohort study. Crit Care 2018;22(1):310.

29. Fernando SM, Qureshi D, Sood MM, et al. Suicide and self-harm in adult survivors of critical illness: population based cohort study. BMJ 2021;373:n973.

30. Davydow DS, Desai SV, Needham DM, et al. Psychiatric morbidity in survivors of the acute respiratory distress syndrome: a systematic review. Psychosom Med 2008;70(4):512–9.

31. Hopkins RO, Key CW, Suchyta MR, et al. Risk factors for depression and anxiety in survivors of acute respiratory distress syndrome. Gen Hosp Psychiatry 2010;32(2):147–55.

32. Huang M, Parker AM, Bienvenu OJ, et al. Psychiatric symptoms in acute respiratory distress syndrome survivors: a 1-year national multicenter study. Crit Care Med 2016;44(5):954–65.

33. Wade DM, Howell DC, Weinman JA, et al. Investigating risk factors for psychological morbidity three months after intensive care: a prospective cohort study. Crit Care 2012;16(5):R192.

34. Girard TD, Shintani AK, Jackson JC, et al. Risk factors for post-traumatic stress disorder symptoms following critical illness requiring mechanical ventilation: a prospective cohort study. Crit Care 2007; 11(1):R28.

35. Choi J, Tate JA, Rogers MA, et al. Depressive symptoms and anxiety in intensive care unit (ICU) survivors after ICU discharge. Heart Lung 2016; 45(2):140–6.

36. Franks ZM, Alcock JA, Lam T, et al. Physical restraints and post-traumatic stress disorder in survivors of critical illness. a systematic review and meta-analysis. Ann Am Thorac Soc 2021;18(4): 689–97.

37. Myhren H, Ekeberg O, Toien K, et al. Posttraumatic stress, anxiety and depression symptoms in

patients during the first year post intensive care unit discharge. Crit Care 2010;14(1):R14.

38. Ohtake PJ, Lee AC, Scott JC, et al. Physical impairments associated with post-intensive care syndrome: systematic review based on the world health organization's international classification of functioning, disability and health framework. Phys Ther 2018;98(8):631–45.

39. Latronico N, Herridge M, Hopkins RO, et al. The ICM research agenda on intensive care unit-acquired weakness. Intensive Care Med 2017;43(9):1270–81.

40. Stevens RD, Marshall SA, Cornblath DR, et al. A framework for diagnosing and classifying intensive care unit-acquired weakness. Crit Care Med 2009;37(10 Suppl):S299–308.

41. Vanhorebeek I, Latronico N, Van den Berghe G. ICU-acquired weakness. Intensive Care Med 2020;46(4):637–53.

42. Kress JP, Hall JB. ICU-acquired weakness and recovery from critical illness. N Engl J Med 2014; 370(17):1626–35.

43. Fan E, Dowdy DW, Colantuoni E, et al. Physical complications in acute lung injury survivors: a two-year longitudinal prospective study. Crit Care Med 2014;42(4):849–59.

44. Hermans G, Van Mechelen H, Clerckx B, et al. Acute outcomes and 1-year mortality of intensive care unit-acquired weakness. A cohort study and propensity-matched analysis. Am J Respir Crit Care Med 2014;190(4):410–20.

45. Wieske L, Dettling-Ihnenfeldt DS, Verhamme C, et al. Impact of ICU-acquired weakness on post-ICU physical functioning: a follow-up study. Crit Care 2015;19:196.

46. Ali NA, O'Brien JM Jr, Hoffmann SP, et al. Acquired weakness, handgrip strength, and mortality in critically ill patients. Am J Respir Crit Care Med 2008; 178(3):261–8.

47. Ferrante LE, Pisani MA, Murphy TE, et al. Functional trajectories among older persons before and after critical illness. JAMA Intern Med 2015; 175(4):523–9.

48. Hopkins RO, Suchyta MR, Kamdar BB, et al. Instrumental activities of daily living after critical illness: a systematic review. Ann Am Thorac Soc 2017;14(8): 1332–43.

49. Jackson JC, Pandharipande PP, Girard TD, et al. Depression, post-traumatic stress disorder, and functional disability in survivors of critical illness in the BRAIN-ICU study: a longitudinal cohort study. Lancet Respir Med 2014;2(5):369–79.

50. Roch A, Wiramus S, Pauly V, et al. Long-term outcome in medical patients aged 80 or over following admission to an intensive care unit. Crit Care 2011;15(1):R36.

51. Needham DM, Wozniak AW, Hough CL, et al. Risk factors for physical impairment after acute lung injury in a national, multicenter study. Am J Respir Crit Care Med 2014;189(10):1214–24.

52. Iwashyna TJ, Ely EW, Smith DM, et al. Long-term cognitive impairment and functional disability among survivors of severe sepsis. JAMA 2010; 304(16):1787–94.

53. Haas JS, Teixeira C, Cabral CR, et al. Factors influencing physical functional status in intensive care unit survivors two years after discharge. BMC Anesthesiol 2013;13:11.

54. Cox CE, Carson SS, Lindquist JH, et al. Differences in one-year health outcomes and resource utilization by definition of prolonged mechanical ventilation: a prospective cohort study. Crit Care 2007;11(1).

55. Fan E, Cheek F, Chlan L, et al. An official American thoracic society clinical practice guideline: the diagnosis of intensive care unit-acquired weakness in adults. Am J Respir Crit Care Med 2014;190(12): 1437–46.

56. Clavet H, Hebert PC, Fergusson D, et al. Joint contracture following prolonged stay in the intensive care unit. CMAJ 2008;178(6):691–7.

57. Altman MT, Knauert MP, Pisani MA. Sleep disturbance after hospitalization and critical illness: a systematic review. Ann Am Thorac Soc 2017; 14(9):1457–68.

58. Wilcox ME, McAndrews MP, Van J, et al. Sleep fragmentation and cognitive trajectories after critical illness. Chest 2021;159(1):366–81.

59. Neufeld KJ, Leoutsakos JS, Yan H, et al. Fatigue Symptoms during the first year following ARDS. Chest 2020;158(3):999–1007.

60. McHugh LG, Milberg JA, Whitcomb ME, et al. Recovery of function in survivors of the acute respiratory distress syndrome. Am J Respir Crit Care Med 1994;150(1):90–4.

61. Zuercher P, Schenk NV, Moret C, et al. Risk factors for dysphagia in ICU patients after invasive mechanical ventilation. Chest 2020;158(5):1983–91.

62. Brodsky MB, Pandian V, Needham DM. Post-extubation dysphagia: a problem needing multidisciplinary efforts. Intensive Care Med 2020;46(1):93–6.

63. Kelmenson DA, Quan D, Moss M. What is the diagnostic accuracy of single nerve conduction studies and muscle ultrasound to identify critical illness polyneuromyopathy: a prospective cohort study. Crit Care 2018;22(1):342.

64. Kress JP, Pohlman AS, O'Connor MF, et al. Daily interruption of sedative infusions in critically ill patients undergoing mechanical ventilation. N Engl J Med 2000;342(20):1471–7.

65. Girard TD, Kress JP, Fuchs BD, et al. Efficacy and safety of a paired sedation and ventilator weaning protocol for mechanically ventilated patients in intensive care (Awakening and Breathing Controlled trial): a randomised controlled trial. Lancet 2008; 371(9607):126–34.

66. Brummel NE, Girard TD, Ely EW, et al. Feasibility and safety of early combined cognitive and physical therapy for critically ill medical and surgical patients: the activity and cognitive therapy in ICU (ACT-ICU) trial. Intensive Care Med 2014;40(3):370–9.

67. Zhao J, Yao L, Wang C, et al. The effects of cognitive intervention on cognitive impairments after intensive care unit admission. Neuropsychol Rehabil 2017;27(3):301–17.

68. Kamdar BB, King LM, Collop NA, et al. The effect of a quality improvement intervention on perceived sleep quality and cognition in a medical ICU. Crit Care Med 2013;41(3):800–9.

69. Girard TD, Exline MC, Carson SS, et al. Haloperidol and ziprasidone for treatment of delirium in critical illness. N Engl J Med 2018;379(26):2506–16.

70. Hodgson CL, Bailey M, Bellomo R, et al. A binational multicenter pilot feasibility randomized controlled trial of early goal-directed mobilization in the ICU. Crit Care Med 2016;44(6):1145–5112.

71. Schweickert WD, Pohlman MC, Pohlman AS, et al. Early physical and occupational therapy in mechanically ventilated, critically ill patients: a randomised controlled trial. Lancet 2009;373(9678):1874–82.

72. Denehy L, Skinner EH, Edbrooke L, et al. Exercise rehabilitation for patients with critical illness: a randomized controlled trial with 12 months of follow-up. Crit Care 2013;17(4):R156.

73. Morris PE, Berry MJ, Files DC, et al. Standardized rehabilitation and hospital length of stay among patients with acute respiratory failure: a randomized clinical trial. JAMA 2016;315(24):2694–702.

74. Devlin JW, Skrobik Y, Gelinas C, et al. Clinical practice guidelines for the prevention and management of pain, agitation/sedation, delirium, immobility, and sleep disruption in adult patients in the ICU. Crit Care Med 2018;46(9):e825–73.

75. Yao L, Li Y, Yin R, et al. Incidence and influencing factors of post-intensive care cognitive impairment. Intensive Crit Care Nurs 2021;103106. https://doi.org/10.1016/j.iccn.2021.103106.

76. Sun X, Huang D, Zeng F, et al. Effect of intensive care unit diary on incidence of posttraumatic stress disorder, anxiety, and depression of adult intensive care unit survivors: a systematic review and meta-analysis. J Adv Nurs 2021;77(7):2929–41.

77. McIlroy PA, King RS, Garrouste-Orgeas M, et al. The effect of ICU diaries on psychological outcomes and quality of life of survivors of critical illness and their relatives: a systematic review and meta-analysis. Crit Care Med 2019;47(2):273–9.

78. Garrouste-Orgeas M, Flahault C, Vinatier I, et al. Effect of an ICU diary on posttraumatic stress disorder symptoms among patients receiving mechanical ventilation: a randomized clinical trial. JAMA 2019;322(3):229–39.

79. Jones C, Backman C, Capuzzo M, et al. Intensive care diaries reduce new onset post traumatic stress disorder following critical illness: a randomised, controlled trial. Crit Care 2010;14(5):R168.

80. Kredentser MS, Blouw M, Marten N, et al. Preventing posttraumatic stress in ICU Survivors: a single-center pilot randomized controlled trial of ICU diaries and psychoeducation. Crit Care Med 2018;46(12):1914–22.

81. Hosey MM, Jaskulski J, Wegener ST, et al. Animal-assisted intervention in the ICU: a tool for humanization. Crit Care 2018;22(1):22.

82. Chapman DK, Collingridge DS, Mitchell LA, et al. Satisfaction with elimination of all visitation restrictions in a mixed-profile intensive care unit. Am J Crit Care 2016;25(1):46–50.

83. Rosa RG, Falavigna M, da Silva DB, et al. Effect of flexible family visitation on delirium among patients in the intensive care unit: the ICU visits randomized clinical trial. JAMA 2019;322(3):216–28.

84. Khan SH, Wang S, Harrawood A, et al. Decreasing Delirium through Music (DDM) in critically ill, mechanically ventilated patients in the intensive care unit: study protocol for a pilot randomized controlled trial. Trials 2017;18(1):574.

85. Sevin CM, Bloom SL, Jackson JC, et al. Comprehensive care of ICU survivors: development and implementation of an ICU recovery center. J Crit Care 2018;46:141–8.

86. Bakhru RN, Davidson JF, Bookstaver RE, et al. Implementation of an ICU recovery clinic at a tertiary care academic center. Crit Care Explor 2019;1(8):e0034.

87. Khan S, Biju A, Wang S, et al. Mobile critical care recovery program (m-CCRP) for acute respiratory failure survivors: study protocol for a randomized controlled trial. Trials 2018;19(1):94.

88. McPeake J, Shaw M, Iwashyna TJ, et al. Intensive care syndrome: promoting independence and return to employment (ins:pire). early evaluation of a complex intervention. PLoS One 2017;12(11):e0188028.

89. Schmidt K, Worrack S, Von Korff M, et al. Effect of a primary care management intervention on mental health-related quality of life among survivors of sepsis: a randomized clinical trial. JAMA 2016;315(24):2703–11.

90. Hua M, Gong MN, Brady J, et al. Early and late unplanned rehospitalizations for survivors of critical illness. Crit Care Med 2015;43(2):430–8.

91. Prescott HC, Langa KM, Iwashyna TJ. Readmission diagnoses after hospitalization for severe sepsis and other acute medical conditions. JAMA 2015;313(10):1055–7.

92. Hodgson CL, Haines KJ, Bailey M, et al. Predictors of return to work in survivors of critical illness. J Crit Care 2018;48:21–5.

93. McPeake J, Mikkelsen ME, Quasim T, et al. Return to employment after critical illness and its association with psychosocial outcomes. a systematic review and meta-analysis. Ann Am Thorac Soc 2019;16(10):1304–11.

94. Hauschildt KE, Seigworth C, Kamphuis LA, et al. Financial toxicity after acute respiratory distress syndrome: a national qualitative cohort study. Crit Care Med 2020;48(8):1103–10.

95. Prescott HC, Sjoding MW, Langa KM, et al. Late mortality after acute hypoxic respiratory failure. Thorax 2017. https://doi.org/10.1136/thoraxjnl-2017-210109.

96. Wunsch H, Guerra C, Barnato AE, et al. Three-year outcomes for Medicare beneficiaries who survive intensive care. JAMA 2010;303(9):849–56.

97. Maley JM, Mark. What happens to critically ill patients after they leave the ICU? Evidence-Based Pract Crit Care 2020;11–6.e1.

98. Maley JH, Brewster I, Mayoral I, et al. Resilience in survivors of critical illness in the context of the survivors' experience and recovery. Ann Am Thorac Soc 2016;13(8):1351–60.

99. Gori A, Topino E, Sette A, et al. Pathways to post-traumatic growth in cancer patients: moderated mediation and single mediation analyses with resilience, personality, and coping strategies. J Affect Disord 2021;279:692–700.

100. Cheng SKW, Chong GHC, Chang SSY, et al. Adjustment to severe acute respiratory syndrome (SARS): roles of appraisal and post-traumatic growth. Psychol Health 2006;21(3):301–17.

101. Biehl M, Sese D. Post-intensive care syndrome and COVID-19 - implications post pandemic. Cleve Clin J Med 2020. https://doi.org/10.3949/ccjm.87a.ccc055.

Supporting Professionals in Critical Care Medicine
Burnout, Resiliency, and System-Level Change

Alexander S. Niven, MD[a],*, Curtis N. Sessler, MD[b],*

KEYWORDS

- Burnout • Moral injury • Moral distress • Resilience • Critical care • Well-being • ICU

KEY POINTS

- Burnout is common among physicians and other health-care professionals in the intensive care unit setting.
- Burnout has significant negative consequences for the individual health-care professional, the interprofessional team, and for hospitals, patients, and health-care systems.
- The COVID-19 pandemic has produced enormous stress on health care broadly, and critical care in particular, further magnifying the problem of burnout.
- Key drivers of burnout in critical care include the quantity and timing (nights, weekends) of work, inadequate resources, requirements to perform menial tasks that contribute little to clinical care, shortfalls in team-based culture and communication, moral distress, and end-of-life issues.
- System-level strategies to address these key drivers, build unit-based cohesion, and support individual resiliency are critical to improve patient safety and outcomes.

Burnout has been recognized as a major and growing problem in health care during the past several decades, with dramatically higher rates compared with US workers in other fields.[1–4] The chronic stress and emotionally intense work makes burnout particularly common in critical care, with roughly one-half of intensive care unit (ICU) physicians and a third of nurses reporting severe symptoms.[5–10] The consequences are significant, including a high personal and professional price for many, decreased productivity and greater conflict among teams, and increased medical errors and staff turnover within health-care systems.

Change in this area, however, has been slow. In 2016, the Critical Care Societies Collaborative (CCSC) issued a broad call to action to address the epidemic of burnout within critical care,[8] but subsequent work has been challenging, with solutions more often focused on the individual than organizational interventions. ICU teams have played a frontline role during the COVID-19 pandemic. Not surprisingly, initial reports depict further surges in burnout, yet likely, fail to fully capture the full impact that this experience will have on the well-being, mental health, and posttraumatic stress that many in our community will face in the months and years ahead.[11–13]

The purpose of this review is to summarize our current understanding of the scope and driving factors of burnout in frontline critical care teams, and its impact on their well-being, performance, and patient outcomes. We will also examine the current best-supported approaches to address this pervasive problem in health care, and the

---

a Division of Pulmonary and Critical Care Medicine, Department of Medicine, Mayo Clinic, 200 First Street, Southwest, Rochester, MN 55905, USA; b Division of Pulmonary and Critical Care Medicine, Department of Internal Medicine, Virginia Commonwealth University, 417 North 11th Street, Richmond, VA 23219, USA
* Corresponding authors.
E-mail addresses: niven.alexander@mayo.edu (A.S.N.); curtis.sessler@vcuhealth.org (C.N.S.)

Clin Chest Med 43 (2022) 563–577
https://doi.org/10.1016/j.ccm.2022.05.010
0272-5231/22/© 2022 Elsevier Inc. All rights reserved.

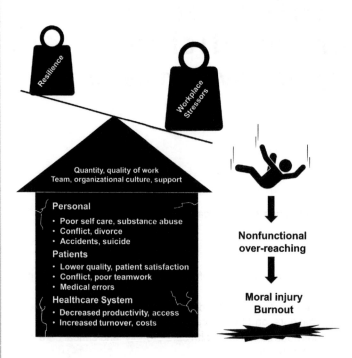

Fig. 1. Imbalance between workplace stressors and individual grit, resilience and organizational support, and solutions can lead to nonfunctional over-reaching, which over time can progress to a "cloud" of negative consequences for workers, patients, and the healthcare system.

urgent need for organizational commitment and systems level change to protect and support the critical care community and the patients they serve.[14]

DEFINITIONS AND BACKGROUND

Because the terms burnout, moral injury, resilience, and grit are often used with variable accuracy, we briefly define them and offer a conceptual framework for their interplay (**Fig. 1**).

"Burnout" is a work-related syndrome characterized by emotional exhaustion, depersonalization, and a low sense of personal accomplishment.[15] Emotional exhaustion is common but depersonalization—callousness and treating patients like objects—may align more strongly with the most negative consequences of this syndrome.[16,17] A low sense of personal accomplishment can manifest as reduced productivity, feelings of clinical ineffectiveness, or a more general perception that patient care or professional achievements are not valuable.[18] The terms "moral distress" and "moral injury" describe the feelings that health-care workers can experience from perpetrating, failing to prevent, or bearing witness to acts that transgress their deeply held moral beliefs and expectations.[19,20] The principles of beneficence and nonmalfeasance are core to the practice of medicine, and events that violate these principles—especially when repeated and due to circumstances beyond their control—place health-care workers at risk for a syndrome similar

in severity to posttraumatic stress disorder (PTSD). PTSD is a mental health condition triggered by experiencing or witnessing a terrifying event and is characterized by flashbacks, nightmares, severe anxiety, and uncontrollable thoughts about the event that results in avoidance behaviors, excessive arousal, and mood disorders.[21] ICU workers may manifest isolated or overlapping manifestations of burnout, moral injury, and PTSD.

"Resilience" generally refers to an individual's ability to adapt or "bounce back" from stressful or negative emotional experiences.[22] Resilience is an inherent attribute of "grit," which is defined as perseverance, passion, and sustained commitment to complete a specific endeavor or long-term goals despite failure, setbacks, and adversity.[23] Common solutions often focus on personal resilience as a primary strategy to combat burnout but these approaches oversimplify the issue. Grit is a complex concept influenced by multiple individual characteristics, only some of which are modifiable using personal resilience strategies. Challenge is a necessary part of professional development, but a balance between stress and recovery is essential to sustain high performance and to avoid injury from "overuse." Without a healthy organizational climate and solutions for support, chronic, excessive demands at work can cause "nonfunctional overreaching"—a short-term reduction in performance that only returns to normal after a period of sustained rest—moral injury, or burnout. The result is a "cloud" of negative consequences for health-care workers and the patients and health-care systems they serve (see **Fig. 1**).

MEASURING THE PROBLEM OF BURNOUT

Although burnout is associated with job dissatisfaction, fatigue, occupational stress, and depression, it is a separate syndrome. There are well-established tools that can help leaders and organizations to define the scope of the problem they face, and the impact of their interventions over time.

The Maslach Burnout Inventory (MBI) is the most widely accepted standard for burnout assessment and includes a Human Services Survey applicable to health-care professionals. Scores for emotional exhaustion of 27 or greater (range 0–54), depersonalization of 10 or greater (range 0–30), and personal accomplishment of 33 or lesser (range 0–48) suggest high levels of burnout in each domain for physicians.[24] As the length of the MBI can limit its utility outside of research studies, several shorter tools with 1 or 3 questions from each MBI domain have been developed with moderate-to-strong correlations with the full MBI.[25–27] A 10 question mini-Z instrument that assesses the 3 domains and 7 drivers of burnout has also been validated against the MBI.[28,29] Other measures separate from the MBI framework include the Copenhagen and Oldenburg Burnout Inventories (CBI, OLBI). The CBI consists of 3 scales measuring personal, work, and client-related burnout. The CBI has been found to be a reliable predictor of future work absence due to illness or resignation, sleep problems, and use of prescription pain medication in a large cohort of human service sector employees.[30] The OLBI was designed to apply to a broad cross section of German workers in a variety of occupations. It includes items that address the core MBI dimensions of emotional exhaustion and depersonalization and has also been adapted for students in academic settings Oldenburg Burnout Inventory for Students (OLBI-S).[31]

BURNOUT IN THE INTENSIVE CARE UNIT TEAM

Estimating the prevalence of burnout among health-care professionals has been hindered by the use of different tools, varying threshold criteria, and considerable variability among specialties and practice settings.[32] Experts estimate that 35% to 45% of nurses and 40% to 54% of physicians in the United States have burnout.[14] Shanafelt and colleagues demonstrated a higher rate of burnout among physicians (37.9%) compared with a broad mix of other workers (27.8%), and less satisfaction with work–life balance (58.8% vs 77.8%, respectively).[4] Serial surveys of US physicians demonstrate persistent, high rates of at least one symptom of burnout, ranging from 45.5% in 2011% to 54.4% in 2014% and 43.9% in 2017.[2]

Burnout is common in critical care compared with other specialties, with reported rates of 28% to 42% for ICU nurses and 25% to 71% for intensivists during the past 15 years.[5–10] In a 2021 Medscape physician survey, intensivists reported the highest symptoms of burnout among all 29 physician specialties.[33] Delivering direct frontline patient care is a common theme among specialties with high rates of burnout, including critical care, emergency medicine, internal medicine, and neurology.[2,4,33]

CONSEQUENCES OF BURNOUT

The negative impact of burnout in health care is far-reaching. The direct physical and emotional manifestations in health-care workers are personally experienced and accordingly most widely recognized. However, the magnitude of downstream consequences for colleagues, critical care teams, hospitals, health care in general—and most importantly patients—is substantial and less well appreciated.

Poncet and colleagues found that nurses with burnout have higher rates of personal health complaints, including sleep disruption, eating disorders, mood and libido disturbances, memory impairment, and depressive symptoms.[6] There is an association between burnout, anxiety, and depression, and sadly physicians and nurses have significantly elevated rates of suicide compared with the general working population.[16,34,35] Burnout doubled the prevalence of suicidal ideation among physicians in one large study.[35]

There is an unmistakable connection between burnout and job performance—with adverse consequences for the worker, patients, and health-care systems. Common themes include lack of empathy, caring, and professionalism; suboptimal communication; and impaired attention to detail and follow-through that can contribute to harm. Nursing burnout is correlated with negative patient perceptions including poor quality of communication, lower overall satisfaction ratings, and a lower likelihood to recommend the hospital.

There is strong evidence linking burnout to increased medical errors and shortfalls in other health-care quality measures.[36,37] Nursing burnout levels correlate with lower quality, safety, and higher rates of nosocomial infections.[38] In a large national study by Tawfik and colleagues, physicians who reported committing a major medical error in the prior 3 months were more likely to have symptoms of burnout, fatigue, and recent suicidal ideation.[39] These errors were independently associated with burnout, fatigue, and work unit safety grade. Certain underlying factors—severe understaffing, for example,—could worsen all 3 of these independent drivers. We suspect that the association between burnout and medical error is bidirectional, with exhaustion and low professionalism contributing to increased errors—and errors in turn compounding feelings of negativism—and reduced professional efficacy.[40]

Burnout is strongly associated with reduced job satisfaction and the intent to reduce work effort or to leave one's current job or career. The quantity and quality of work delivered by burned out health-care workers can suffer due to increased absenteeism, reduced effort, and suboptimal performance.[41] Physician distress has been linked to physician prescribing habits, test ordering, the risk of malpractice suits, and patient adherence with provider recommendations.[42] Several large studies have found striking and strong correlations between physician burnout and plans to reduce clinical hours, leave their current practice, and leave health care, including a survey of nearly 1000 intensivists.[5,43] Reports also demonstrate that burned out physicians leave their organizations at double the frequency. Considered together, these data provide a compelling business case for burnout as a driver of reduced quality and quantity of work, patient and health care worker (HCW) harm, and increased costs related to employee turnover.[44–46]

Although the scope and impact of the COVID-19 pandemic has yet to be fully realized, the consequences of this on the critical care community is undoubtedly severe and will only magnify these problems. Reports from around the globe describe a high prevalence of anxiety, depression, and other mental health issues among health-care workers broadly including the ICU setting.[11,47,48] The long-term personal health consequences of the widespread and now persistent challenges that ICU health-care workers have faced remain undefined. Although only time will determine the impact of these complex issues on the ICU workforce, it is reasonable to speculate that attrition will present increasing health system challenges with critical care delivery in the months and years to come.

DRIVING FACTORS FOR BURNOUT

The driving factors for burnout are a complex network of workplace and organizational factors, which can affect health-care workers differently based on their personal characteristics, coping skills, and the quality of their personal and professional relationships. The literature studying the driving factors for burnout is heavily focused on physicians and nurses and defining the different forces that influence burnout, job satisfaction, and well-being in other members of the health-care team remains an opportunity for future research.

Individual and work environment factors commonly associated with health-care worker burnout and well-being and potential solutions are listed in **Table 1**. Four core categories have been described in ICU workers, including personal characteristics, organizational factors, exposure to end-of-life issues, and the quality of working relationships.[8] Personal characteristics associated with a greater risk of burnout include certain personality types, and idealistic perfectionists who tend to overcommit or engage in frequent self-criticism.[49] A limited support system outside of work, including being single, living without family, and earning a lower household income, are also risk factors.[50] Younger physicians have nearly twice the prevalence of burnout than their older colleagues, although the influences of training, experience, and early work force departure on this finding are not well delineated.[51] Although evidence suggests women intensivists may be at greater risk for burnout, other experts have argued that higher levels of provider empathy and insufficient support for family caregiver responsibilities may be more important than gender differences alone.[5,52]

Excessive workload is a consistent theme among organizational factors, although its definition varies by ICU discipline.[5,8–10,40,53] Intensivists share the burden of long hours, high-intensity shifts that include nights and weekends, and strain from simultaneous admissions and deteriorating patients.[40,53] ICU strain—the result of imbalance between the supply of available beds, staff, and/or resources and the demand to provide high-quality care—is considered an important driver of provider stress and burnout.[54] The number of consecutive shifts and burden of night duty—with its associated sleep disruption—is clearly associated with burnout in critical care physicians.[5] Working a continuous 14-day period of clinical time, for example, was associated with increased burnout symptoms compared with a system that provided weekend coverage by another physician.[55] Quan and colleagues found that one-third of a large cohort of health-care workers screened positive for insomnia, obstructive sleep apnea, or shift work sleep disorder,

Table 1
Driving factors that lead to clinician burnout or professional engagement and well-being, and previously identified, modifiable conditions that contribute the current high rate of burnout within critical care

Driving Factors	Individual	Work Environment
Meaning, purpose in work	Inability to prioritize professional interests Challenging patient, family, and staff interactions Certification, maintenance requirements	Limited time, resources for professional development, certification requirements, innovation and research Limited provider support, processes for patient, family centered care, communication Licensing, institutional regulatory training requirements
Workload, job demands	High patient volume, acuity, turnover High unit mortality rate Ethical dilemmas, moral distress Compensation (salary vs productivity model)	Inadequate staffing, experience Poor consult support, palliative care integration Productivity models, targets
Personal risk	Risk of clinical activity to self, family (COVID-19, workplace violence)	Inadequate personal protective equipment Limited safety culture, processes
Efficiency	Work demands, skills mismatch Excessive administrative burden Time with electronic medical record (EMR) vs patients Workflow interruptions Documentation requirements	Inadequate staffing, experience Ineffective team structure, collaboration Technology, work system inefficiencies Poor teamwork, communication systems Internal, external barriers to integrated, patient-centered care Limited autonomy, opportunities to engage in quality improvement
Control, flexibility at work	High patient acuity, volume with unpredictable workload Inability to deliver appropriate care Little control, flexibility of personal calendar Difficulty requesting days off, finding coverage	Limited options for additional support, redistribution of patients during surges Supply chain issues, health-care network and insurance barriers Insufficient schedule flexibility for vacations, medical appointments, unexpected absences Overreliance on learners to meet service requirements
Work-life integration	Long work hours Multiple consecutive shifts Excessive night responsibilities Sleep disruption Inability to select days off, poor self-care habits Limited time for personal, family responsibilities	Unrealistic practice expectations, culture Burdensome call schedules Schedules allow insufficient time for rest, recovery Limited backup systems, options for part-time work Limited child care, social support systems

(continued on next page)

Table 1 (continued)		
Driving Factors	**Individual**	**Work Environment**
Social support, community	Limited coping skills for stress Poor social support, isolation Conflict with peers, consultants, supervisors Deteriorating personal relationships Effort/recognition imbalance	Limited coaching, mentorship Limited opportunities to build professional relationships, community Toxic work environment Insufficient peer, occupational health support Negative reinforcement, insufficient rewards
Alignment of culture, values	Evolving personal, professional values Mismatch between expectations, responsibilities Variable altruism, commitment to organization	Limited leadership vision, behaviors, and staff empowerment Equitable health-care delivery for all not clearly prioritized, lack of alignment with organizational vision Decisions are not just, transparent, or clearly communicated

and these individuals had almost a 4-fold increased risk of burnout.[56]

In contrast, the inability to choose days off, rapid patient turnover, and limited opportunities to participate in ICU team discussions were major driving factors for burnout in ICU nurses.[6] Ethically challenging decisions and feeling "forced" to deliver futile care for prolonged periods can also increase the normal stressors of critical care practice. Factors related to end-of-life care, including caring for dying patients or witnessing decisions to decline or withdraw life-sustaining treatment, have more consistently been identified as risk factors for burnout in ICU nurses than physicians.[6,8,50]

Inefficient work processes and excessive administrative tasks have been identified as common stressors across physician specialties, especially when they do not meaningfully support clinical work.[57] Computerized physician order entry, for example, has been associated with a 29% greater rate of physician burnout.[57] Among intensivists, increases in documentation time contribute to packed shifts with less time for direct patient care and minimal opportunity for personal recovery.[53] Lack of autonomy, flexibility, or ability to control and improve one's personal work environment seems to increase the impact of these factors.[58] The drivers of burnout begin in training, and include challenging grading schema, poor peer collaboration, inadequate preparation and support for clinical experiences, excessive workload, and poor supervision with less opportunities for autonomy.[14,59]

Poor working relationships, interpersonal conflict, and strained patient and family interactions are strong risk factors for burnout in both nurses and physicians.[5,6,8,60,61] Psychologists have described a phenomenon called "mood contagion," which occurs when unintentional imitation of another person's emotional behavior activates a congruent mood state in the observer, potentially amplifying a negative work environment.[62] Stress is also higher when staff have high work demands but little control over their work environment, which saps both motivation and performance—and schedule control can be protective.[6] Poor teamwork, planning, preparation, and communication from local leadership only compounds this problem, especially within a culture that favors negative reinforcement.[63]

The unexpected and significant strain of the COVID-19 pandemic has highlighted the weaknesses of our health-care delivery system and intensified these driving factors for burnout. Insufficient numbers of frontline critical care staff have faced overwhelming volumes of critically ill patients, leading to excessive workload, inadequate recovery time, and exhaustion in many. Fear of being infected, an inability to rest or care for family, struggles with difficult emotions, regrets about restricted visitation policies, and witnessing hasty end-of-life decisions are modifiable risk factors that have been associated with anxiety, depression, and peritraumatic dissociation in ICU workers caring for COVID-19 patients. Worker concerns about optimal care delivery, lack of

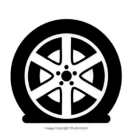

HEALTHCARE WORKER CHALLENGES	PRINCIPLE
Insufficient planning, communication and timely updates	Prepare Me
Negative work environment Longer, more intense shifts	Support Me
Threat of occupational COVID-19 exposure due to limited hospital resources	Protect Me
Risk of personal illness, family COVID-19 exposure due to clinical duties	Care for Me
Disruption of work-life balance Neglect of personal, family needs	Honor Me

Image Copyright Shutterstock

Fig. 2. Health-care worker challenges areas in need of organizational support during COVID-19 pandemic with directed principles.

control, and involuntary deployment to work with COVID-19 patients have also negatively influenced health-care outcomes.[64] Past experiences suggest that nonmedical "essential personnel" such as janitors, food service, and health-care administrators also represent an at-risk population in this setting.[65] Focus group interviews with interprofessional health-care workers at a major academic medical center early in the pandemic identified 8 major sources of anxiety and 6 broad requests to their organizational leaders. These workers' primary concerns centered around their personal safety, their ability to protect and care for their family, and their ability to synthesize new information and shape organizational changes to continue competent patient care delivery. They looked for organizational support to help them meet their increased work demands and to care for them if they became ill (**Fig. 2**).

Shanafelt and colleagues has proposed grouping the long list of driving factors that contribute to burnout, engagement, and well-being into 7 dimensions.[45] Recognizing that each of these drivers is influenced by individual and workplace factors, we have summarized our current understanding of key elements relevant to the critical care community using an adapted version of this framework in **Table 1**.

EVIDENCE-BASED APPROACHES TO COMBAT BURNOUT

It has been more than 20 years since the Institute of Medicine first identified medical error as a leading cause of death in the United States.[66] Despite tireless efforts by health-care organizations and regulatory agencies, the road to close the "quality chasm" has proven longer and more challenging than anticipated.[67] Experts have proposed that the epidemic of burnout in medical

professionals—on whom the US health-care system depends to improve its performance—is a significant contributing factor to this ongoing problem, worthy of systems level attention. Several systematic reviews and meta-analyses provide a framework of evidence-based interventions that have shown generally modest improvements in physician burnout, with organizational approaches demonstrating greater impact compared with interventions focused on individuals.[68,69] Results of a national survey of ICU workers by Kleinpell and CCSC colleagues also provide a snapshot of current organizational and individual measures from various ICU workers.[70]

Individual Strategies

Available evidence suggests that an adequate balance between stress and recovery is essential for humans to sustain a high level of performance, and these concepts are well integrated into high-reliability industries such as aviation and nuclear energy. A summary of the common challenges that individuals face within the health-care environment and frequently cited solutions to foster resilience and recovery are summarized in **Fig. 3**.

The American Academy of Sleep Medicine recently issued a position statement highlighting the importance of sufficient sleep and guiding principles to manage fatigue from the heavy workload, long hours, sleep interruptions, and circadian misalignment commonly seen in health care.[71,72] The benefits of strategic napping and use of caffeine to improve performance during night shifts are well established.[73,74] Although the quality of evidence precludes more specific recommendations, regular exercise improves overall and subjective sleep quality, sleep latency, and apnea-hypopnea index, and has favorable effects on mood, mental health, behavioral and cognitive function, and quality of life.[75,76] Brief breaks that

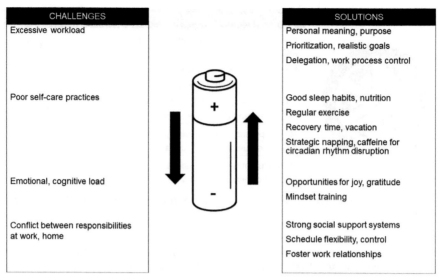

CHALLENGES	SOLUTIONS
Excessive workload	Personal meaning, purpose Prioritization, realistic goals Delegation, work process control
Poor self-care practices	Good sleep habits, nutrition Regular exercise Recovery time, vacation Strategic napping, caffeine for circadian rhythm disruption
Emotional, cognitive load	Opportunities for joy, gratitude Mindset training
Conflict between responsibilities at work, home	Strong social support systems Schedule flexibility, control Foster work relationships

Fig. 3. Common challenges that "drain" health-care workers, and solutions that "charge" individual resilience, recovery, and professional performance.

incorporate light exercise during ICU rounds can relieve stress and buoy team morale.[77] A balanced diet is a commonly accepted component of many well-being programs, and the National Institutes of Health has identified the role of nutrition in health promotion and disease prevention as a research priority.[78] Mindfulness-based interventions are associated with positive effects on physician well-being and performance, although the evidence supporting these findings is heterogeneous.[79,80] Presence of high emotional intelligence, a trait that can be learned, has also been linked to less burnout.[81]

In a cross-sectional survey of nurses working in high stress areas including the ICU, spiritual well-being, hope, resilience, and meaning were found to be protective factors against burnout.[82] Meaning at work requires alignment of personal and organizational values, a sense of personal accomplishment, and opportunities for joy, gratitude, and professional relationships. In a prospective randomized trial, volunteer physicians who participated in a facilitated small group curriculum to promote mindfulness, reflection, and share experiences for 1 hour every 2 weeks reported significant and sustained improvements in engagement, empowerment, and meaning at work compared with peers who received the same amount of protected time without any structured activities.[68]

Work Unit/Team Approaches

Strong teamwork is important in any modern health-care environment, and critical for ICU

teams and complex care delivery. Experts highlight the central role interprofessional interactions play in practitioner well-being, particularly in the ICU.[61] Many health-care organizations have turned to well-established teamwork curricula to improve safe care delivery, and recent reviews have highlighted the importance of successful multidisciplinary teams to both ensure health care quality and combat burnout.[83–85] Experts suggest that high-performing teams must be able to both work together interdependently and support individual growth and well-being using 5 core principles (**Box 1**). A variety of assessment tools is available to measure baseline team performance and progress over time.[86,87]

There is compelling evidence that challenging relationships, conflict, incivility, and workplace violence are powerful drivers of burnout and turnover, and offer key targets for intervention.[88] A variety of interventions that emphasize collaborative teamwork, leadership, and communication have been demonstrated to decrease burnout among ICU and acute care workers in prospective trials.[89–91] Health-care staff have among the highest risk of workplace violence,[92] with rates at least 5-fold higher than the average US worker and rising.[93] Psychiatric and emergency department workers are at greatest risk, followed by ICU and other in-patient staff. Results of a multihospital randomized controlled intervention addressing environmental, administrative, and behavioral issues significantly reduced violent events.[94] Earlier this year, US House of Representatives passed the Workplace Violence Prevention for Health Care

Box 1
Core principles of effective teamwork to maximize health-care quality and reduce burnout

Shared Goals: The team establishes shared goals that all members can clearly articulate, understand, and support.

Clear Roles: Each team member has clear expectations for their function, responsibilities, and accountability. Role clarity helps to determine adequate staffing, which is associated with improved clinician well-being and decreased risk of burnout.

Mutual Trust: Team members must trust each other and feel safe to admit mistakes, ask questions, offer new ideas, or try new skills without fear of embarrassment or punishment. A strong team climate promotes clinician well-being and retention.

Effective Communication: Consistent, efficient, bidirectional, collaborative communication is associated with decreased clinician burnout.

Measurable Processes, Outcomes: The team should receive reliable, ongoing assessment of their structure, function, and performance with actionable feedback to improve performance, drive results, and combat the emotional exhaustion and burnout that comes with low personal accomplishment.

has been challenging. Common identified themes have included attention to basic physiologic and personal needs including personal protective equipment, realistic training, strong and agile leadership to foster staff trust and engagement, and regular, clear communication.[13,95,96] Building community, connectedness, and team cohesion have been cited as important practice interventions to prevent burnout, including staff member shift pairings to foster peer support, shift huddles to prepare for and debrief clinical experiences, and ready and varied opportunities for emotional and behavioral health support to address the reactions commonly expected from exposure to severe stress.[71,97,98] (**Fig. 4**).

Organizational Approaches

Health-care organizations have a critical role to play in the battle against burnout. Although individual-focused strategies may be beneficial and effective components of larger organizational efforts, the available evidence suggests that personal interventions alone are insufficient. The collective experience during the COVID-19 pandemic has highlighted the critical need for organizations to appropriately support their staff to sustain their performance during prolonged periods of significant stress. Stress is compounded by reductions in available staffing due to quarantine of exposed and infected health-care workers. The goal must be to fix the work environment, rather than to prepare people to tolerate a broken system (**Fig. 5**).

A primary goal of our health system transformation must be to enable clinical teams to compassionately care for patients and their families as human beings while honoring the need for worker health. Organizations must create positive work and learning environments that prevent and reduce burnout; foster professional well-being

and Social Services Workers Act, calling for the Occupational Safety and Health Administration to strengthen its current health-care workplace safety standards.

The COVID-19 pandemic has placed even greater demands on critical care teams. Many health-care systems have been forced to augment staffing to meet surge demands, and integrating these workers into the ICU practice and culture

Challenges		Solutions
Workload demands		Appropriate staffing, work system redesign
Difficult patient & family encounters		Goal concordant care & communication
Workplace violence		Prevention plans, post-event intervention
Ethical dilemmas, end of life care		Palliative care, ethics consult integration
Varied job performance, standards		Strong & agile leadership
Inefficient teamwork, work processes		Staff-led QI, empowerment
Poor communication, collaboration		Teamwork training
Administrative burden		Workflow, technology solutions
Isolation, interpersonal conflict		Peer support, huddles & debriefing
Medical errors, moral distress		Safety culture, mutual trust & support
Effort reward imbalance		Recognition programs, awards

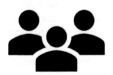

Fig. 4. Challenges and solutions to foster high team performance and a positive work environment.

CHALLENGES	SOLUTIONS
Workload demands	Appropriate staffing, system redesign
Difficult patient, family encounters	Goal concordant care, communication
Workplace violence	Prevention plans, post-event intervention
Ethical dilemmas, end of life care	Palliative care, ethics consult integration
Varied job performance, standards	Strong, agile leadership
Inefficient teamwork, work processes	Staff-led QI, empowerment
Poor communication, collaboration	Teamwork training
Administrative burden	Workflow, technology solutions
Isolation, interpersonal conflict	Peer support, huddles & debriefing
Medical errors, moral distress	Safety culture, mutual trust & support
Effort reward imbalance	Recognition programs, awards

Fig. 5. Organizational challenges and solutions to support and sustain staff performance.

and a culture that allows individuals to seek help without barriers or stigma; and ensure high-quality care delivery through established strategies that use interprofessional teamwork, workflow efficiency, and health information technology to reduce administrative burden.[14] Such a major transformation requires leader engagement at every level, and broadening systems commitment to the "quadruple aim"—enhancing patient experience, improving population health, reducing cost, and improving the work life of health-care providers.[99] Recognizing that there are many areas in this field that require further research, organizations should measure burnout prevalence and establish it as a routine institutional performance metric to determine the impact of continuous quality improvement efforts on staff well-being within their learning health-care system.

Professional societies also have a role to play. The CCSC recently summarized existing well-being initiatives among 17 professional societies serving the interprofessional critical care community and developed specific recommendations in this area based on this information and a series of semistructured interviews.[100] Society representatives agreed that professional societies have a moral imperative to address burnout and to share well-being initiatives. The authors developed a roadmap with recommendations to acknowledge the problem of burnout, to commit to supporting member well-being, to create collaborations to promote well-being, to educate and advocate for change, to foster innovation through research, and to support organizational and individual solutions. The authors also argued that societies should create sustainable collaborative models to integrate well-being considerations throughout society activities to provide a safe space for members to discuss challenges without fear of professional ramifications, to raise public awareness, and to advocate for system-based change.

SUMMARY AND FUTURE RECOMMENDATIONS

There is a moral and ethical imperative to address burnout in health care. Burnout starts during training and affects approximately half of our colleagues and coworkers, placing them at risk for broken relationships, alcoholism, substance abuse, and suicide. It degrades the meaning of our daily work and the effectiveness of our interprofessional teams, damages the safety and quality of care that our patients receive, and increases staff turnover and cost in our health-care systems. The COVID-19 pandemic will only intensify the scope of this problem among frontline ICU workers, and the collateral damage could threaten the viability of critical care delivery platforms in many regions of the United States and beyond.

Our journey toward a strong, viable health-care system—a system that provides an exceptional clinician and patient experience with outstanding clinical outcomes at lower cost—has significant consequences for patients, clinicians, health-care organizations, and society. Closing the "quality chasm" will require learning systems that take a systematic approach to the epidemic of burnout, using continuous quality improvement and existing knowledge to immediately improve learning and work environments and investing in research to answer the many unanswered questions that remain in this field.

Immediate Priorities	Strategic Goals
Develop a community, conversation about well-being	Define epidemiology of burnout across professions
Integrate well-being concepts within organizational activities	Clarify sources of professional fulfillment, well-being, impact on personal, professional, and societal outcomes
Foster a culture of support, with ready access to behavioral health services when needed	Evaluate systems interventions to mitigate burnout, promote interprofessional well-being
Identify sustainable funding to speed current, future efforts	Create a sustainable learning system that delivers quality care in a positive, supportive work environment
Clarify work system, learning environment, individual factors that promote burnout, implications	Advocate for major changes in health-care delivery, regulatory incentives, and reimbursement
Reduce administrative burden using systems engineering, technology, regulatory changes	
Support interprofessional development, team training	

Table 2
Immediate priorities and strategic goals to combat burnout and its detrimental consequences in health care based on current evidence and expert recommendations

Using the evidence compiled in this review and other expert recommendations, we suggest the following immediate priorities and strategic goals (**Table 2**).[14] Increasing burnout awareness and integrating proven best practices into the critical care practice environment are obvious and urgent first steps given the challenges that our frontline ICU teams continue to face. This will require organizational commitment, leadership emphasis, a culture of support, and necessary resources to sustain and protect ICU teams as they meet the current unprecedented demand for critical care services.

The next steps are more challenging but still achievable; we need to free our providers and

care team from their computers and grant them the privilege of spending more time at the bedside with their patients. There is already significant will to reduce the current costly inefficiencies and administrative burden within our health-care system but this will require meaningful funding, organizational and regulatory support. Reshaping our practice will require strengthening our team-based practices to deliver true collaborative, interprofessional care, and leveraging health information technology and systems engineering to develop an "intelligent" clinical environment that supports clinical reasoning and efficient delivery of evidence-based best practices.

The remaining listed goals are longer term but equally as important. The absence of data in this review on the prevalence and driving factors of burnout in critical care pharmacists, respiratory therapists, ICU support staff, and other members of the multidisciplinary team underlines an important area in need of epidemiologic studies. In addition to advancing our understanding of the barriers and drivers to burnout and well-being within the context of the ongoing COVID-19 pandemic and beyond, we must design meaningful prospective trials that will inform the necessary systems interventions to transform our current culture and health-care platform into a sustainable, learning system that delivers the "quadruple aim." This is the ultimate challenge that we face, and it will require both research funding and major revisions in our current health-care delivery model, regulatory incentives, and reimbursement to achieve long-term, sustainable change.

CLINICS CARE POINTS

- Burnout is a major problem that impacts every level of the healthcare system, including the safety and quality of care that our patients receive.
- Available evidence suggests that the COVID-19 pandemic has only increased the scope of burnout challenges, underlining the need for urgent action to address this growing threat to healthcare access and delivery in critical care and beyond.

DISCLOSURE

The authors have nothing to disclose.

REFERENCES

1. Linzer M, Visser MR, Oort FJ, et al. Predicting and preventing physician burnout: results from the United States and The Netherlands. Am J Med 2001;111(2):170–5.
2. Shanafelt TD, West CP, Sinsky C, et al. Changes in burnout and satisfaction with work-life integration in physicians and the general US working population between 2011 and 2017. Mayo Clin Proc 2019; 94(9):1681–94.
3. Shanafelt TD, Hasan O, Dyrbye LN, et al. Changes in burnout and satisfaction with work-life balance in physicians and the general US working population between 2011 and 2014. Mayo Clin Proc 2015; 90(12):1600–13 [published correction appears in Mayo Clin Proc. 2016 Feb;91(2):276].
4. Shanafelt TD, Boone S, Tan L, et al. Burnout and satisfaction with work-life balance among US physicians relative to the general US population. Arch Intern Med 2012;172(18):1377–85.
5. Embriaco N, Azoulay E, Barrau K, et al. High level of burnout in intensivists: prevalence and associated factors. Am J Respir Crit Care Med 2007; 175(7):686–92 [published correction appears in Am J Respir Crit Care Med. 2007 Jun 1;175(11): 1209-10].
6. Poncet MC, Toullic P, Papazian L, et al. Burnout syndrome in critical care nursing staff. Am J Respir Crit Care Med 2007;175(7):698–704.
7. Garcia TT, Garcia PC, Molon ME, et al. Prevalence of burnout in pediatric intensivists: an observational comparison with general pediatricians. Pediatr Crit Care Med 2014;15(8):e347–53.
8. Moss M, Good VS, Gozal D, et al. An official critical care societies collaborative statement-burnout syndrome in critical care health-care professionals: a call for action. Chest 2016;150(1):17–26.
9. Pastores SM, Kvetan V, Coopersmith CM, et al. Workforce, workload, and burnout among intensivists and advanced practice providers: a narrative review. Crit Care Med 2019;47(4):550–7.
10. Chuang CH, Tseng PC, Lin CY, et al. Burnout in the intensive care unit professionals: a systematic review. Medicine (Baltimore) 2016;95(50):e5629.
11. Azoulay E, Cariou A, Bruneel F, et al. Symptoms of anxiety, depression, and peritraumatic dissociation in critical care clinicians managing patients with COVID-19. A cross-sectional study. Am J Respir Crit Care Med 2020;202(10):1388–98.
12. Karnatovskaia LV, Johnson MM, Varga K, et al. Stress and fear: clinical implications for providers and patients (in the time of COVID-19 and beyond). Mayo Clin Proc 2020;95(11):2487–98.
13. Shechter A, Diaz F, Moise N, et al. Psychological distress, coping behaviors, and preferences for support among New York healthcare workers during the COVID-19 pandemic. Gen Hosp Psychiatry 2020;66:1–8.
14. National Academies of Sciences, Engineering, and Medicine. Taking action against clinician burnout: a systems approach to professional well-being. Washington, DC: The National Academies Press; 2019. https://doi.org/10.17266/25521.
15. Freudenberger HJ. Staff burnout. J Soc Issues 1974;30:159–65.
16. Maslach C, Leiter MP. Understanding the burnout experience: recent research and its implications for psychiatry. World Psychiatry 2016;15(2):103–11.
17. Maslach C, Leiter MP. Early predictors of job burnout and engagement. J Appl Psychol 2008; 93(3):498–512.
18. West CP, Dyrbye LN, Shanafelt TD. Physician burnout: contributors, consequences and solutions. J Intern Med 2018;283(6):516–29.
19. Litz BT, Stein N, Delaney E, et al. Moral injury and moral repair in war veterans: a preliminary model and intervention strategy. Clin Psychol Rev 2009; 29(8):695–706.
20. Talbot SG, Dean W. Physicians aren't 'burning out.'They're suffering from moral injury. Stat. July 26, 2018. Available at: https://www.statnews.com/2018/07/26/physicians-not-burning-out-they-are-suffering-moral-injury/. Accessed July 17, 2021.
21. Bryant RA. Post-traumatic stress disorder: a state-of-the-art review of evidence and challenges. World Psychiatry 2019;18(3):259–69.
22. Herrman H, Stewart DE, Diaz-Granados N, et al. What is resilience? Can J Psychiatry 2011;56(5): 258–65.
23. Duckworth AL, Peterson C, Matthews MD, et al. Grit: perseverance and passion for long-term goals. J Pers Soc Psychol 2007;92(6):1087–101.
24. Maslach C, Jackson SE, Leiter MP. Maslach burnout inventory manual. 3rd edition. Palo Alto (CA): Consulting Psychologists Press; 1996.
25. Williams ES, Manwell LB, Konrad TR, et al. The relationship of organizational culture, stress, satisfaction, and burnout with physician-reported error and suboptimal patient care: results from the MEMO study. Health Care Manage Rev 2007; 32(3):203–12.
26. Dolan ED, Mohr D, Lempa M, et al. Using a single item to measure burnout in primary care staff: a psychometric evaluation. J Gen Intern Med 2015; 30(5):582–7.
27. Waddimba AC, Scribani M, Nieves MA, et al. Validation of single-item screening measures for provider burnout in a rural health care network. Eval Health Prof 2016;39(2):215–25.
28. Linzer M, Konrad TR, Douglas J, et al. Managed care, time pressure, and physician job satisfaction: results from the physician worklife study. J Gen Intern Med 2000;15(7):441–50.

29. Linzer M, Smith CD, Hingle S, et al. Evaluation of work satisfaction, stress, and burnout among US internal medicine physicians and trainees. JAMA Netw Open 2020;3(10):e2018758.

30. Kristensen TS, Borritz M, Villadsen EV, et al. The Copenhagen burnout inventory: a new tool for the assessment of burnout. Work Stress 2005;19(3): 192–207.

31. Reis D, Xanthopoulou Tsaousis I. Measuring job and academic burnout with the Oldenburg Burnout Inventory (OLBI): Factorial invariance across samples and countries. Burnout Res 2015;2(1):8–18.

32. Rotenstein LS, Torre M, Ramos MA, et al. Prevalence of burnout among physicians: a systematic review. JAMA 2018;320(11):1131–50.

33. Available at: https://www.medscape.com/slideshow/2021-lifestyle-burnout-6013456#1. accessed August 1, 2021.

34. Davidson JE, Proudfoot J, Lee K, et al. Nurse suicide in the United States: analysis of the center for disease control 2014 national violent death reporting system dataset. Arch Psychiatr Nurs 2019;33(5):16–21.

35. Shanafelt TD, Balch CM, Dyrbye L, et al. Special report: suicidal ideation among American surgeons. Arch Surg 2011;146(1):54–62.

36. Salyers MP, Bonfils KA, Luther L, et al. The relationship between professional burnout and quality and safety in healthcare: a meta-analysis. J Gen Intern Med 2017;32(4):475–82.

37. West CP, Tan AD, Habermann TM, et al. Association of resident fatigue and distress with perceived medical errors. JAMA 2009;302(12):1294–300.

38. Cimiotti JP, Aiken LH, Sloane DM, et al. Nurse staffing, burnout, and health care-associated infection. Am J Infect Control 2012;40(6):486–90 [published correction appears in Am J Infect Control. 2012 Sep;40(7):680].

39. Tawfik DS, Profit J, Morgenthaler TI, et al. Physician burnout, well-being, and work unit safety grades in relationship to reported medical errors. Mayo Clin Proc 2018;93(11):1571–80.

40. Sessler CN. Intensivist burnout: running on empty? Chest 2019;156(5):817–9.

41. Shanafelt TD, Mungo M, Schmitgen J, et al. Longitudinal study evaluating the association between physician burnout and changes in professional work effort. Mayo Clin Proc 2016;91(4):422–31.

42. Balch CM, Oreskovich MR, Dyrbye LN, et al. Personal consequences of malpractice lawsuits on American surgeons. J Am Coll Surg 2011;213(5): 657–67.

43. Sinsky CA, Dyrbye LN, West CP, et al. Professional satisfaction and the career plans of US physicians. Mayo Clin Proc 2017;92(11):1625–35.

44. Shanafelt T, Sinsky C. The business case for investing in physician well-being. JAMA Intern Med 2017;177(12):1826–32.

45. Shanafelt TD, Noseworthy JH. Executive leadership and physician well-being: nine organizational strategies to promote engagement and reduce burnout. Mayo Clin Proc 2017;92(1):129–46.

46. Han S, Shanafelt TD, Sinsky CA, et al. Estimating the attributable cost of physician burnout in the United States. Ann Intern Med 2019;170(11): 784–90.

47. Pappa S, Ntella V, Giannakas T, et al. Prevalence of depression, anxiety, and insomnia among healthcare workers during the COVID-19 pandemic: a systematic review and meta-analysis [published correction appears in Brain Behav Immun. 2021 Feb;92:247]. Brain Behav Immun 2020;88:901–7.

48. Lai J, Ma S, Wang Y, et al. Factors associated with mental health outcomes among health care workers exposed to coronavirus disease 2019. JAMA Netw Open 2020;3(3):e203976.

49. Cañadas-De la Fuente GA, Vargas C, San Luis C, et al. Risk factors and prevalence of burnout syndrome in the nursing profession. Int J Nurs Stud 2015;52(1):240–9.

50. Merlani P, Verdon M, Businger A, et al. Burnout in ICU caregivers: a multicenter study of factors associated to centers. Am J Respir Crit Care Med 2011; 184(10):1140–6.

51. Shanafelt TD, Sloan JA, Habermann TM. The well-being of physicians. Am J Med 2003;114(6):513–9.

52. Azoulay E, Herridge M. Understanding ICU staff burnout: the show must go on. Am J Respir Crit Care Med 2011;184:1099–100.

53. Lilly CM, Cucchi E, Marshall N, et al. Battling intensivist burnout: a role for workload management. Chest 2019;156(5):1001–7.

54. Opgenorth D, Stelfox HT, Gilfoyle E, et al. Perspectives on strained intensive care unit capacity: a survey of critical care professionals. PLoS One 2018; 13(8):e0201524.

55. Ali NA, Hammersley J, Hoffmann SP, et al. Continuity of care in intensive care units: a cluster-randomized trial of intensivist staffing. Am J Respir Crit Care Med 2011;184(7):803–8.

56. Quan SF, Weaver MD, Barger LK. Interim findings from a sleep health and wellness program to reduce occupational burnout. Sleep 2019; 42(suppl_1):A401.

57. Shanafelt TD, Dyrbye LN, Sinsky C, et al. Relationship between clerical burden and characteristics of the electronic environment with physician burnout and professional satisfaction. Mayo Clin Proc 2016;91(7):836–48.

58. Swenson S, Kabcenell A, Shanafelt T. Physician-organization collaboration reduces physician burnout

and promotes engagement: the Mayo Clinic experience. J Healthc Manag 2016;61(2):105–27.

59. Dyrbye LN, Harper W, Durning SJ, et al. Patterns of distress in US medical students. Med Teach 2011; 33(10):834–9.

60. Azoulay E, Timsit JF, Sprung CL, et al. Prevalence and factors of intensive care unit conflicts: the conflicus study. Am J Respir Crit Care Med 2009; 180(9):853–60.

61. Dow AW, Baernholdt M, Santen SA, et al. Practitioner wellbeing as an interprofessional imperative. J Interprof Care 2019;33(6):603–7.

62. Neumann R, Strack F. Mood contagion": the automatic transfer of mood between persons. J Pers Soc Psychol 2000;79(2):211–23.

63. Pollock A, Campbell P, Cheyne J, et al. Interventions to support the resilience and mental health of frontline health and social care professionals during and after a disease outbreak, epidemic or pandemic: a mixed methods systematic review. Cochrane Database Syst Rev 2020;11(11): CD013779.

64. Stuijfzand S, Deforges C, Sandoz V, et al. Psychological impact of an epidemic/pandemic on the mental health of healthcare professionals: a rapid review. BMC Public Health 2020;20(1):1230.

65. DePierro J, Lowe S, Katz C. Lessons learned from 9/11: mental health perspectives on the COVID-19 pandemic. Psychiatry Res 2020;288:113024.

66. Institute of Medicine Committee on Quality of Health Care in, A. To err is human: building a safer health system. In: Kohn LT, Corrigan JM, Donaldson MS, editors. To Err is human: building a safer health system. Washington, DC: National Academies Press (US) Copyright 2000 by the National Academy of Sciences. All rights reserved; 1999.

67. Institute of Medicine 2001. Crossing the Quality Chasm: A New Health System for the 21st Century. Washington, DC: The National Academies Press.

68. West CP, Dyrbye LN, Rabatin JT, et al. Intervention to promote physician well-being, job satisfaction, and professionalism: a randomized clinical trial. JAMA Intern Med 2014;174(4):527–33.

69. Panagioti M, Panagopoulou E, Bower P, et al. Controlled interventions to reduce burnout in physicians: a systematic review and meta-analysis. JAMA Intern Med 2017;177(2):195–205.

70. Kleinpell R, Moss M, Good VS, et al. The critical nature of addressing burnout prevention: results from the critical care societies collaborative's national Summit and survey on prevention and management of burnout in the ICU. Crit Care Med 2020; 48(2):249–53.

71. Kancherla BS, Upender R, Collen JF, et al. Sleep, fatigue and burnout among physicians: an

72. American Academy of Sleep Medicine position statement. J Clin Sleep Med 2020;16(5):803–5.

73. American Academy of Sleep Medicine. Tip sheet for health care providers: prioritizing sleep & managing fatigue. Available at: https://j2vjt3dnbra3ps7ll1clb4q2-wpengine.netdna-ssl.com/wp-content/uploads/2021/05/Prioritizing-Sleep-and-Managing-Fatigue.pdf. Accessed August 4, 2021.

74. Purnell MT, Feyer AM, Herbison GP. The impact of a nap opportunity during the night shift on the performance and alertness of 12-h shift workers. J Sleep Res 2002;11(3):219–27.

75. Urry E, Landolt HP. Adenosine, caffeine, and performance: from cognitive neuroscience of sleep to sleep pharmacogenetics. Curr Top Behav Neurosci 2015;25:331–66.

76. Kelley GA, Kelley KS. Exercise and sleep: a systematic review of previous meta-analyses. J Evid Based Med 2017;10(1):26–36.

77. Matta Mello Portugal E, Cevada T, Sobral Monteiro-Junior R, et al. Neuroscience of exercise: from neurobiology mechanisms to mental health. Neuropsychobiology 2013;68(1):1–14.

78. Armas M, Aronowitz D, Gaona R, et al. Active breaks initiative during hospital rounds in the Surgical ICU to improve wellness of healthcare providers: an observational descriptive study. World J Surg 2021;45(4):1026–30.

79. Rodgers GP, Collins FS. Precision nutrition-the answer to "what to eat to Stay healthy. JAMA 2020;324(8):735–6.

80. Scheepers RA, Emke H, Epstein RM, et al. The impact of mindfulness-based interventions on doctors' well-being and performance: a systematic review. Med Educ 2020;54(2):138–49.

81. Sood A, Prasad K, Schroeder D, et al. Stress management and resilience training among Department of Medicine faculty: a pilot randomized clinical trial. J Gen Intern Med 2011;26(8):858–61.

82. Lin DT, Liebert CA, Tran J, et al. Emotional intelligence as a predictor of resident well-being. J Am Coll Surg 2016;223(2):352–8.

83. Rushton CH, Batcheller J, Schroeder K, et al. Burnout and resilience among nurses practicing in high-intensity settings. Am J Crit Care 2015; 24(5):412–20.

84. Agency for healthcare research and quality TeamSTEPPS 2.0 curriculum. Available at: https://www.ahrq.gov/teamstepps/index.html. Accessed June 6, 2022.

85. Parker K, Jacobson A, McGuire M, et al. How to build high-quality interprofessional collaboration and education in your hospital: the IP-COMPASS tool. Qual Manag Health Care 2012;21(3):160–8.

86. Welp A, Manser T. Integrating teamwork, clinician occupational well-being and patient safety -

development of a conceptual framework based on a systematic review. BMC Health Serv Res 2016; 16:281.

86. Malec JF, Torsher LC, Dunn WF, et al. The mayo high performance teamwork scale: reliability and validity for evaluating key crew resource management skills. Simul Healthc 2007;2(1):4–10.

87. Boet S, Etherington N, Larrigan S, et al. Measuring the teamwork performance of teams in crisis situations: a systematic review of assessment tools and their measurement properties. BMJ Qual Saf 2019; 28(4):327–37.

88. Duan X, Ni X, Shi L, et al. The impact of workplace violence on job satisfaction, job burnout, and turnover intention: the mediating role of social support. Health Qual Life Outcomes 2019;17(1):93.

89. El Khamali R, Mouaci A, Valera S, et al. Effects of a multimodal program including Simulation on job strain among nurses working in intensive care units: a randomized clinical trial. JAMA 2018; 320(19):1988–97.

90. Monroe M, Morse E, Price JM. The relationship between critical care work environment and professional quality of life. Am J Crit Care 2020;29(2): 145–9.

91. Deneckere S, Euwema M, Lodewijckx C, et al. Better interprofessional teamwork, higher level of organized care, and lower risk of burnout in acute health care teams using care pathways: a cluster randomized controlled trial. Med Care 2013;51(1): 99–107.

92. Speroni KG, Fitch T, Dawson E, et al. Incidence and cost of nurse workplace violence perpetrated by hospital patients or patient visitors. J Emerg Nurs 2014;40(3):218–95.

93. U.S. Government Accountability Office. Workplace safety and Health: additional efforts needed to help protect health care workers from workplace violence. 2016. Available at: https://www.gao.gov/products/gao-16-11. Accessed August 14, 2021.

94. Arnetz JE, Hamblin L, Russell J, et al. Preventing patient-to-worker violence in hospitals: outcome of a randomized controlled intervention. J Occup Environ Med 2017;59(1):18–27.

95. Catania G, Zanini M, Hayter M, et al. Lessons from Italian front-line nurses' experiences during the COVID-19 pandemic: a qualitative descriptive study. J Nurs Manag 2021;29(3):404–11.

96. Rangachari P, L Woods J. Preserving organizational resilience, patient safety, and staff retention during COVID-19 requires a holistic consideration of the psychological safety of healthcare workers. Int J Environ Res Public Health 2020;17(12):4267.

97. Brooks S, Amlôt R, Rubin GJ, et al. Psychological resilience and post-traumatic growth in disaster-exposed organisations: overview of the literature. BMJ Mil Health 2020;166(1):52–6.

98. Yörük S, Güler D. The relationship between psychological resilience, burnout, stress, and sociodemographic factors with depression in nurses and midwives during the COVID-19 pandemic: a cross-sectional study in Turkey. Perspect Psychiatr Care 2021;57(1):390–8.

99. Bodenheimer T, Sinsky C. From triple to quadruple aim: care of the patient requires care of the provider. Ann Fam Med 2014;12(6):573–6.

100. Rinne ST, Shah T, Anderson E, et al. Professional societies' role in addressing member burnout and promoting well-being. Ann Am Thorac Soc 2021; 18(9):1482–9.

Moving?

Make sure your subscription moves with you!

To notify us of your new address, find your **Clinics Account Number** (located on your mailing label above your name), and contact customer service at:

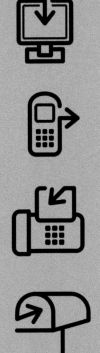

Email: **journalscustomerservice-usa@elsevier.com**

800-654-2452 (subscribers in the U.S. & Canada)
314-447-8871 (subscribers outside of the U.S. & Canada)

Fax number: **314-447-8029**

Elsevier Health Sciences Division
Subscription Customer Service
3251 Riverport Lane
Maryland Heights, MO 63043

*To ensure uninterrupted delivery of your subscription, please notify us at least 4 weeks in advance of move.

9780323896825